Psychological
Disorders
of Children
and
Adolescents

Little, Brown and Company   *Boston/Toronto*

Psychological Disorders of Children and Adolescents

Judith Page Van Evra

St. Jerome's College, University of Waterloo

Library of Congress Cataloging in Publication Data

Van Evra, Judith Page.
   Psychological disorders of children & adolescents.

   1. Child psychopathology.   2. Child psychotherapy.   3. Adolescent
psychopathology.   4. Adolescent psychotherapy.   I. Title.   [DNLM: 1. Mental
disorders—In infancy and childhood.   2. Mental disorders—In adolescence.
3. Psychotherapy—In infancy and childhood.   4. Psychotherapy—In adolescence.
WS 350 V217p]
RJ499.V34   1983   618.92′89   82-18011
ISBN 0-316-89606-3

Library of Congress Catalog Card Number 82-18011

ISBN 0-316-89606-3

9 8 7 6 5 4 3 2 1

MV

Published simultaneously in Canada
by Little, Brown & Company (Canada) Limited

Printed in the United States of America

Acknowledgments

   Excerpt from Virginia Axline, *Play Therapy* (New York: Ballantine Books, Inc.,
1947), pp. 16–17, reprinted by permission of the author.
   Excerpt from C. E. Schaefer and H. L. Millman, *Therapies for Children* (San

Francisco: Jossey-Bass, 1978), pp. 448–49, reprinted by permission of the publishers.

Excerpt reprinted by permission of the publishers from *The Golden Cage: The Enigma of Anorexia Nervosa* by Hilde Bruch, Cambridge, Mass.: Harvard University Press. Copyright © 1978 by the President and Fellows of Harvard College.

Excerpts from L. Kanner, *Child Psychiatry*, Fourth Edition, 1972. Courtesy of Charles C Thomas, Publisher, Springfield, Illinois.

Excerpt from William C. Rhodes and J. L. Paul, *Emotionally Disturbed and Deviant Children* (Englewood Cliffs, N.J.: Prentice-Hall, 1978), p. 45, reprinted by permission of the author.

Excerpt from S. Chess and M. Hassibi, *Principles and Practice of Child Psychiatry* (New York: Plenum Publishing Corporation, 1978), pp. 241–42, reprinted by permission of the publisher and author.

Excerpt from D. J. Cohen, B. Caparulo, and B. Shaywitz, "Primary Childhood Aphasia and Childhood Autism: Clinical, Biological, and Conceptual Observations," *Journal of American Academic Child Psychiatry* 1976, 15:4, pp. 604–45. Copyright © 1976 American Academy of Child Psychiatry. Reprinted by permission of the Williams & Wilkins Company and the author.

Excerpt from Benjamin B. Wolman, *Children Without Childhood* (New York: Grune & Stratton, Inc., 1970), pp. 97–98, reprinted by permission of the publishers and the author.

Excerpt from R. Simmons, in *Psychological Problems of the Child and His Family* by P. D. Steinhauer and Quentin Rae-Grant, © Macmillan of Canada 1977. Reprinted by permission of Gage Publishing Limited.

To my husband, Jim,
and our daughters,
Stephanie, Susan, and Jennifer

Preface

The study of psychological disorders in children and adolescents has mushroomed over the past few decades. Attempts to describe and define symptoms and disorders more precisely and to understand them more fully have continued alongside efforts to treat them more effectively. There has been increasing emphasis on the need to take into account the important differences between childhood and adult problems in terms of nature, study, and treatment, and to discover in what ways relevant developmental and environmental variables interact to produce those differences. Along with the development of new and highly varied techniques to treat childhood disorders have come many diverse and complex ethical and clinical issues which demand attention.

One of my primary purposes in writing this book was to present as comprehensive, balanced, accurate, and timely a theoretical and conceptual picture of the field as possible. This book introduces students to the many facets of this area of study, and it is appropriate for undergraduate and beginning graduate courses in child and adolescent disorders. Diverse theoretical viewpoints and perspectives are presented, along with discussion of how they complement and supplement one another. Empirical evidence is discussed throughout the book as it bears on various viewpoints, either lending support to or refuting claims regarding etiology, symptomatology, and remediation. A developmental perspective is maintained throughout to emphasize the significant differences between adult and child symptoms and behaviors and the problems that are encountered in attempts to study and understand children as they develop and mature. Sections on the advantages and limitations of various research designs are included to provide students with greater means by which to critically read and evaluate the research literature.

A second major aim of this work is to present students with a view that balances theoretical perspectives and models with issues that arise in an applied, clinical setting—issues all practicing clinicians must address, regardless of their theoretical persuasion. Ethical considerations involved in research and clinical work are discussed, as are the myriad diagnostic and remedial questions which practicing clinicians face daily. Many case studies are included, as well as analyses of the concrete decision-making steps which clinicians take in the course of evaluating and treating children. The discussion questions which are included at the end of each chapter to stimulate further thought and discussion reflect both theoretical and clinical concerns.

Part I of the book deals with the historical background of the field of childhood disorders and the various theoretical perspectives, as well as how they have interacted and influenced one another. The clinical models which developed from each of the theoretical perspectives are described, and general research issues are discussed.

Part II deals with many diagnostic issues, including the dimensions along which behavior can be evaluated as to its "normality" or "abnormality." A section on classification systems includes clinically derived systems such as the DSM-III and empirically or factor-analytically based systems. There is also a brief discussion of various etiological factors (more extended discussions of causality are included in later sections on specific disorders). A wide array of specific diagnostic instruments and techniques are covered in Part II, along with examples of how they are selected and used in clinical practice.

Part III focuses on treatment. Representative samples of the many remedial interventions available are described, and examples are given of how specific treatments might be selected and implemented. An entire chapter is devoted to the question of the relative effectiveness of various treatments: research designs that can facilitate the evaluation of effectiveness are presented, as well as many of the research findings from such evaluations.

With this knowledge as background, the student is introduced in Part IV to a wide range of specific psychological disorders. Theoretical explanations, clinical descriptions, and treatment approaches are included, along with case studies, to illustrate both theoretical and clinical aspects of the disorders. Research data bearing on differing theoretical points of view and on the efficacy of various treatment methods appear throughout.

Part V focuses on prevention and advocacy. There has been increasing emphasis on the importance of preventive work, in the hope that such efforts may avert much needless suffering as well as great economic cost. Child advocacy efforts have been expanding as well and promise not only to benefit children with various problems but to improve the quality of life for all children and adolescents.

I would like to acknowledge the contributions and assistance of many individuals who facilitated and supported the writing of this book, only a small number of whom are named below.

Many thanks go to George Bergquist for his encouragement, support, and direction in the early stages of the manuscript's development, to Tom Pavela for his very able editorial assistance and suggestions, and to the anonymous reviewers whose insightful comments and suggestions contributed significantly to the book. Thanks go also to Molly Faulkner, Julie Winston, and Nikki Sklare, of the editorial and production departments at Little, Brown and Co., and to Sally Lifland, for their many contributions and suggestions and for their ready assistance in so many ways. Support from my colleagues and from the administration of St. Jerome's College, University of Waterloo, is also gratefully acknowledged, with a special word of appreciation to Laura Moyer for her good-natured and very capable secretarial and typing assistance. Finally, many thanks to my husband for all of his help with successive drafts and for his continual support and encouragement. My genuine affection and heartfelt gratitude go to him and to all of my family for their unerring interest and patience and for the sacrifices they so willingly made during the writing of this book.

Contents

Contents

Contents

Contents

Chapter 7

Part IV

Types of Disorders

Chapter 8

Chapter 9 *Mental Retardation* 187

Chapter 10 *Learning Disabilities* 211

Contents

Contents

Chapter 13 — *Psychosomatic Disorders* 285

Chapter 14 — *Juvenile Delinquency* 305

Contents

Part V   **Prevention and Advocacy**

Chapter 15   *Prevention*   331

Chapter 16   *Child Advocacy*   343

Contents

PART I

Historical and
Theoretical Issues

CHAPTER 1   Historical Background

As we know it today, the study of children with psychological problems has a relatively short history. This is not surprising when one considers that the scientific study even of normal children was begun relatively recently, with most of the work having been done in this century.

Early Views of Children

Before the seventeenth century, children as human beings were not perceived as a separate group and were therefore given no special status. Rather, they were seen as completely dependent before about the age of three and were thereafter considered simply a smaller version of adults. According to Aries (1962), for example, at the end of the sixteenth and into the seventeenth century, "coddling" provoked criticism. By the end of the seventeenth century, however, there was a growing tendency to view childhood as a separate, albeit imperfect, time of life (Aries, 1962). The dissemination of John Locke's seventeenth-century concept of the child as a "tabula rasa" and Rousseau's, in the eighteenth-century, of the child as a "noble savage" began to draw attention to the influence, both positive and negative, that adults could have on a child's behavior and development. Locke suggested that when the child is born his or her mind is, in effect, a clean slate, upon which all experience is subsequently written to form the child's personality. Rousseau's idea was that children are inherently good and become corrupted only as the result of adult interference. Both of these viewpoints, in addition to promoting a highly environmentalist concept of children's problems, were important in focusing attention on children as individuals and on the relevance of childhood experiences.

Eighteenth-century humanitarians also were beginning to encourage differential treatment of children and adults, and greater concern was developing over the welfare of children generally. Protection and guidance were increasingly seen as more appropriate treatment than the customary severe punishment; more concern began to be shown for the child's physical health and hygiene, and children were being elevated to a more central place in the family (Aries, 1962).

Origins of Scientific Study

This growing concern, however, was only very gradually translated into scientific study, and little was published before the nineteenth

4

century, when educators began to focus on children (Kolansky, 1973). Dennis's (1949) review turned up only forty-two articles circulated before 1882. The earliest, appearing in 1787, was a scientific record of the behavior of the author's son. Following that account, there was a gap of forty-one years during which there were apparently no publications dealing with normal behavior in children (Dennis, 1949). During the latter part of the nineteenth century, interest in the subject began to grow, with most of the initial efforts taking the form of intensive case studies. Preyer's (1882) baby bibliography, a chronicling of his own child's development, is probably the best known; but Darwin's (1877) diary concerning his son also appeared in the late nineteenth century. In addition, Hall's questionnaire, which solicited answers from both parents and children on a wide choice of topics, broadened the range of research techniques and the scope of the information to be gleaned, and thus extended the field of study (Kanner, 1976).

From these rather modest beginnings in the nineteenth century, interest in the study of normal children increased rapidly in the twentieth, with growing focus among the scientific community on various developmental processes, particularly in the areas of socialization, language, and cognition. Many of these early findings were well publicized, and there followed many, many books on child-rearing approaches and on techniques to help parents produce healthy, happy, well-adjusted children. One need only browse through any bookstore today to see the mushrooming of interest and the plethora of books on children and parenting, heralded by Dr. Benjamin Spock's best-selling child care manual, *Baby and Child Care* (1957), first printed in 1946. Some have even suggested that the transmission to parents of findings in sciences such as psychology and pediatrics has led to an obsession with children's problems (Aries, 1962).

Approaches to Childhood Disorders

It stands to reason that the increased scientific study of normal children and a recognition of childhood's importance as a separate state of development, with characteristic behaviors and problems, was a necessary first step before there could be any concerted effort or interest directed toward specific problems and abnormalities in that development. Deviance from the normal developmental processes and the less than optimal functioning of some children began to attract greater attention. It seemed increasingly important to find ways to alleviate their unhappiness, to remove developmental obstacles, and to facilitate their maximal functioning. Like the study of normal children, most of the work with problem children has been done in the current century, although important groundwork had been laid much earlier.

Early Foundations

Most of the work before 1900 was centered on retarded children (Rubinstein, 1948). One of the first systematic looks at retarded children was Jean Itard's classic efforts with *The Wild Boy of Aveyron* (1962), an account of which was first printed in 1801. Itard took on the challenge of trying to treat a wild child found near a forest who could not speak and who was considered hopelessly retarded by others. Seguin's efforts to train the retarded also drew considerable attention in the nineteenth century (Achenbach, 1974). The emphasis at that time on moral treatment of deviant behavior (Ullman and Krasner, 1969) gradually yielded to the notion that abnormal behavior was an illness. Thus was born the medical model, which has had a very significant and far-reaching effect on the whole field of psychological disturbances. (The medical model will be described more fully in the next chapter.) With the exception of Maudsley (1867), who included in his book a chapter on "Insanity of Early Life" (Kanner, 1976) and thus was one of the first to study serious disorders in children, few people wrote about insanity before 1900, and its treatment was discussed little if at all (Rubinstein, 1948).

Twentieth-Century Changes

Most of the work, then, has been done in the twentieth century. The early part of the century saw primarily cultural and social changes and changes in attitudes toward children (Kanner, 1972). Gradually, probation, special classes, and protective institutions such as foster homes were created, especially for the seriously mistreated (Kanner, 1972). The mental hygiene movement also grew during the first quarter of this century, largely to the credit of Clifford Beers and his classic book, *A Mind That Found Itself* (1908). Because of his own experience—his obsessive fear of epilepsy had culminated in a suicide attempt, and he

6

had suffered persecutory delusions—Beers was instrumental in forming the National Committee for Mental Hygiene in 1909.

Gradually, more facilities such as child guidance clinics and services such as visiting teacher programs were instituted, aimed at improving the home and school environments of children (Eisenberg, 1969; Kanner, 1972, 1976). Binet's (1916) intelligence testing in the early part of the twentieth century, with its introduction of standardized norms and its emphasis on assessment, also contributed to a better understanding of children with problems. In addition, there was growing enthusiasm for multidisciplinary work, exemplified by the formation of the American Orthopsychiatric Association, an organization of social workers, psychologists, and psychiatrists. Kanner's 1935 book on child psychiatry is reportedly the first American book on the subject (Rubinstein, 1948).

INFLUENCE OF PSYCHOANALYTIC THOUGHT

The decade from 1930 to 1940 was a most important one (Kolansky, 1973) because of the great psychoanalytic influence of Sigmund Freud and such followers as Adolph Meyer (1915), with his "commonsense psychiatry." Both men maintained that the seeds of adult disorders were sown in childhood (Kanner, 1976). Freud's theories on the unconscious influences on behavior, unconscious motivation, irrational behavior, and the importance of early parent-child relationships and conflicts added new dimensions to the study of disorders in children. These will be discussed more fully in Chapter 2.

Not all of Freud's ideas, of course, were accepted smoothly, and he was strongly challenged on a number of fronts. His tenets were criticized as untestable as well as too reliant on inference, which introduced possible distortion and inaccuracy; and he was seen as too deterministic and too pessimistic.

DEVELOPMENT OF HUMANISM

The humanistic school of thought arose in the 1940s. Maslow's (1968) "third force" psychology and Carl Rogers's (1951) nondirective psychotherapy, based on the humanistic emphasis on each individual's capacity for growth and change, added yet another significant dimension to the field of childhood disorders. The humanistic perspective focused on empathic warmth and unconditional acceptance from the therapist in order to facilitate growth, rather than emphasizing underlying dynamics and unconscious motivation, as Freud's analytic approach had done. Thus, it tended also to be more positive and optimistic. Many of the therapeutic approaches that arise from this school, however, such as existential and phenomenological therapies, are better suited to adults, and hence there is less emphasis on those therapies in this book. However, Axline (1947) and Moustakas (1959) are clear exceptions, and the use of their nondirective relationship therapy with children is described in detail in Chapter 6.

GROWTH OF BEHAVIORISM

Another major trend which began in the early part of this century, partly as a reaction against Freud's influence, was the increasing use of learning theory principles to explain behavior. Credit for this development is usually given to John B. Watson (1925, 1928), who was very much dissatisfied with the dependence of psychoanalytic explanations on unobserved phenomena. According to Watson (1928), scientific studies of children were slow to start because of strong pressure against laboratory work with children. But by 1912 behaviorists had decided they could no longer work with the intangible aspects of psychology and the introspective study of consciousness (Watson, 1925), and Freud's postulation of the unconscious was attacked as "voodooism" (Watson, 1928a, p. 94). According to Watson, the only legitimate object of study was what could be observed, and he emphasized scientific methodology and careful observation of how behaviors were acquired. He listed and studied hundreds of infant responses in the laboratory and in doing so discovered that even emotional responses could be conditioned (Watson and Rayner, 1920).

Use of these techniques and emphases took a big jump forward with Skinner's work in the 1930s (Kirschenbaum, 1968), which stressed operant conditioning over classical conditioning. Skinner's name became associated with still more recent work in the area, particularly after publication of *Walden Two* (1948), which delineated his concept of an ideal society, and *Beyond Freedom and Dignity* (1971); he also tried to promote the application of his techniques in the educational field.

INFLUENCE OF COGNITIVE PSYCHOLOGY

The most recent trend in the behavioral field is the growing emphasis on cognitive behavior modification and therapy (Beck et al., 1979; Mahoney, 1974; Meichenbaum, 1977), in which cognitive processes and verbal mediation (rather than external contingencies and reinforcements) are used to modify behavior.

The use of cognitive and behavioral techniques with various disorders, although relatively new, has significantly affected clinical practice. Attention was drawn to the practical applications of this rapidly expanding field of interest by Wolpe and Lazarus (1966) and Lazarus (1971), with their work on systematic desensitization, and by Lovaas and many others, with their studies of the use of behavioral techniques with severely disturbed children (Lovaas, 1966; Lovaas et al., 1973; Lovaas, Schreibman, and Koegel, 1976). The relative recency of this approach and its rapid growth are underscored by the fact that the first behavioral journal appeared in 1963 (Craighead, Kazdin, and Mahoney, 1976), to be followed in the last fifteen or twenty years by hundreds of behavior modification articles in various journals and dozens of books on behavior therapy and its use in clinical practice.

For more detailed histories of the development of this area of study, the reader is referred to Kanner's (1972) overview of trends and changes, or to Kolansky (1973) and Ullman and Krasner (1969).

Current Trends

There has been increasing emphasis on a developmental approach to childhood disorders. Psychological researchers have found that it is necessary to address the additional variables that arise because of the fact that children change rapidly as they grow and because of the " ... overwhelming significance of developmental processes for all aspects of child behavior, normal or pathological" (Achenbach, 1974, p. 3). Problems that are normal at certain developmental stages are not normal at others. The continual process of change in a maturing child must be taken into account in order to adequately diagnose and treat the child. Moreover, common symptom patterns have been known to change or improve spontaneously simply as a function of maturation, which further confounds the study of childhood disorders.

Other more current emphases include a search for neurobiological factors underlying psychological disorders and for the physiological correlates of many symptom patterns. Another thrust involves studying family interaction systems rather than individual children in an attempt to understand the development and maintenance of various disorders and to generate the most effective remedial interventions possible.

In many ways, a developmental perspective can help to unify diverse points of view (Boverman and French, 1979). Moreover, there is growing evidence that many of the approaches and interventions can be integrated significantly to provide a more comprehensive understanding of the problems of children and adolescents.

Because of increasing knowledge about both the psychological antecedents of disturbances and the influence of the environment on normal development, there has been increasing emphasis on children's rights to proper and concerned care. Legislation has been passed and federal funding initiated over the past two decades to protect those rights, and parents' organizations have sprung up to apply pressure to governmental agencies to provide certain basic services. Passage in 1975 of Public Law 94-142, for example, which guarantees handicapped children an appropriate education in as normal an environment as possible, reflects the progress that has been made in this century toward understanding and helping children with various kinds of disabilities.

Many people have advocated a broader role for psychology as a health, rather than mental health, profession, calling for psychological research in areas such as heart disease, cancer, stroke, and accidents (Schofield, 1969). There has also been more emphasis recently on behavioral health, or the maintenance of health and prevention of illness (Matarazzo, 1980), which was graphically demonstrated by the formation in 1978 of a Division of Health Psychology in the American Psychological Association.

Vestiges of many of the earlier views and approaches are still evident in the practice of present-day clinicians. Garfield (1981) maintains that there have been no significant breakthroughs in psychotherapy over the past forty years, although more stress has been placed on effectiveness and accountability. There are, however, signs

10

of growing rapprochement and integrative efforts between the major approaches; these are discussed more fully in Chapter 6 on treatment techniques. In keeping with this trend toward accepting the positive aspects of several viewpoints, this book presents as broad a view as possible, including treatment techniques from several approaches and, whenever possible, research literature to support the differing views and techniques.

Discussion Questions

1. Discuss the reasons why the study of childhood disorders had to await important changes in society's attitudes toward and about children.
2. Discuss the contributions of various theoretical outlooks to the developing field of child study.
3. Try to predict which aspects of this field of study will be emphasized in the next ten to fifteen years. Give reasons for your predictions.

CHAPTER 2   # Theoretical Perspectives and Models of Disturbance

Depite many attempts to conceptualize psychological disorders in children, no one perspective or orientation has yet gained universal acceptance or definitively addressed all or even most of the questions in this field. There are many ways to categorize and discuss theoretical models. One can divide them into intrapsychic and environmental, or organismic and mechanistic, or medical and psychological. Within each of these groupings, further differentiations can be made. Thus, among environmental models one might include sociocultural, learning, and humanistic approaches. But since these classifications are hard to separate and distinguish and there is little agreement in the area, only the five major approaches will be discussed here. A working familiarity with these major approaches and theoretical views not only will enable students to read and evaluate the relevant research literature more critically, but also will facilitate the work of clinicians with clients. Although each of the perspectives continues to change and evolve, the central concepts, tenets, and philosophical outlooks remain essentially the same. In addition, each theoretical perspective has led to characteristic conceptual models of disturbance, methods of assessment, and remedial strategies.

Psychoanalytic Approach

Theoretical Perspective

The beginnings of psychoanalysis date back to the nineteenth century with the emergence of the medical model, in which deviant or abnormal behavior was seen as an indication of an underlying disorder, most often of an organic nature. Although the medical model was later expanded to include psychological or intrapsychic factors (and hence the term "quasi-medical model" appeared), the model still appears to be most appropriate where organic and physiological factors are clearly involved. The basic tenet holds that underlying pathology, whether physical or psychological, causes the surface behavior which is deemed disturbed or "pathological." According to this view, simple treatment of symptoms will result in only short-term benefits at best, unless one also removes the underlying pathology.

The strongest proponent of the analytic view, and the most vocal, was clearly Sigmund Freud. Freud's theories of psychopathology and personality development have had a profound influence on study in

14

this area. His greatest contributions were his emphases on unconscious motivation, the development of defense mechanisms, and the importance of characteristic conflicts between children and their parents during the early years of development.

It was Freud's contention that children normally go through certain conflictual periods with their parents which are anxiety-provoking and potentially pathogenic. How these early conflicts are handled and resolved is of paramount importance for the child's later development and psychological well-being, as they have a cumulative, pyramiding effect. Unresolved conflicts or poorly managed psychological situations during the early years can lay the foundation for future psychopathology, unless there is systematic and intensive investigation and resolution of these conflicts in a therapeutic context.

Freud's view, and that of other classical analysts, is a highly deterministic one, with major personality characteristics and potential problems developing very early and remaining highly resistant to change, especially spontaneous change.

Although an in-depth analysis of Freud's theory of personality development is beyond the scope of this book and can be found in virtually any developmental text or book on theories of personality or psychopathology, certain key concepts need to be reviewed here. For more extensive discussions, the reader is referred to Achenbach (1974) or Kessler (1966) for an excellent summary of psychoanalytic theory.

One of the most influential of Freud's tenets was, of course, that of unconscious influences on behavior, including the development of defense mechanisms which are used to cope with unacceptable impulses and the anxiety that they generate. Freud described a universal progression in which children go through a number of stages of psychosexual development, including oral, anal, phallic, and genital, each accompanied by characteristic feelings and conflicts. Sexuality in Freud's sense, however, is far broader than the usual notion of sexuality, the latter being part of Freud's later, more mature, genital stage. In earlier stages, sexuality for Freud refers to pleasure associated with specific areas of the body, or erogenous zones. Thus, in the oral stage, the infant derives pleasure from activities centered around the mouth—for example, sucking; in the anal phase, pleasure is derived from eliminative functions; and so on.

It was a further contention of Freud that if a child is either too severely frustrated or too much indulged in pleasure-seeking at a particular stage, the child becomes fixated, or arrested, at that stage, and normal developmental progression is disrupted. In addition, pleasure-seeking at each stage brings about a reaction from the environment (usually parents) which may include censure, restrictions, and conflicting demands, all of which generate anxiety in the child. The child also develops a superego (conscience), an internalization of parental prohibitions, through which self-criticism replaces parental criticism. This superego too opposes the expression of certian impulses. There is then a conflict between expression of impulses and the possible punishment or loss of love from parent figures, as well as anxiety generated as a result of violation of conscience if such impulses are expressed. That is, there is conflict among id (impulses), ego (reality factors), and superego (conscience).

In order to avoid such negative consequences, the child develops certain defensive maneuvers or compromise behaviors which are intended either to give partial expression to the impulses, but in a disguised or indirect way, or to prevent their expression altogether. The child might, for example, *repress* unacceptable impulses. When this happens, the impulses are pushed into the unconscious and the child no longer has to deal with them. On the surface this may appear to be a fairly good solution to the problem. However, according to Freud, repressed impulses continue to seek expression, and the child is obliged to use considerable psychic energy to prevent their expression. Assuming the psychic makeup is a kind of hydraulic system with a finite quantity of energy which is continually shifting, the energy a child uses to repress such impulses is unavailable for other, more constructive activities; and so the person's life becomes constricted and development is adversely affected.

A child might also project those impulses onto others in the environment. Individuals who use *projection* first deny that the impulses are theirs or exist within them (that is, they repress them); then they project them onto others in the environment. For example, the classic dynamic in paranoid individuals, according to the analysts, is denial of hostile impulses in themselves and projection of them onto others, so that they then feel that others are hostile toward them.

Another way to handle unacceptable impulses is through *reaction formation*. In this defense mechanism, an individual overcompensates by following denial of impulses with behavior that is diametrically opposed to the unacceptable impulse. For example, a mother who feels

16

extremely hostile toward a child but finds such hostility completely unacceptable may instead behave very solicitously toward the child and become overprotective.

Regression is a defensive maneuver in which a child or adult reverts to an earlier level of functioning when confronting extreme anxiety or stress or other difficult psychological states, as when a previously trained three-year-old reverts to bed-wetting when his mother gives much attention to a new sibling. Or a normally active six-year-old may become very whiny and clingy when she is faced with a new and stressful situation.

Individuals may also use *intellectualization* to protect themselves from anticipated psychological threat. Affect or potential emotional expression is channeled into intellectual and cognitive activities. The latter then become the be-all and end-all; the former may disappear, or may be dismissed with a pejorative label such as "silly" or "stupid."

Displacement as a defense refers to a change in the object of an emotion. A man who is furious with his boss but dare not express it directly may come home and fight with his wife. He has then displaced his anger from boss onto wife, which offers a partial expression of an impulse but in a distorted form.

Rationalization is another, fairly normal mechanism used by most individuals at various times to handle anxiety. If they have acted in a way that causes them to feel uncomfortable or guilty, they may rationalize their behavior by coming up with a good reason or an alibi for it. "He deserved it" and "It was good for my blood pressure" are examples of statements used to help excuse what is felt to be unacceptable behavior or expression of impulses.

A defense mechanism considered to constitute a positive and healthy expression of impulses is *sublimation*. With sublimation, one channels an otherwise unacceptable impulse into socially acceptable behavior. For example, an individual might channel very hostile, aggressive impulses into a competitive attitude and become a very effective courtroom lawyer or a successful athlete.

In any case, such defense mechanisms are used to some extent by everyone at various times and in varying degrees. Students interested in pursuing their normal use would probably find Freud's *Psychopathology of Everyday Life* (1952) or his discussion of errors (1935) most intriguing. Excessive use of defenses, however, requires considerable energy, and one's surface behavior may appear to be quite irrational when it is influenced and distorted by unconscious forces. Thus over-reactions or irrational behavior may occur as a result of environmental events that have triggered underlying conflicts.

Clinical Model

The foregoing ideas led to a psychodynamic model of diagnosis and treatment. In this model, diagnosis consists of finding out what psychological conflicts are responsible for the individual's symptoms; in other words, determining the "cause." The therapist needs to become aware of the individual's underlying conflicts, unconscious influences, unexpressed impulses, and early childhood experiences. Free association is one of the methods by which analysts typically try to find out more about someone's unconscious processes. The patient is asked to say whatever comes to mind without censoring any thoughts. The substance of the thoughts and the way in which one thought leads to another are considered to be important clues to the understanding of unconscious processes. Dreams are frequently interpreted similarly. Child analysts such an Anna Freud (1946) and Melanie Klein (1932) have used play itself and the symbolic nature of play activities to establish the nature of a child's conflicts. Projective testing, which is discussed more fully in Chapter 5 on diagnostic techniques, represents still another avenue to reach the unconscious.

Once the therapist understands the inner dynamics of the patient, those dynamics can be explained to the patient, leading to the development of "insight" on the part of the patient. Such insight is a central goal of psychodynamic therapies. Presumably, if patients can confront their conflicts and defensive behaviors in the safety of the therapeutic relationship, they can give vent to their unacceptable impulses and thus free up their personalities and their psychic energy. The emphasis is clearly on the interpretation of present behavior in terms of past events, and this requires extensive—and expensive—forays into an individual's psychic functioning, a process which can often take years.

Critique

It is for these very basic tenets that Freud and the classical analysts have received the most criticism. The behaviorists, in particular, find fault with the psychoanalytic perspective on the grounds that it includes too many unobservable and therefore untestable concepts. Too much needs to be inferred, and there is too little opportunity for empirical validation of theories. The classical analysts have also been taken to task for being too pessimistic about human development and a person's capacity for change and growth and too "gloomy" in their view of people (McCandless, 1976). They have been accused of attaching too much importance to pathology and conflict while giving relatively little attention to the positive and healthy aspects of personality development.

This emphasis, however, mirrors and is based on the medical model, which by definition has traditionally been problem- or disease-oriented. Only recently has the medical field begun to stress more positive aspects of physical functioning, such as preventive medicine and maintenance of fitness. As a medical doctor in the late nineteenth and early twentieth century, Freud was simply reflecting the nature of his discipline and the emphasis of his era in his focus on conflict as it effects pathology. The medical model, however, can be misleading when the underlying processes are psychological states, which generally can only be inferred.

The medical model has also been criticized for giving inadequate attention to other factors affecting the child, such as particular aspects of the environment, although in truth the Neo-Freudians or the more contemporary analytic theorists have given more attention to such factors. Erikson's (1963) discussion of developmental stages, for example, has a much more sociocultural and interpersonal emphasis. Others have shown an increased interest in short-term therapy (Barten, 1971; Wolberg, 1965) in which the therapists draw on analytic concepts but are more efficient and therefore can reach a greater number of the people who need their services. Still others interpret some behavior in psychodynamic or analytic terms, but borrow from other theoretical perspectives as well. Although there are many different emphases among therapists who take a psychodynamic or "intrapsychic" (Craighead, Kazdin, and Mahoney, 1976) approach, the focus is still primarily on internal factors or intrapsychic conflicts and events.

Behavioral Approach

Theoretical Perspective

The learning theorists, beginning with John Watson (1930), were highly dissatisfied with Freud's approach to the study of deviant behavior. They were critical of his untestable tenets and explanations and his unmeasurable constructs. They insisted that only behavior which could be observed, empirically tested, and reliably investigated should be the subject matter of psychology. Although investigators could not observe or measure directly a construct such as "hostile impulses," they could measure and count such behaviors as hitting and fighting. More recently others have included some unobservable, inferred constructs or mediating variables such as cognition or perception as legitimate objects of study. They are careful, however, to distinguish such unobserved and inferred variables from intrapsychic ones (Craighead, Kazdin, and Mahoney, 1976) by the fact that behavioral or physiological indices of the former can be found by which to assess them objectively, and attempts are made to relate such covert events to observable behavior.

Behaviorists do not consider specific behaviors as "symptoms" of underlying disorders or syndromes, but rather as maladaptive behavior that needs to be changed, and hence they are very much against a medical model. Diagnostic labels are denounced as highly subjective and misleading because such labels assume an underlying coherence or diagnostic entity which may not exist and in any case is untestable. Furthermore, labeling a child's behavior as "normal" or "abnormal," "disturbed" or "healthy," constitutes a value judgment that is influenced by cultural and social factors, personal biases, and theoretical orientation and that cannot be empirically validated (Bandura and Walters, 1963).

This theoretical perspective emphasizes learned behavior. If deviant behaviors have been acquired by means of regular learning theory principles and follow the same laws as normal behavior, they can be unlearned and new behaviors learned. Change can occur at any time throughout one's life, according to the behaviorists, and therefore theirs is a less deterministic view than the analytic one. There is less need to know the early history of the child, or what specific stages the child has gone through; more weight is given to the possibility of change.

According to the learning theorists, behavior can be studied scientifically, with controlled experimental methods and observation, and the results can therefore be more easily agreed upon and replicated.

The early behaviorist theorizing was given a social learning emphasis through the work of such people as Sears (1951) and Bandura and Walters (1963). There is newer emphasis on cognitive behavior mod-

20

ification (Beck, 1976; Mahoney, 1974; Meichenbaum, 1974) and the use of the cognitive processes involved in learning.

Clinical Model

What the behaviorists stress is the need to observe and measure problem behavior; to determine the antecedent conditions for specific behaviors and correlates of those behaviors (Bandura and Walters, 1963); and to single out the environmental factors that are reinforcing and maintaining that behavior. The objective is to help the child learn more adaptive behaviors, through the use of classical or operant conditioning techniques and a variety of other behavioral techniques. The main goal is actual behavior change rather than mere insight.

Some of the tools and techniques used in the assessment of problem behavior are quite different from those used by psychodynamic workers. Careful observation, counting, and charting are important aspects of behavioral assessment when one is trying to identify target behaviors for intervention and to obtain baseline data against which to measure change. An assessment of the environment of the child, the context in which particular behaviors occur, and the contingencies and reinforcements that sustain the undesirable or deviant behavior is also necessary. Once these factors are identified, a course of action can be developed.

Many new behavioral techniques have been developed as the popularity of the behavioral model has increased. Extinction procedures and counterconditioning techniques have been used (Bandura and Walters, 1963). In the former, the undesirable behavior is not reinforced and consequently decreases; in the latter, responses incompatible with the undesirable behavior are elicited and reinforced, thus reducing the undesirable behavior. Social imitation or modeling, where desired behavior is exhibited by a model in the presence of the child showing deviant behavior (Bandura and Walters, 1963), has been used to shape prosocial responses which are incompatible with previously exhibited undesirable behavior. In fact, according to Bandura and Walters, some client changes which were previously attributed to specific therapeutic techniques or interactions may actually have been due to the client's learning of certain therapeutic values and attitudes through observation and modeling of the therapist. Other techniques include systematic desensitization (Wolpe and Lazarus, 1966), assertiveness training (Wolpe, 1958), relaxation training, and operant conditioning. (Many of these will be discussed in more detail in later chapters, where their use in clinical practice with specific disorders can be demonstrated.)

Finally, not only the techniques but the types of personnel required differ significantly for psychodynamic and behavioral approaches. The former approaches call for long-term professional training, whereas behavioral techniques can fairly easily be taught to parents, teachers, and others involved on a day-by-day basis with a child and family. Thus, the number of individuals who can work to implement the behavioral programs is much greater.

Critique

One of the most frequent criticisms of the behavioral methods is that they deal only with symptoms, not with underlying causes, and that if such underlying causes are not eliminated, other symptoms will develop. This notion of *symptom substitution* is a very controversial one. Most behaviorists maintain that there is little evidence of negative effects after treatment of specific behaviors, especially if alternative desirable behaviors are taught (Bandura and Walters, 1963; Craighead, Kazdin, and Mahoney, 1976). In addition, some positive side effects frequently follow through a process of generalization (Craighead, Kazdin, and Mahoney, 1976), although changes in a person following symptom removal are hard to predict (Blom, 1977).

One could better predict a person's behavior following behavior modification if one knew that individual's response hierarchy and could then determine which behavior was most likely to occur after an undesirable one had been eliminated (Bandura and Walters, 1963). If the new behavior was deviant also, symptom substitution would seem to have occurred; whereas that would not be the case if the next response on the hierarchy was an adaptive or desirable one. Although there is no evidence that substitution of other deviant responses for the eliminated ones occurs, neither does elimination of an undesirable one ensure that positive ones will follow (Bandura and Walters, 1963). Therefore, it is important to include procedures intended to elicit and maintain positive behaviors that are incompatible with the undesirable ones (Bandura and Walters, 1963; Craighead, Kazdin, and Mahoney, 1976).

Behavioral methods have also been criticized on the grounds that insufficient attention is given to the complexity of human behavior and motivation or to the influence of inner states on behavior (Blom, 1977). Internal conditions such as anxiety and relaxation are important components of many behavior therapies, however; and with the increasing emphasis on cognitive behavior modification (to be discussed in the next section), there is much more focus on internal activity, covert verbalization, and cognitive processes. Thus, this criticism appears to be less valid here than it was in regard to the earliest applications of learning principles to intervention techniques. In addition, although environmental events are emphasized and are thought to be most amenable to intervention, behavioral therapists also acknowledge the interaction of the environmental influences with genetic and constitutional characteristics of the child (Ross, 1980). However, affective components of such complex motivational states as jealousy, guilt, and ambition are still not generally included in discussions of behavioral therapy.

Finally, although behavior modification has frequently been criticized on ethical grounds as infringing on the freedom of others by exerting behavioral control, one must realize that *all* forms of therapy exert some control over the clients' lives (Graziano, 1978).

Efforts to integrate the analytic and behavioral perspectives and models, or to restate analytic concepts in learning theory terms, such as in the classic work of Dollard and Miller (1950), have generally had little impact (Garfield, 1981). Fundamental differences in view of reality, in focus, in likelihood of change, and in therapeutic emphasis (Messer and Winokur, 1980) hinder such integration. At a more applied, clinical level, however, behavior modification techniques have been combined with more psychodynamic techniques in the treatment of children (Blom, 1977; Weinberger, 1971). Blom argued against a single paradigm in approaching behavior problems and suggested a set of guidelines to help clinicians determine when behavior modification techniques might be useful and when they would be less appropriate. Among the situations warranting a consideration of behavior modification, according to Blom, are those where single symptoms exist, with little indication of general disturbance; where the situation is urgent; where behavior modification can be a corollary to other interventions; where alternative skills must be developed; where relationship problems need to be bypassed; and where there is a need for structure and predictability. Situations for which Blom feels such techniques would not be appropriate include those where emotions need to be expressed and worked through (as in grief, for instance); where relationship problems need to be addressed directly; where inner conflict persists; where goals other than removal of symptoms exist; where insight is possible; or where feelings interfere with the application of other procedures. Blom cautions that these are guidelines and as such are not totally inclusive, but they do indicate circumstances in which a clinician might draw on both approaches.

Such attempts at integration can be helpful and stimulating theoretically and can aid clinicians who are faced with a wide variety of problems to choose the most appropriate intervention for individual clients. The various approaches need not be mutually exclusive; they can often be used concurrently and in various combinations.

Cognitive-Developmental Approach

Theoretical Perspective

The cognitive-developmental approach, based largely on the work of Jean Piaget, stresses the central importance of the child's increasing ability to understand and experience the world through such cognitive processes as memory, perception, interpretation of stimuli, and abstract thought and through the use of symbols, information processing, problem-solving strategies, and language, all of which mediate and influence behavior. These processes determine interactions between the individual and events in the environment. They are critical determinants of behavior, since it is one's perception of and interpretation of events rather than the events themselves that often determines behavior and that accounts for individuality of reaction to similar situations (Craighead, Kazdin, and Mahoney, 1976).

Piaget's work has stimulated voluminous research, and a thorough review of his theories is beyond the scope of this book. Good summaries can be found in most developmental texts; Piaget and Inhelder's *The Psychology of the Child* (1969) is recommended for students interested in doing more extensive reading of Piagetian theory. However, a brief discussion of some of his ideas as they relate to the growing emphasis on the role of cognitive processes in psychological disorders is necessary. For a very extensive discussion of such cognitive

24

processes as perception, memory, learning, problem-solving, reasoning, and language, the reader is referred to Anderson (1980).

One of the basic tenets of Piagetian theory is that the process of cognitive development is an interactive one which progresses or develops as the child matures and as objects and events in the environment are experienced. In the infant stage, most learning is accomplished through sensorimotor activities. However, the maturing child becomes increasingly capable of more complex cognitive functioning, which culminates in the development of a capacity for symbolic thought, usually during early adolescence.

Piaget's overriding interests were in how children *organize* their experience and how they *adapt* to their environment. Cognitive abilities increasingly replace motor activity, but both are adaptive (Tuddenham, 1966). As Tuddenham put it, Piaget helped to describe " . . . how the unanalyzed 'bloom of confusion' of the infant becomes the world of the child—in which not only objects, but time, space, causality, and the rest acquire a coherent organization" (Tuddenham, 1966, p. 217).

The organism's adaptation is accomplished either through assimilation (fitting new experiences into existing ideas or schema) or through accommodation, whereby a child changes ideas or concepts to accommodate or incorporate the new experience. Thus, the child develops as a result of ongoing assimilation and accommodation. This process occurs as a function both of forces and drives within an individual and of the individual's interactions with the environment. These forces and interactions result in changes in the child's *capacity* to understand.

The child's route from infancy to the advanced cognitive levels, according to Piaget, proceeds through regular and universal stages. Piaget's studies led him to investigate the qualitative differences in cognitive structures existing at successive stages which allow a child to solve problems at one stage that he or she was unable to solve at previous stages.

Piaget held that mental growth cannot be separated from physical growth and that study of developmental processes cannot be restricted to biological maturation, as experience is considered to be of equal importance (Piaget and Inhelder, 1969). Individuals are active beings, with change an inherent part of their lives (Papalia and Olds, 1982), and the cognitive structures that develop are action structures or organized actions on objects (Kohlberg, 1969). Cognitive theory assumes that the first step in the development of a behavior is the construction of a cognitive representation of the individual's environment. "The cognitive representation thus acts as the effective environment which arouses motives and emotions, and guides overt behavior toward its target or goal" (Baldwin, 1969, p. 326). The cognitive function or mechanism, then, according to Baldwin, is the first step in the progression from stimuli to response, in which stimuli are processed to extract information (Baldwin, 1969). Kohlberg (1969) describes it well:

> Cognitive structure refers to rules for processing information or for connecting experienced events. Cognition (as most clearly reflected in thinking) means putting things together or relating events, and this relating is an active connecting process. . . . In part this means that connections are formed by selective and active processes of attention, information-gathering strategies, motivated thinking, etc. More basically, it means that the process of relating particular events depends upon prior general modes of relating developed by the organism." (Kohlberg, 1969, pp. 349–350)

Thus, development is not a function solely of reinforcement or lack of reinforcement from external forces in the environment, nor is it a result solely of maturation. Rather, development involves maturational forces *and* exploration and activity of the child, in an interaction of organism and environment.

Clinical Model

These theoretical views regarding cognitive development and the importance of cognitive processes in all areas of functioning have had a pronounced influence on the assessment of, and intervention with, children manifesting a wide range of academic and behavior problems, as well as on the education of normal children. For example, attuning educational efforts to the thought patterns that are natural for the child's age makes those educational efforts more effective and allows children to be taught more than was previously expected (Tuddenham, 1966). What the child learns and how that learning is assimilated depends not only on environmental influences but also on what is already known by the child (Reid and Hresko, 1981). When these concepts are applied educationally, the learner is clearly the most important piece in the learning puzzle. "Effective instruction provides activities (in the broadest sense) to facilitate the *learner's ability to construct meaning from experience*," including modeling, observation, action, discussion, and other experiences (Reid and Bresko, 1981, p. 49).

The emphasis is on the *processes* involved in learning, and on the different problem-solving strategies employed by different children. For example, whether a child is reflective or impulsive affects selection and evaluation of hypotheses involved in problem-solving (Kagan, 1966). Therefore, the poorer intellectual performance of brain-damaged and reading-retarded children, who are more likely to be impulsive, may be due to impulsivity more often than to inadequate resources (Kagan, 1966). This suggestion has clear implications for remediation, because training in reflection as a specific habit, independent of content, then may be valuable (Kagan, 1966).

Cognitive theory is also important clinically in understanding the development of various disorders. Cognitive development, for example, sets limits on the kinds of thought processes children can use and the strategies they employ to cope with stress (Achenbach, 1978a). At certain stages children can rationally distinguish real from imagined danger (Achenbach, 1978a), whereas they may not have been able to do so in the previous stage.

The Piagetian progression through cognitive stages has also been linked to psychodynamic theorizing in the suggestions of Elkind (1976) regarding the relationship between cognitive stages or levels and specific clinical symptoms. He suggests, for example, that certain kinds of defensive thought processes can be related to successive Piagetian cognitive stages, such as the derivation of magical thinking from the preschool period, denial and rationalization from the elementary school period, and rejection (as he defines it) and projection from the formal operations stage. He also suggests that a child must be at a certain level of cognitive development before specific syndromes can be manifested, and that the nature of a problem changes as cognitive development proceeds. For example, when loss is experienced during infancy, according to Elkind, the infant has no defenses and may develop anaclitic depression; whereas the elementary school–aged child can rationalize, deny, and use other cognitive mechanisms to cope with loss. With the expanded cognitive development of adolescence, however, depression may be most difficult to overcome, because new aspects of the problem can now be grasped as a result of developed cognitive structures, and old defenses such as denial may no longer be effective.

Clearly the diagnostic problem is to determine the kinds of cognitive functions of which a child is capable (Flavell, 1977) and how they are used in interaction with environmental influences and events. However, since the relationship between behavioral expression and mental processes is not certain, Flavell prefers to speak of a "working hypothesis." For example, children may have cognitive ability and not show it for a number of reasons. Such ability may be masked by emotional and motivational factors, or the child may not understand the instructions, or the child may have the cognitive skill but not the necessary language to express it (Flavell, 1977). Moreover, the task may actually be demanding a different cognitive operation from the one the experimenter assumes is involved. For example, a child may fail to demonstrate a particular skill not because she is incapable of that skill but because some other aspect of the task—for example, memory of component parts—is posing a difficulty.

Diagnosis can be difficult also for the reason that the functions being measured change as the child matures (Flavell, 1977). Moreover, cognitive psychology is inferential in that the clinician must observe behavior on intellectual tasks and then infer aspects of underlying mechanisms or internal processes on the basis of that overt behavior (Anderson, 1980). However, research efforts appear to be focusing increasingly on cognitive functioning and ability at specified developmental points rather than on efforts to give cognitive tasks which predict later ability (Stein, 1982). Computer models of cognitive processes have been used to try to increase understanding of how people learn (Stein, 1982).

Treatment or intervention in the cognitive-developmental model depends on the alteration of cognitive processes which determine or mediate behavior rather than on changing environmental reinforcement contingencies. For example, individuals might learn problem-solving skills which can be generalized to many kinds of problems, rather than training for one deficit area (Craighead, Kazdin, and Mahoney, 1976). Intervention strategies emphasize the client's cognitive skills for problem-solving and help to develop component skills such as weighing alternatives and considering consequences to various alternatives (Craighead, Kazdin, and Mahoney, 1976). Interventions to alter cognitive functions include training in specific cognitive skills and involve rehearsal, modeling, self-instruction, and other techniques, many of which are discussed later in this text in relation

28

to specific problems. Intervention may also involve more closely matching educational and therapeutic input to a child's level of cognitive development and capacity to organize and use that input. Craighead and colleagues (1976) provide a good discussion of the ways in which cognitive processes mediate behavior and the ways in which they can be used clinically.

Critique

The cognitive-developmental approach is highly significant and influential. It emphasizes changes in cognitive structure that cannot be explained by simple learning theory (Kohlberg, 1969). It supplements learning theory in its concern with language and cognitive events and the ways in which they mediate a wide range of behavior. Recent work on what are called metaprocesses extends this interest a step further to include the study of how individuals acquire information or think *about* cognitive processes. Metacognition, for example, refers to the acquisition of information about one's own cognitive functioning, such as how one monitors and uses such processes as checking and planning (Meichenbaum and Asarnow, 1979).

This approach is represented in such current interventions as cognitive behavioral modification, which seeks to modify behavior as a result of alterations in cognitive processes and thus combines behavioral principles with cognitive developmental perspectives. Thus, it serves to integrate many of the valuable concepts of learning theory and extends the utility of such concepts by applying them to highly complex cognitive functions. It also emphasizes the role of language, including self-verbalization, and imagery in the mediation of behavior (Craighead, Kazdin, and Mahoney, 1976). In addition, its emphasis on both organismic and environmental variables provides a means by which biological and learning or behavioral approaches can be synthesized to provide a more comprehensive understanding of how children develop and how disorders might arise.

Most of the criticism of this approach appears to center on the amount of inference that is required regarding internal, unobservable processes such as verbal mediation of behavior. That is, observable behavior is assumed to reflect underlying cognitive processes. At times this can lead to inaccurate conclusions, as when one infers a specific cognitive event when in fact other cognitive events are responsible for the behaviors observed. In addition, much of the research in this area is relatively new and requires verification and elaboration with respect to the generalization and maintenance of changes observed. Finally, some suggest that more research is needed in non-cognitive areas of behavior such as aggression and dependency (Craig, 1979), though cognitive theorists would likely argue that such behaviors are mediated by and determined by the cognitive processes they study. Moreover, children's perceptions are interrelated with and influence all their other cognitive processes, including reasoning and memory, which affect the way in which they interpret and respond to environmental events; and moods and emotions affect how they perceive, remember, attend, think, and learn (Bower, 1982).

In general, it appears that this approach holds substantial promise both theoretically and clinically and that it will be useful in integrating other points of view.

Neurobiological Approach

Theoretical Perspective

Many aspects of behavior and development point up the importance and relevance of biological factors both in normal development and in the development of psychological disorders. A biological perspective is important to include because it emphasizes what individuals bring to life situations—a composite of genetic, chromosomal, biochemical, neurological, and physiological characteristics and predispositions which directly and indirectly affect behavior and development. Aspects of an infant's temperament and "biological clock," for instance, can affect very early parent-child interactions. Moreover, particular children may be predisposed genetically to manifest certain behaviors (Thomas, 1979). In addition, overall health and stamina, the presence or absence of physical or neurological abnormalities and handicaps, and even such characteristics as size and hair color all affect individuals' feelings about themselves and their reactions to and interactions with others.

A biological or neurobiological approach also takes into consideration prenatal and postnatal influences and events that can cause neurological impairment or other dysfunction. Biological or physiological events during the prenatal and postnatal period can have highly significant effects on behavior, learning, and overall development. For example, asphyxia due to insufficient oxygen at birth can lead to mental retardation, brain damage, and possibly cerebral palsy (Windle, 1973).

A neurobiological approach can help to explain the normal development of such functions as language and locomotion, and other behaviors which develop in predictable ways and cannot be explained solely by psychodynamic or learning theory principles.

The biological concept of maturation, for example, explains an individual's development as an unfolding of inner potential and capability, provided there is not serious interference with the natural maturational and developmental sequence. The *rate* of maturation, however, is likely determined by hereditary influences. Moreover, although maturation prepares individuals for much behavior, the actual development of that behavior is influenced in important ways by environmental and learning factors (Alexander, Roodin, and Gorman, 1980). As certain levels of maturation are necessary before some specific behaviors are possible (e.g., sphincter control), interference with or delays in maturation will also result in delays in related behaviors. Thus, a child who has good neurological and genetic potential at birth may not receive adequate stimulation to fully develop his or her genetically determined intellectual potential. Biological timing, however, affects the consequences for development of certain environmental events or even whether they have any effects (Bower, 1979). Conversely, although one cannot separate clearly biological or innate from learned behavior, much learning that is influenced by the environment is also genetically determined (Gould and Gould, 1981). The fact that development does not occur by chance but rather according to an orderly and innately determined sequence is central to Piaget as well as to ethologists (Alexander, Roodin, and Gorman, 1980).

Much research has been done on cerebral dominance (the dominance of one hemisphere of the brain over the other) and its effect on such functions as handedness. Moreover, there is considerable research available regarding specialization of function and control by the two hemispheres of the brain. The left hemisphere is generally regarded as associated primarily with language acquisition and function, and the right with nonverbal and spatial skills. Adequate brain functioning is clearly involved in the acquisition and integration of written and spoken information, often referred to as the central processing function of the brain. Behavior, then, depends on functional input and output systems and a brain that mediates and controls both (Bower, 1979). Damage or problems in any area of the brain can lead to skill deficits and impairments (Bower, 1979). Dysfunctions in central processing are then manifested in reading or learning problems, for example. (These are discussed in more detail in Chapter 10 on learning disabilities.) However, the presence of specific learning disabilities does not necessarily indicate cerebral dysfunction.

Emphasis on an organic or biological view leads to explanations of many disorders in terms of developmental lags or immaturity of brain development. Studies of the electrical activity of the brain recorded on graphs known as electroencephalograms (EEGs) indicate developmental changes in brain function as a result of maturation (Achenbach, 1974). The graphs may also reveal a high incidence of EEG abnormalities in some children who are experiencing various disorders; their EEGs may be similar to those of younger children (Anthony, 1970) and may thus suggest maturational delays. Some investigators, such as Wender and Klein (1981), have argued that research evidence supports a central role for biological dysfunction in many disorders, including some "neurotic" ones, and that drugs can provide long-term relief in some cases where psychoanalysis and behavior therapy have been ineffective. They argue further that studies of children in adoptive homes have challenged the view that most disorders are psychogenically caused. They stress, rather, the importance of genetic factors in a wide range of problems, where psychological factors could trigger disorders in individuals who were thus biologically predisposed.

The whole area of psychosomatic or psychophysiological disorders also relies heavily on biological factors in its suggestions of genetic or constitutional predisposition or vulnerability, as well as in its findings of varying individualized physiological responses to stimuli. In addition, the medical aspects of a biological or neurobiological approach interact with cognitive developmental events, as when drugs sedate an individual and distort perception, hence affecting cognitive processes and development.

32

Ethologists have contributed to this perspective by extending their ideas and methodology from animals to humans. The emphasis on innately determined or inherited patterns of behavior and their function in an organism's adaptation, as well as their methods of observing in naturalistic surroundings, have been useful in the study of child development.

Specific details regarding biological development and growth can be obtained elsewhere, but the importance of that perspective needs emphasis here. The significance of the biological aspects of psychological disorders will become clearer in the context of specific disorders and their etiology and progression.

For a thorough and detailed discussion of genetic, neurochemical, neurological, and other biological aspects of behavior, the reader is referred to the *Comprehensive Textbook of Psychiatry II*, Vol. 1 (Freedman, Kaplan, and Sadock, 1975).

Clinical Model

A determination of the biological and physiological processes associated with psychological disorders dictates to a large extent the flavor of the diagnostic and treatment procedures to be used. The goal of an assessment in such an approach is to discover the underlying physiological, neurological, or biochemical abnormalities or deficits. To that end, such diagnostic procedures and techniques as blood chemistry analyses, neuropsychological assessments, or a search for EEG abnormalities might be undertaken. In addition, behavioral observations and interviews might be used to evaluate background factors and to elicit information concerning such events as frequent high fevers, falls, or specific diseases which may have resulted in neurological damage or other physiological dysfunction. Some of this damage or dysfunction would be inferred on the basis of behavioral observation, as, for example, in the case of a child whose behavior suggested neurological damage but whose EEGs were normal. The goal is to relate behavioral problems to a physiological or biochemical substrate or base.

Intervention from this point of view can encompass several modes of attack. First, where possible, chemical or hormonal imbalances or deficits would be treated directly with medication, hormonal supplements, or diet, as with diabetics, for example. However, failure to respond to biological treatment does not necessarily mean that the problems are psychological, as the proper biological treatment may not yet have been developed; nor does failure with psychotherapy necessarily mean that the problem is biological (Wender and Klein, 1981). Second, in addition to medication and diet, other treatment, such as biofeedback and relaxation techniques, may be used to alter physiological functions, as with anxious clients, for example. Such techniques may allow an individual greater control over the physiological aspects of anxiety and hence reduce the subjectively experienced distress. Third, where underlying dysfunction has been inferred but has not been confirmed or cannot be treated directly, intervention efforts might be concentrated on educational and behavioral aspects of the problem to help the child cope with existing problems.

Critique

Although the biological aspects of development and the neurobiological and neurological mechanisms underlying disordered behavior are important and can add immeasurably to our understanding of children, they are not adequate as explanatory tools. That is, they alone cannot explain all aspects of psychological disorders. Nor is the approach without problems. For one thing, considerable inference is often required to deduce brain function from behavioral observation. For example, sometimes brain dysfunction is inferred on the basis of such behavioral indices as poor coordination or problems with symbolic thought. These are sometimes referred to as "soft signs" because they are behavioral and do not show up on such instruments as EEGs. Thus, neurological dysfunction is often inferred rather than demonstrated objectively or conclusively. Second, a biological emphasis may lead to a tendency to underestimate environmental events and influences on a child's functioning, either generally or in response to actual neurological damage or other biochemical or hormonal deficits or abnormalities. Third, there is always the problem of possible misdiagnosis and resultant ineffective handling. For example, until we understand more fully the relationship between organic function and behavior, we risk treating some children without organic problems as

34

if they in fact do have them, which often results in a more pessimistic outlook; or we mistakenly implicate parents or internal conflict in behavior problems when in fact organic dysfunction is present (Achenbach, 1974). Moreover, the fact that medication can alter some behaviors does not tell us much about the processes involved (Anthony, 1970). Finally, the connection between various physiological events and disordered behavior is often correlational and is therefore not definitive regarding cause-and-effect relationships (Knopf, 1979).

Humanistic Approach

Theoretical Perspective

The humanistic movement in psychology arose as a "third force" because of dissatisfaction with both the psychoanalytic and the behavioral schools of thought. The two names most closely associated with this perspective are Carl Rogers and Abraham Maslow. Maslow's studies, dealing chiefly with normal persons, and Rogers's, based primarily on therapeutic work with clients, emphasize the capacity within the individual for growth and change. Their work depends largely on the subjective experience of the person, and emphasizes growth and evolution of the person's self: self-actualization (Maslow, 1968). Freedom and permissiveness are stressed to allow a child to grow, to "let him *be*" (Maslow, 1968, p. 199), and, according to Rogers, to allow active interaction with the environment in order to facilitate self-enhancement (Ullman and Krasner, 1969). According to Maslow, people are intrinsically good rather than innately evil, and negative behaviors and characteristics result when that intrinsic good is frustrated. Rather than being interpreted in terms of illness or a medical model, deviant behavior is interpreted in terms of " ... the loss of human potentialities and capacities" (Maslow, 1968, p. 204) when a person lives in fear of growth and change.

Because of its strong emphasis on the capacity of people to change, and the assumption that people have the ability to solve their own problems given the right environmental conditions, the humanistic perspective, like the behavioristic one, is very optimistic and positive.

Humanists introduced the study of a number of areas of human functioning, such as creativity, love, and will, and of other purposeful and prosocial behaviors, such as altruism, which had been largely overlooked or ignored by the other theoretical views. These areas had not been addressed in any significant way by the pathology-oriented analytic school or by the behaviorists, who saw them as unobservable, untestable, and unscientific.

Clinical Model

The nondirective model of therapeutic intervention which reflects the humanistic perspective and has been most vocally espoused and formulated by Carl Rogers (1951, 1961), is one in which the client (not a patient, as in a medical model) feels accepted—unconditionally. The therapist develops a warm, uncritical, nonjudgmental context within which the person can feel free to experience and explore certain feelings. As a result, the person is able to grow, to solve his or her own problems, and to attain a higher level of self-fulfillment. Rogers insisted that the therapist remain "nondirective"—that the therapist refrain from giving advice, asking questions, persuading, or otherwise influencing the client (Ullman and Krasner, 1969). The individual has the capacity to move toward maturity and to understand what is causing dissatisfaction (Rogers, 1961) and can do so if the proper therapeutic atmosphere is provided.

This approach to the treatment of children is best exemplified in the work of such child psychotherapists as Virginia Axline (1947) and Clark Moustakas (1959b), but nondirective techniques are a part of the repertoire of many other therapists in the course of their daily work with children and their families. These techniques and their use with children will be discussed in greater detail in Chapter 6 in the section on play therapy.

Critique

The humanists' forays into the areas of functioning not extensively explored previously have constituted an important contribution to the study of human development and behavior. Their ideas and concepts regarding human nature and the internal forces that shape behavior have been used and applied in various ways by many clinicians. Since humanists have traditionally been less concerned with deviant than with normal children or adults (McCandless, 1976), however, and since they abhor labels in the same way as behaviorists do, there is little to be found in the literature on their diagnoses or interpretations of the specific behavioral and emotional disorders discussed in this text.

Concluding Comments

There has been considerable discussion of a family systems approach to psychological disorders. Rather than viewing a referral problem as strictly the child's problem, the therapist views the child as one component in a family system of interactions. The emphasis is on the *interactions* between the child and other members of the family, and the patterns of interaction are related to specific problems (Hetherington and Martin, 1979). The family is seen as a system in which dyads (two members in an interaction) and triads (three members in an interaction) interact in specific sequences which need to be changed in order to resolve presenting problems (Haley, 1976). As these theories can have psychodynamic or behavioral emphases, however, they are discussed more fully in Chapter 6 in the section on family therapy.

Other models discussed by various writers include sociological, educational, and statistical models (Achenbach, 1974), which can be very useful for specific purposes or when conceptualizing more limited areas of disturbance. However, the approaches discussed in this chapter have dominated the research literature and provide a broad backdrop against which to view childhood disorders. Much of the discussion concerning specific disorders throughout the text will be concentrated on the first two—the psychodynamic and behavioral models—simply because they have exerted the most pervasive influence for the longest period of time and have generated the most research on the assessment and treatment of specific disorders. However, cognitive and biological approaches have also spawned considerable research and are essential components of any comprehensive look at psychological problems in children and adolescents. In many ways they represent the most current emphases in the literature as well as perhaps an indication of future directions. Moreover, they may provide the soundest basis on which to build more integrated and comprehensive views of psychological disorders in children and ado-

T A B L E 2.1 *A comparison of the basic principles and practices of the five major approaches*

	Psychodynamic	Behavioral
Causes of deviant behavior	Underlying conflict	Faulty learning
	Unconscious forces	Environmental reinforcement of maladaptive behavior
Assessment techniques	Projective techniques	Observation
	Dream analysis	Rating scales
	Free association	Charting
	Personality tests	Interview
	Clinical interview	
Goals of intervention	Develop insight	Decrease maladaptive behaviors
	Decrease need for defenses	Increase positive behaviors
	Resolve conflicts	
Therapeutic techniques	Individual or group psychotherapy	Operant and classical conditioning
	Play therapy	Relaxation and systematic desensitization
	Family therapy	Modeling
		Implosive therapy
Criticisms	Pessimistic	Possible symptom substitution
	Untestable	Insufficiently complex

lescents. For this reason they are well represented throughout the discussions of specific disorders in later chapters.

Lugo and Hershey's (1979) summary of the basic concepts, tools, processes, and methods involved in each of these perspectives is highly recommended.

Table 2.1 summarizes very briefly the basic tenets and tools of each major perspective.

Cognitive-developmental	Neurobiological	Humanistic
Faulty or distorted cognitive processes	Neurobiological damage or dysfunction	Frustration of growth, self-fulfillment
Inaccurate perceptions	Biochemical or hormonal imbalances	
Stimuli poorly matched to child's cognitive level	Genetic defects	
Inadequate experiences	Maturational lags	
Intelligence tests	EEG	Interview
Tests of various cognitive skills	Neurological examination	
	Neuropsychological assessment	
	Interviews regarding developmental history	
	Observation	
Alter cognitive process to effect change	Alter physiological, neurological, or biochemical functioning	Remove obstacles to growth and self-fulfillment
Problem resolution		
Cognitive-behavioral intervention	Medication	Establish accepting, permissive atmosphere
Self-instruction	Biofeedback	Nondirective psychotherapy
Modeling	Relaxation techniques	
Training in verbal mediation strategies		
Too much reliance on inference regarding internal processes	Insufficient emphasis on environmental influences	Does not address specific disorders
	Requires inference of brain function from behavioral observation	

Discussion Questions

1. How do the major theoretical perspectives reflect different views of human behavior? On what basic issues do they differ?
2. Discuss possible ways in which aspects of the different views might be integrated. How could such efforts affect one's clinical approach to a disorder?
3. Discuss the relative merits of each of the perspectives.

CHAPTER 3   # Research Issues

Basic Types of Research

Research in the area of child psychopathology is generally of two major types, basic and applied, although there is wide variation within each of these types. Research into the nature and etiology of various disorders is basic and process-oriented, its major aim being to acquire new knowledge—to discover the very nature of a disorder. For instance, continuing research into the question of physiological and neurochemical factors in the development of schizophrenia would be categorized as basic research. Research into diagnostic techniques and studies of the relative effectiveness of specific therapeutic interventions, on the other hand, are examples of applied or product-oriented research, which is sometimes referred to as "research utilization" (Lustman, 1968), because its prime purpose is to put knowledge into use. Effective ways actually to treat disorders must be found, as well as practical means of making the resources available to the people who need them. In his report to the U.S. Mental Health Commission, Lustman warned that at times the pressure on social scientists to "do something" when faced with human suffering and need may mask the fact that treatment utilization must be preceded by appropriate basic research. Further, decisions grounded in such basic research have a much higher probability of success than those guided only by a consensus of apparent need; in other words, agreeing that there is a need in no way guarantees successful handling of a problem (Lustman, 1968).

Within the two broad areas of basic and applied research, there are many differences in research method, in location or site of the research, and in temporal dimension. Some of these differences will be reviewed here briefly.

Methods

The two fundamental approaches to research problems are correlational and experimental. In *experimental* studies, children are randomly assigned to a group which receives a particular kind of treatment (independent variable), and their behavior and/or their responses are compared along the dimension being studied (dependent variable) with those of a control group which does not receive the treatment. The experimental and control groups in such a study

42

are matched on other variables that could affect results, such as age, sex, and IQ. For example, a new teaching method (independent variable) could be introduced to one (experimental) group, and the established method continued with another (control) group, both groups having been matched as to age, IQ, sex, socioeconomic level, and whatever other variables seem relevant. Assignment to the experimental group must be random to avoid confounding or contaminating the results with subtle biases or other factors. The effect of the new teaching method on the reading level (dependent variable) is noted by comparing the reading levels of the two groups after the experimental group has been exposed to the new method. If there is a substantial improvement in the performance of the experimental group, one may conclude, with a certain measure of confidence, that the treatment received (the new teaching method in this case) by one group did in fact cause the behavior or response (that is, improved reading or higher reading level) which was noted following the treatment.

It is also important, even necessary, to study any interaction effects which might exist among the variables. For example, a new teaching method may be more effective at one age than another. That is, age and teaching method interact, and such an effect needs to be studied as well. Similarly, poverty and a single-parent home may not, separately, be critical factors in the development of a disorder, but together the two may produce a very different set of circumstances and exercise a much greater influence than either factor would exert singly.

In *correlational* studies, the association between certain variables or behaviors in selected samples or populations of children is studied. Subjects are chosen and groups are matched on as many related variables as possible—age and IQ, for example—to yield the most meaningful data. Since assignment to experimental and control groups is not random, however, as in the experimental method, causal directions cannot be inferred. If, for example, a positive correlation were found between height and reading levels, one could conclude neither that tallness causes good reading nor that good reading causes tallness. There is a relationship or association, but not necessarily causation. This is very important to remember when considering less extreme and more realistic problems. One variable could possibly cause the other, or both could be caused by other variables which have not been taken into account. In addition, one must guard against circular reasoning in the interpretation of correlations, as when, for example, a

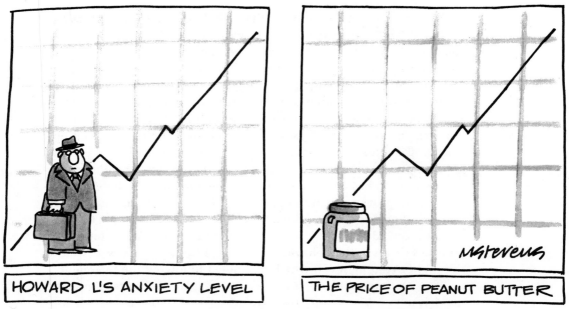

HOWARD L'S ANXIETY LEVEL   THE PRICE OF PEANUT BUTTER

FIGURE 3.1   *Coincidence or what?* Drawing by M. Stevens; © 1981 The New Yorker Magazine, Inc.

disorder is inferred from symptoms and then the symptoms are said to be produced by the disorder (Lefkowitz and Burton, 1978).

The cartoon in Figure 3.1 clearly demonstrates the hazards of drawing conclusions about causation from simple correlation. In this situation, both variables are quite possibly affected by a third factor, such as general economic conditions or financial stress.

Although causation cannot be inferred from correlational studies, such studies are enormously helpful in indicating how behaviors or characteristics covary, and they are fruitful grounds for hypotheses which can then be tested in a more experimental situation. Correlational studies are *exploratory* in nature; data are observed and organized, patterns noted, and hypotheses suggested. In addition, some statistical techniques, such as cross-lag analysis (Lewin, 1979), allow one to increase the predictive ability of correlational data. Many of the specified hypotheses derived from such studies can then be tested with a more rigorous experimental method, in *confirmatory research* (Achenbach, 1974; Chess and Hassibi, 1978). Correlational studies are the only way, ethically, to pursue many questions, because there are certain conditions, such as child abuse and poverty, that obviously cannot be introduced experimentally into a child's life to study their effects.

Location

Research studies are usually conducted in laboratory, naturalistic, or semicontrolled settings. The laboratory setting has traditionally been considered the most productive because its experimental rigor allows for more adequate control of confounding variables. Because of its greater precision and direction, such research is also easier for others to replicate. The price that must be paid for this control and replicative possibility, however, is an artificiality which some feel limits generalizability of the results or predictive accuracy.

The study of children in a naturalistic setting has the advantage of including many more variables and offers an opportunity for observing the child in an actual or real-life situation. However, control of the many possibly confounding variables is much more difficult, if not impossible. Although children in such a study can be matched on such variables as age, sex, and achievement levels, there are many other variables that are beyond the experimenter's control but can confound the results. These include number of siblings, extraneous distractions, activity of others, subtle cues, and a seemingly endless list of other possibilities. It is obviously impossible to achieve the rigor and control of the laboratory.

The most satisfactory setting for the study of many problems is one which includes as many positive characteristics as possible of both the laboratory and natural settings. For example, to study task behavior in children, one might well observe children within an actual classroom, subject to the presence of the teacher, other students, and hallway noise—the usual classroom environment—but at the same time incorporate such experimental factors as careful matching and random assignment to groups receiving different kinds of reinforcement, varying teaching methods, or whatever other independent variable is being studied.

Duration

The time span involved in research projects varies widely. It is a more important variable with children than with adults because of the rapid rate of development in children. In a *longitudinal* approach, the same children are studied at different ages over a long period of time. It is in many ways a preferred method because it gives a more accurate picture of developmental processes and therefore, perhaps, a better view of the development of psychopathological processes. However, it is harder to keep an entire sample intact over a long time period, and samples that were representative in the beginning may become biased when subjects or their families drop out nonrandomly (Vasta, 1979). Also, it is not easy to incorporate improved instruments and changed measures into one's longitudinal design.

In a *cross-sectional* approach, children from various age groups are studied simultaneously, and the incidences of various behaviors and disorders at different ages are compared. Although it is not possible to gauge the development of an individual child over a period of time, some developmental trends can be noted in the changing rates of certain behaviors in the various age groups. The cross-sectional approach has two distinct advantages: it is less time-consuming and easier to arrange. By studying several age groups simultaneously, researchers can acquire much data quickly and efficiently, and new samples are available to verify earlier data. However, more approximation and estimation are involved in the interpretation of the data. As single individuals have not been followed over a long period of time, one is obliged to rely more on inferences regarding developmental processes. In addition, variables other than the ones the experimenter has controlled can confound the data.

A third approach, involving a *short-term or cross-sectional longitudinal* method, combines the advantages of the other two. Separate groups are studied simultaneously, as is done for a cross-sectional study, but the ages of the groups studied overlap, and they are also studied over a period of time. Information is thus obtained on the development of children within the groups, and observations are made regarding the progression and other characteristics of several age groups simultaneously (Achenbach, 1974; Vasta, 1979).

Table 3.1 provides a simplified summary of the basic method and location variables, any of which could be used in either cross-sectional or longitudinal studies, although the practical difficulties inherent in some combinations would be greater than in others.

The research methods outlined in this chapter are illustrated throughout the book as the literature related to specific topics is discussed. Additional research designs used specifically to assess treat-

TABLE 3.1   *A comparison of basic research design characteristics*

	Location	
Method	*Laboratory*	*Naturalistic*
Experimental: Causal inferences can be made if certain conditions are met	Most controlled, precise Least like actual life situation	Most difficult to design Hard to control relevant variables
Correlational: Causation cannot be inferred	Can prearrange laboratory conditions to study groups with various existent characteristics Can control for some variables through matching	Most like actual life Only way to study some problems of children

ment effectiveness are examined in more detail in Chapter 7. For more thorough and extensive discussions of various research designs and methodological problems, the reader is referred to Vasta's (1979) introduction to research methods, or to Achenbach's (1974) excellent chapter on "scientific strategies."

Problems in Research with Children

Research into disorders in children—and the interpretation of the research—differs in important ways from that with adults. First, children rarely volunteer to participate in research projects. The parents usually offer the children to the researcher or, if they are part of a clinic or school population, consent to the children's participation in a project. Although cooperation is promised by the parents, the child's actual feeling about involvement could conceivably affect the results of the research in a way that might not be true of a subject who has volunteered. Second, a child is a rapidly maturing and developing organism whose rate of growth and development is changing and whose progress in various skill areas may be uneven. Some behaviors that are quite normal developmental problems may be mistaken for pathological behavior, or they may interact with other factors to produce disordered behavior. While some of this fluidity can be corrected for through the proper use of control groups, random assignment, and other experimental procedures, developmental differences and imbalances add one more variable for the researcher to consider in interpreting the data. Third, the investigator must know something of the level at which the child is functioning linguistically, cognitively, emotionally, and socially and must be acquainted with the child's cultural and socioeconomic background, in order to ensure that the research instruments being used are appropriate for and are understood fully by the child.

In addition, there are methodological problems to reckon with, such as inconsistent criteria, problems of sampling and definition, subjective ratings of intensity and severity, and other factors (Chess and Hassibi, 1978).

There is also the important and difficult matter of adequate controls in experimental research with children. In addition to matching experimental and control groups on such relevant variables as age, sex, intellectual functioning, and socioeconomic level, an experimenter must also try to anticipate the possible influence of other variables on the data. These include number and ages of siblings, developmental history, parent handling techniques, past academic experiences, teacher styles, effects of medication, and many, many others, the control of which may be extremely difficult, if not impossible. Some of these problems are discussed in more detail in Chapter 7.

Ethical Issues

Research with any human subject, adult or child, involves numerous ethical considerations. However, because of the above-mentioned problems as well as others that are peculiar to children, certain ethical questions require special emphasis.

Careful consideration of the risk/benefit ratio is imperative. That is, an investigator must assess whether the benefits expected from the research outweigh the potential physical or psychological risks to the child or the family. For example, how upset might children who already feel like failures become if they are asked to do a reading task of which they are not capable? Or what might be the effect of asking fearful children to fill in a checklist that accentuates and emphasizes the number of things that bother them? Although everything will be explained later, should children be placed in a situation that is threatening to them, even temporarily? And under what conditions, if any, would this be acceptable? How threatening is too threatening? And at what age? How much liberty should researchers have to involve institutional children with severe handicaps or disorders in experiments? What is the risk to them? And are they capable of understanding procedures sufficiently to give informed consent to participation?

In the area of treatment, children have less freedom than adults to influence the goals of treatment, or to refuse or terminate it if there is something they don't like (Ross, 1980). Moreover, as Ross points out, a child can resist verbal therapies by not talking or by giving a repetitive "I don't know"; but if adults are rearranging reinforcement contingencies in a behavioral program, the child may not even know treatment is going on, let alone be able to refuse it, and behavioral methods are effective means of changing behavior. Some of these issues are also discussed in Chapter 16 on child advocacy.

Many questions remain, and unfortunately there are no easy or pat answers, but children need to be protected against manipulation and against exploitation of their age, innocence, willingness, or even their disturbance. Certain suggested procedures may not be warranted, despite the intensity of the researcher's investigative zeal, because the level of risk outweighs the possible benefits, or because the risk involved cannot be adequately assessed.

Another area of ethical consideration is that of information and feedback. The children and their families have a right to receive reasonable explanations beforehand about the intent of the research, what they will be asked to do, and, to the greatest possible extent, what the goals are (without confounding the experiment). After the study, interested children, parents, and/or participating schools have a right to feedback or information concerning the findings, and these must be communicated in a clear and understandable way. The ethics of the matter aside, the good will of the participants is essential to further research, and public cooperation and understanding are contingent on researchers conducting themselves in an ethical and professional manner. Subjects should never end up feeling coerced, manipulated, tricked, exploited, or "used."

A third area which is important enough to be emphasized repeatedly is the need for confidentiality and for respect for the privacy of subjects. They should be assured that their achievements, problems, feelings, income levels, behavioral characteristics, and inner con-flicts—and any other information they have provided about them-selves—will remain absolutely confidential and will not be released to any other persons or agencies without their express written and informed consent.

Future Directions

Although there are many aspects of childhood disorders which require more research, certain questions have acquired greater salience and higher priority in recent years and have spawned consid-erable research activity. One intriguing area that is receiving increased attention is the study of the "invulnerables" or stress-resis-tant children (Pines, 1977/78; Garmezy, 1979). These are children who have come from very disturbed, multiple-problem backgrounds but who still develop with surprisingly few problems and may even thrive and make exceptional contributions to society.

Solid, methodologically sound studies are needed into the effective-ness of different kinds of treatment; into the use of paraprofessionals and the training of people within their own roles to deliver services in a more natural way, that is, an ecological approach (Van Evra, 1974); into narrowing the existing gaps between our present knowledge and our delivery of effective help in order to make the best use of availa-ble, often shrinking, resources; into the etiology of many disorders; into the special problems and vulnerabilities of defined age groups, including early infancy, preschool, school-age, and adolescence; and into the myriad types of parent-child interactions and the range of effects these interactions can have on developing children. These and many other questions demand innovative thinking and creative research if our knowledge of various disturbances and disorders is to be advanced and their prevention or remediation facilitated.

Discussion Questions

1. Give examples of the problems that would fit best and be most effectively studied in each cell of Table 3.1.
2. Design a study based on a single area of disturbance or a single question, using the following format:

50

    a. State the problem.
    b. Generate hypotheses about your study.
    c. Discuss which research method would be most appropriate.
    d. Discuss any problems you might encounter in carrying out the study.
3. Discuss ways in which the rights of a young child and an adolescent may differ. What concrete steps could be taken to protect their rights?

PART II

Diagnostic Considerations and Practices

Basic Principles of Disturbance

A careful, thorough diagnostic or behavioral assessment is of central importance in the overall treatment plan for a child, regardless of one's theoretical persuasion. In general, behavioral therapists avoid the word "diagnosis" (i.e., the classification of disorders according to a nosology or classificatory system) because it implies a medical model and a search for underlying causes of overt behavior. Rather, they speak of behavioral assessment, which involves evaluating the conditions under which a child's current behavior arose and is maintained so that they can plan for as effective an intervention as possible. In these chapters, however, the terms "diagnosis" and "assessment" will be used interchangeably to refer to efforts of clinicians to fully understand the nature of the problems with which they are dealing, whatever their theoretical persuasion.

Before the discussion in Chapter 5 of the specific diagnostic tools and techniques at the clinician's disposal, it is important to mention some basic issues which are central to a good evaluation. For example, it is vital to consider the difficulties inherent in trying to differentiate normal from abnormal or adaptive from maladaptive behavior, and in trying to classify disordered behavior. It is also important to consider how and why symptoms develop and what general factors may play a causal role in that development.

Normality and Abnormality

One of the problems both parents and clinicians face is that of distinguishing troublesome but normal behavior from difficult behavior which is considered "disturbed" or suggests the need for professional intervention.

One question related to this issue involves the continuity or discontinuity of abnormal and normal behavior. In a continuity view, abnormal behavior is seen as occupying a different point on a continuum of functioning from normality or health at one end to irreversible illness at the other (Eisenberg, 1966). A discontinuity view, on the other hand, postulates qualitative differences between healthy and disordered individuals. According to this view, individuals with a disorder have something that normal individuals do not have or lack something that normal individuals have, rather than having more or less of a quality that normal individuals have.

There are a number of ways in which normal and abnormal behav-

56

ior are defined. The most commonly used standards against which to compare problem behaviors include statistical norms, cultural norms, and developmental norms. If one compares behavior against *statistical norms*, one is looking at the frequency with which a behavior occurs in a given population. If it appears often or is engaged in by a large proportion of that population, it is considered "normal." If it occurs only rarely in a given population, it is considered "abnormal." There are obvious difficulties with such a definition of abnormality, however. For example, some behaviors or problems that are observed relatively frequently, such as school failure, might by this definition be classified as "normal." Other less frequently observed but highly desirable behaviors, such as genuinely altruistic acts or exceptional musical talent, for example, might be classified as abnormal. In other words, with statistical normality as a criterion it is difficult to distinguish between deviations that are positive or desirable and those that are negative or undesirable (Kessler, 1966). Thus, statistical norms are clearly inadequate as a basis for defining abnormality, although they can be helpful in making specific observations or comparisons for particular purposes.

When *cultural norms* are used as a criterion for defining normality and abnormality, specific behaviors are viewed within the *context* of the child's environment and the expectations of others, whether those are expectations of the family, the community, the larger society, or certain subcultural groupings. By this definition, a behavior is considered abnormal if it deviates significantly from a particular subgroup's standards and expectations. It follows, then, that some behaviors that are acceptable within a specific family or community or cultural group might be considered quite deviant in another or in the larger society.

The use of *developmental norms* as criteria for distinguishing between abnormality and normality will be emphasized throughout this text. The lines between normality and abnormality are less clear in children than in adults (Anthony, 1970), and most child problems do not fit well into adult categories (Achenbach, 1974). As maturational processes are of central significance for all aspects of normal and disordered behavior (Achenbach, 1974), a developmental framework is necessary (Anthony, 1970).

Developmental norms place specific behaviors in the context of a child's ongoing change and maturation. Specific behaviors can be assessed from various perspectives, but idiosyncratic aspects of a child's development (particular stress, system of rewards) affect how the child perceives and responds to developmental challenges (Achenbach, 1978a). Moreover, developmental considerations and changes enter in in a way that is not true of adults. For one thing, some of a child's symptoms may disappear with maturational changes and development; many "disturbances" may simply be temporary exaggerations of common reactions. Or the nature of the symptoms may change with age, as in the case of anxiety, which is characteristically manifested differently at different ages in a process known as "developmental symptom substitution" (Levitt, 1971).

In addition, Achenbach (1978a) and others have suggested that certain disorders characterize specific developmental stages or periods. For example, during infancy disorders are more likely to be organically based or to reflect problems of biological adaptation, whereas problems during preschool are more likely to be related to a child's integration into a larger environment, including language acquisition. Children of elementary school age are more likely to manifest school-related problem behaviors, while adolescents more frequently experience school refusal or depression (Achenbach, 1978a). Thus, common symptom pictures in children are not consistent but shift with the child's situation, so that one set of symptoms may be replaced by a completely different one or acute and very severe symptom pictures may be reversed (Anthony, 1970).

Some of these issues are discussed in more detail in Chapter 7, where the methodological problems involved in evaluating treatment effectiveness are addressed.

Such developmental considerations are an essential part of any discussion of normality and abnormality, as many behaviors which are normal at one developmental stage may indicate a serious disturbance at another. No one thinks twice about a one-year-old wetting the bed every night, but most would consider it highly abnormal as a nightly event at age fourteen. Therefore, one dimension along which behaviors are evaluated is that of *age-appropriateness*. Second, one must consider the *duration* of the behavior. Virtually all children go through periods in their development during which their behavior is very difficult to cope with, whether in reaction to specific life events or because of the stress that is a function of a particular developmental period that is traditionally difficult for most children. These are usually relatively short-lived, however, and are often clearly related to the child's current situation or to a particular developmental stage. If, on the other hand, such behavior persists for an extended period of time, or if there are indications that it is becoming a chronic part of the child's repertoire, outside intervention may be necessary. Third, the *intensity* of a child's upset or symptomatic behavior must be assessed. Mild compulsive behavior in children, for example, is not uncommon. However, if it interferes significantly with such children's functioning or nearly incapacitates them, it can be considered to be abnormal or maladaptive and "disturbed." Fourth, the *frequency* of a behavior may be useful in determining where on a continuum of normality it would fall. A child who occasionally gets into a fight at school would probably be considered a normally developing child. One, however, who is consistently and almost daily involved in physically or verbally aggressive confrontations at school may need professional intervention to discover why this behavior persists in spite of presumably negative reinforcement from teachers and peers. If problem behaviors are very frequent, they are also likely to be more pervasive and to interfere with functioning in many areas. Fifth, Kanfer and Grimm (1976) stress the importance of knowing what demands are characteristically being made of a child or what is expected and reinforced by the environment—that is, the *context* or setting for the behavior—before it is judged to be deviant. Unusual behaviors in unusual circumstances may even be quite adaptive, as in the case of a child who became severely inhibited and withdrawn to avoid further punishment by an alcoholic father (Kanfer and Grimm, 1976).

Many behaviors seen in clinic children are also seen in normal children, but either they do not interfere with the normal child's development (Ross, 1980) or they are tolerated by the parents (Kanner, 1972). As there are no absolute criteria for normal and abnormal behavior, an additional significant determinant of a judgment as to whether behavior is disordered, then, is often the outlook of the *person evaluating* the behavior (Kanner, 1972).

Thus, although there are no standard or precise guidelines agreed on by everyone, many clinicians would evaluate the normality or abnormality of a child's behavior along the dimensions of age-appropriateness, duration, intensity, frequency, and context of the symptoms. The expectations and tolerance of people in the environment who are doing the evaluating and the child's developmental level also affect the classification of behavior as normal or abnormal. According to these criteria, the most disturbed children would be those who regularly and over a long period of time engage in highly inappropriate behavior which causes great anxiety or unhappiness in almost all areas of their lives. However, children whose disturbed behavior is less obvious are more common, and it is those children who present the most troublesome diagnostic difficulties and disagreements.

Symptom Development

Specific symptoms characteristic of various disorders will be dealt with in future chapters, but some general statements about symptom development and the function of symptoms are appropriate here. Again, there is controversy in the field about the significance of symptoms, depending on one's theoretical perspective. If one uses a medical model, for example, in the conceptualization of children's problems, one might well like Kanner's (1972) statement that " ... a symptom is an indication of 'the existence of a cause of which it is the effect'" (p. 165). That is, the symptom itself is not the problem, but a signal of one, and the cause needs to be determined in order for the therapist to be effective.

Behaviorists usually view the "symptom" as maladaptive behavior that is being reinforced and maintained in the environment and that needs to be extinguished so that new and more desirable behaviors can be learned. This view does not require a search for underlying psychodynamic causal conflicts. Rather, one looks for the environmental events and reinforcers that are maintaining the "disturbed" behavior. Attention should be paid to specific stimuli situations as well as to the person's characteristics (Goldfried and Sprafkin, 1974), as behavior and development depend on the child in interaction with environmental events and influences. Cognitive psychologists, on the other hand, would look at such issues as the child's perception of the environment, the stage of cognitive development at which the child is functioning, and the child's capacity to organize and adapt to the environmental stress being faced.

One's view of disturbed behavior, then, greatly influences one's approach to diagnosis and assessment and one's choice of diagnostic instruments and techniques.

Similar symptoms or behavior can reflect very different problems, and given problems can be manifested in very different ways. For

60

example, a child who is unduly active or agitated in the test situation may be restless because he is highly anxious, neurologically hyperactive, or simply not feeling well. Similarly, a given problem can be manifested in a number of ways, so that a child who is very anxious may show it through restlessness and overactivity, aggressive behavior, or inhibition and withdrawal. Premature conclusions based on insufficient information about a child can lead to serious diagnostic errors. If in addition labels are prematurely and mistakenly applied, they can be very difficult for the child to live down or overcome even after the behavior has changed.

Classification of Disorders

Discussions of diagnostic issues and labels of normality and abnormality also usually involve categorization and classification. The orderly and consistent classification of psychological disorders and symptoms is an arduous and complex task.

There appears to be widespread agreement on the need for some kind of classificatory scheme which will provide clear groupings of children or symptoms that are relatively equivalent in order to facilitate identification of and communication about specific disorders. Moreover, classification systems can be used to guide planning, to establish incidence and prevalence figures for better planning and research, and to establish homogeneous categories for the study of cause and treatment (Eisenberg, 1966). Such classification systems can be helpful to the extent that they are correlated with significant and relevant variables and can be used in a uniform way (Achenbach, 1974).

There is widespread disagreement, however, about the form such schemes should take and about the usefulness of existing classification systems. Criteria for inclusion of specific disorders in given categories are often controversial, reflecting differing views of etiology, prognosis, and treatment. Many classificatory schema have been developed, but none seem to adequately and definitively answer the many questions that arise around the issue of classification of psychological disorders.

Existing classification schemes vary in their emphases, but most fall within two broad groupings. One group, the most commonly used historically, is made up of those with a heavy reliance on clinical judgments of practicing psychiatrists or clinical raters. These have generally been derived from the psychiatric literature and have traditionally been based primarily on a medical model, although newer editions include behavioral aspects as well. Some have been organized along etiological lines (for example, organic versus nonorganic conditions), while others have emphasized clinical descriptions of syndromes. The second broad group comprises those classification systems which rely more heavily on empirical and statistical groupings of specific behaviors and which attempt to analyze clusters of symptoms or behaviors in order to discern underlying factors.

Clinically Derived Systems

Of the first broad type of classification systems, one of the most commonly used and best known systems is the Diagnostic and Statistical Manual of Mental Disorders (DSM), published by the American Psychiatric Association and now in its third edition as DSM-III (APA, 1980). It has increasingly differentiated between child and adult disorders with each edition, and the current classification features the most objective behavioral criteria. The most recent edition has a lesser emphasis on psychoanalytically based terminology and assumptions and a greater behavioral emphasis in order to enhance its reliability as well as its appeal to more diverse theoretical positions (Schwartz and Johnson, 1981).

The DSM-II (1968) had been criticized as unscientific because it was based on a vote of specific psychiatrists rather than on empirical data, and it confounded etiology, symptomatology, and prognosis as bases for diagnostic decisions (Knopf, 1979). The DSM-III, however, is perceived by many as significantly more comprehensive and inclusive than DSM-II and more detailed and objective in its diagnostic criteria (Cantwell et al., 1979; Schwartz and Johnson, 1981). It is considered fairly easy to use and more helpful than DSM-II, although some problems with differential diagnosis have been noted (Cantwell et al., 1979). DSM-III, like some of the other systems, involves classification along several dimensions, or axes, which helps to take into account the complexity of individuals and which addresses to some extent Achenbach's (1974) concerns regarding the "whole child." A portion of the DSM-III is illustrated in Table 4.1.

62

TABLE 4.1 *Outline of DSM-III classification system, with emphasis on disorders of childhood and adolescence*

I. *Disorders usually arising in childhood or adolescence*
  A. *Mental retardation*
    Mild
    Moderate
    Severe
    Profound
  B. *Attention deficit disorder*
    With hyperactivity
    Without hyperactivity
    Residual type
  C. *Conduct disorder*
    Undersocialized, aggressive
    Undersocialized, nonaggressive
    Socialized, aggressive
    Socialized, nonaggressive
    Atypical
  D. *Anxiety disorders of childhood or adolescence*
    Separation anxiety disorder
    Avoidant disorder of childhood or adolescence
    Overanxious disorder
  E. *Other disorders of infancy, childhood, or adolescence*
    Reactive attachment disorder of infancy
    Schizoid disorder of childhood or adolescence
    Elective mutism
    Oppositional disorder
    Identity disorder
  F. *Eating disorder*
    Anorexia nervosa
    Bulimia
    Pica
    Rumination disorder of infancy
    Atypical eating disorder
  G. *Stereotyped movement disorders*
    Transient tic disorder
    Chronic motor tic disorder

Tourette's syndrome
    Atypical tic disorder
    Atypical stereotyped movement disorder
  H. *Other disorders with physical manifestations*
    Stuttering
    Functional enuresis
    Functional encopresis
    Sleepwalking
    Sleep terror
  I. *Pervasive developmental disorders*
    Infantile autism
    Childhood onset pervasive developmental disorder
    Atypical pervasive developmental disorder
  J. *Specific developmental disorders (Axis II)*
    Developmental reading disorder
    Developmental arithmetic disorder
    Developmental language disorder
    Developmental articulation disorder
    Mixed specific developmental disorder
    Atypical specific developmental disorder
II. *Organic mental disorders* (e.g., senile and presenile dementias, substance-induced organic disorder, other organic brain syndrome)
III. *Substance use disorders* (e.g., alcohol abuse, barbiturate abuse, other substance abuse)
IV. *Schizophrenic disorders* (e.g., disorganized, catatonic, paranoid, undifferentiated, residual)

V. *Paranoid disorders*
VI. *Psychotic disorders not elsewhere classified* (e.g., schizophreniform disorder, brief reactive psychosis)
VII. *Affective disorders* (e.g., manic disorders, depressive disorders, mixed cyclothymic disorder)
VIII. *Anxiety disorders* (e.g., phobic disorders, obsessive compulsive disorder, generalized anxiety disorder)
IX. *Somataform disorders* (e.g., conversion disorder, psychogenic pain disorder)
X. *Dissociative disorders* (e.g., psychogenic amnesia, multiple personality)
XI. *Psychosexual disorders* (e.g., transsexualism, gender identity disorder of childhood, sexual sadism, psychosexual dysfunction)
XII. *Factitious disorders* (e.g., factitious illness with physical or psychological symptoms)
XIII. *Disorders of impulse control not elsewhere classified* (e.g., pathological gambling, kleptomania)
XIV. *Adjustment disorder* (e.g., adjustment disorder with depressed mood, with anxious mood, with mixed emotional features)
XV. *Psychological factors affecting physical condition*
XVI. *Personality disorders (Axis II)* (e.g., dependent, passive-aggressive disorder)
XVII. *Conditions not attributable to mental disorders*

Source: American Psychiatric Association, *Diagnostic and Statistical Manual of Mental Disorders*, Third Edition (Washington, D.C.: APA, 1980). Reprinted by permission.

The classification system of the World Health Organization (WHO) is a triple-axis classification which takes into account not only clinical syndrome, but intellectual level and associated etiological factors as well (Rutter et al., 1969). Based on clinical facts, it covers disorders to age twelve.

An alternative classification system was developed by the Committee on Child Psychiatry of the Group for the Advancement of Psychiatry (GAP, 1966, 1974). It is a "clinical-descriptive" system and includes a "healthy responses" category to emphasize a child's strengths. It pays particular attention to developmental variables, with inclusion of critical stages when a child is especially vulnerable to stressful stimuli. It recommends specific diagnoses at different developmental levels and includes criteria for each category (GAP, 1974). A sample from the GAP system is illustrated in Table 4.2.

Despite its claims of maximally operational definitions, however, the degree of inference required varies from category to category (Achenbach, 1974).

Others have tried to use developmental concepts in a general classification scheme based on the main characteristics of normal behavior, in which symptom pictures are related to classes of normal behavior such as functional (for example, eating, sleeping), cognitive, affective, social, and integrative (Anthony, 1970).

Empirically Derived Systems

The second broad group of classification schemes attempts to empirically and statistically identify clusters of symptoms which often occur together. Through the use of factor analysis, hundreds of descriptive statements can be ordered along logical dimensions, identified by the nature of their interrelationship, and thus reduced to manageable numbers (Ross, 1980). For example, Achenbach's (1966) factor analysis of behavioral symptoms in six hundred child psychiatric patients led to his description of two general clusters of internalizing and externalizing symptoms. Internalization refers to a tendency to handle problems "internally" through such symptoms as stomachaches, depression, and withdrawal. Externalization refers to the "acting out" of problems through deviant, aggressive, or antisocial behavior. Factor analytic studies have suggested that children who tend to externalize

64

TABLE 4.2 *Psychopathological disorders in childhood proposed classification*

1. *Healthy Responses*

   This category assesses the positive strengths of the child and tries to avoid the diagnosis of healthy states by the exclusion of pathology. The criteria for assessment are the intellectual, social, emotional, personal, adaptive, and psychosocial functioning of the child in relation to developmental and situational crises.

   Healthy Responses:
   1. Developmental crisis
   2. Situational crisis
   3. Other responses

2. *Reactive Disorders*

   This category is based on disorders in which behavior and/or symptoms are the result of situational factors. These disturbances must be of a pathological degree so as to distinguish them from the healthy responses to a situational crisis.

3. *Developmental Disorders*

   These are disorders in personality development that may be beyond the range of normal variation in that they occur at a time, in a sequence, or in a degree not expected for a given age level or stage in development.

   Developmental Deviations:
   1. Deviations in maturational patterns
   2. Deviations in specific dimensions of development
   3. Moior
   4. Sensory
   5. Speech
   6. Cognitive functions
   7. Social development
   8. Psychosexual
   9. Affective
   10. Integrative
   11. Other developmental deviations

4. *Psychoneurotic Disorders*

   These disorders are based on unconscious conflicts over the handling of sexual and aggressive impulses that remain active and unresolved, though removed from awareness by the mechanism of repression. Marked personality disorganization or decompensation, or the gross disturbance of reality testing is not seen. Because of their internalized character, these disorders tend toward chronicity, with a self-perpetuating or repetitive nature. Subcategories are based on specific syndromes.

   Psychoneurotic Disorders:
   1. Anxiety type
   2. Phobic type
   3. Conversion type
   4. Dissociative type
   5. Obsessive-compulsive type
   6. Depressive type
   7. Other psychoneurotic disorders

6. *Personality Disorders*

   These disorders are characterized by chronic or fixed pathological trends, representing traits that have become ingrained in the personality structure. In most but not all such disorders, these trends or traits are

TABLE 4.2   *Psychopathological disorders in childhood proposed classification*   (*continued*)

not perceived by the child as a source of intrapsychic distress or anxiety. In making this classification, the total personality picture must be considered and not just the presence of a single behavior or symptom.

Personality Disorders:
1. Compulsive personality
2. Hysterical
3. Anxious
4. Overly dependent
5. Oppositional
6. Overly inhibited
7. Overly independent
8. Isolated
9. Mistrustful

Tension-Discharge Disorders:
1. Impulse-ridden personality
2. Neurotic personality disorder

Sociosyntonic Personality Disorders:
1. Sexual deviation
2. Other personality disorders

6. *Psychotic Disorders*

These disorders are characterized by marked, pervasive deviations from the behavior that is expected for the child's age. They are revealed in severe and continued impairment of emotional relationships with persons; loss of speech or failure in its development; disturbances in sensory perception; bizarre or stereotyped behavior and motility patterns; marked resistance to change in environment or routine; outbursts of intense and unpredictable panic; absence of a sense of personal identity; and blunted, uneven, or fragmented intellectual development. Major categories are based on the developmental period, with subcategories in each period for the listing of a specific syndrome, if known.

Psychotic Disorders:
1. Psychoses of infancy and early childhood
    a. Early infantile autism
    b. Interactional psychotic disorder
    c. Other psychoses of infancy and early childhood
2. Psychoses of later childhood
    a. Schizophreniform psychotic disorder
    b. Other psychoses of later childhood
3. Psychoses of adolescence
    a. Acute confusional state
    b. Schizophrenic disorder, adult type
    c. Other psychoses of adolescence

7. *Psychophysiologic Disorders*

These disorders are characterized by a significant interaction between somatic and psychological components. They may be precipitated and perpetuated by psychological or social stimuli of stressful nature. These disorders ordinarily involve those organ systems innervated by the autonomic nervous system.

Psychophysiologic Disorders:
1. Skin
2. Musculoskeletal
3. Respiratory

4. Cardiovascular
5. Hemic and lymphatic
6. Gastrointestinal
7. Genitourinary
8. Endocrine
9. Of nervous system
10. Of organs of special sense
11. Other psychophysiologic disorders

8. *Brain Syndromes*

These disorders are characterized by impairment of orientation, judgment, discrimination, learning, memory, and other cognitive functions, as well as by frequent labile affect. They are basically caused by diffuse impairment of brain tissue function. Personality disturbances of a psychotic, neurotic, or behavioral nature also may be present.

Brain Syndromes:
1. Acute
2. Chronic

9. *Mental Retardation*
10. *Other Disorders*

This category is for disorders that cannot be classified by the above definitions or for disorders we will describe in the future.

Source: Reprinted by permission from *Psychopathological Disorders in Childhood: A Proposed Classification* (New York: Group for the Advancement of Psychiatry, 1966).

their problems often perform poorly in school, come from socially deviant parents, and have a history of previous difficulties; whereas children who tend to internalize problems have " . . . been socialized in such a way that their reactions to stress were manifested in unaggressive symptoms of intraself conflict" (Achenbach, 1974, page 558). Achenbach reported twice as many internalizers as externalizers among girls, with the reverse true for boys.

He found the general clusters to be associated as well with specific syndromes, some of which resemble traditional psychiatric categories and others which are peculiar to particular developmental stages. An illustration of this kind of classification and the behaviors involved is provided in Table 4.3.

Achenbach's two clusters are similar to the two groups—personality problems and conduct disorders—found by Peterson (1961) in a factor analytic study of problem behaviors in kindergarten and elementary-school children. Children in the conduct problem group tended to express antisocial impulses or to act out against society. Those in the

TABLE 4.3   *First-order varimax loadings on behavior problem scales*

Internalizing scales

I. Schizoid

40. Auditory hallucination	.55
70. Visual hallucination	.50
29. Fears	.44
30. Fears school	.41
11. Clings to adults	.37
50. Anxious	.36
47. Nightmares	.31
59. Public masturbation	.30
75. Shy, timid	.30
Eigenvalue	2.53

II. Depressed

35. Feels worthless	.68
52. Feels guilty	.67
32. Needs to be perfect	.58
33. Feels unloved	.55
112. Worrying	.52
103. Sad	.51
31. Fears own impulses	.48
91. Suicidal talk	.46
12. Lonely	.40
14. Cries much	.39
50. Anxious	.39
71. Self-conscious	.39
34. Feels persecuted	.34
88. Sulks	.32
45. Nervous	.31

89. Suspicious	.30
18. Harms self	.30
Eigenvalue	4.94

III. Uncommunicative

65. Won't talk	.61
69. Secretive	.50
75. Shy, timid	.42
103. Sad	.36
80. Stares blankly	.33
71. Self-conscious	.32
13. Confused	.32
86. Stubborn	.30
Eigenvalue	2.97

IV. Obsessive-Compulsive

85. Strange ideas	.52
100. Can't sleep	.52
76. Sleeps little	.45
84. Strange behavior	.43
9. Obsessions	.42
92. Walks, talks in sleep	.40
80. Stares blankly	.40
17. Daydreams	.38
46. Twitches	.37
83. Hoarding	.37
66. Compulsions	.36
54. Overtired	.36
13. Confused	.35

93. Excess talk	.34
47. Nightmares	.33
50. Anxious	.33
Eigenvalue	4.03

V. Somatic Complaints

56f. Stomach problems	.64
56a. Pains	.50
56b. Headaches	.58
56c. Nausea	.56
56g. Vomits	.44
49. Constipated	.41
51. Dizziness	.39
77. Sleeps much	.32
54. Overtired	.31
Eigenvalue	3.08

Mixed scale

VI. Social Withdrawal

48. Unliked	.59
25. Poor peer relations	.59
111. Withdrawn	.56
42. Likes to be alone	.46
38. Is teased	.36
64. Prefers younger children	.33
34. Feels persecuted	.32
102. Slow moving	.31
Eigenvalue	3.05

personality problem group showed a variety of characteristics suggesting withdrawal, low self-esteem, and dysphoric mood.

After reviewing many factor analytic studies, Quay (1979) concluded that most nonpsychotic behavior problems could be subsumed under four major headings (conduct disorders, anxiety/withdrawn, immaturity, and socialized aggression) and suggested, therefore, that perhaps the many subdivisions of traditional systems are not warranted. Ross (1980) reduces the number of dimensions even further, suggesting that disordered behavior falls into one of two major classes: excesses or deficits. According to him, behavior disorders are constituted of behaviors that occur too frequently or too rarely. These two classes are broadly consistent with the previously discussed external-

Externalizing scales			Other problems
VII. *Hyperactive*		68. Screams	2. Allergy
8. Can't concentrate	.65	90. Swears	4. Asthma
1. Acts too young	.58	25. Poor peer relations	5. Acts like opposite sex
61. Poor schoolwork	.56	88. Sulks	6. Encopresis
62. Clumsy	.48	7. Brags	15. Cruel to animals
13. Confused	.45	43. Lies, cheats	24. Doesn't eat well
17. Daydreams	.43	27. Jealous	26. Lacks guilt
41. Impulsive	.40	87. Moody	28. Eats nonfood
64. Prefers younger		19. Demands attention	36. Accident prone
children	.40	93. Excess talk	44. Bites nails
10. Hyperactive	.36	48. Unliked	53. Overeats
79. Speech problem	.31	Eigenvalue	55. Overweight
20. Destroys own things	.30		56d. Eye problems
Eigenvalue	3.75	*IX.* *Delinquent*	56e. Rashes
		82. Steals outside home	58. Picking
VIII. *Aggressive*		81. Steals at home	60. Excess masturbation
3. Argues	.71	21. Destroys things belong-	63. Prefers older children
22. Disobedient at home	.66	ing to others	73. Sex problems
95. Temper tantrums	.64	106. Vandalism	78. Smears feces
86. Stubborn	.63	72. Sets fires	96. Sex preoccupation
37. Fighting	.61	101. Truant	98. Thumb-sucking
16. Cruel to others	.60	67. Runs away	99. Too neat
97. Threatens people	.57	39. Bad friends	105. Alcohol, drugs
94. Teases	.56	43. Lies, cheats	107. Wets self
74. Shows off	.55	20. Destroys own things	108. Wets bed
104. Loud	.51	90. Swears	109. Whining
23. Disobedient at school	.51	23. Disobedient at school	110. Wishes to be opposite sex
57. Attacks people	.50	Eigenvalue	

Note: Items are designated with the numbers they bear on the Child Behavior Checklist (CBCL) and summary labels for their content. For actual wording of items, see the CBCL. Other Problems items were excluded from scales because of low frequency or low loadings.

Source: T. M. Achenbach, "The Child Behavior Profile: I. Boys aged 6–11," *Journal of Consulting Clinical Psychology* 1978(b): 46, pp. 478–488. Copyright 1978 by the American Psychological Association. Reprinted by permission of the author.

izing-internalizing and conduct disorder–anxiety/withdrawal dimensions.

Such multivariate studies have also led to the development of more objective measurement instruments (Quay, 1979). However, some judgment is still involved in deciding how to label specific clusters and in selecting items for the original data-gathering instruments (Ross, 1980). Thus, behavioral dimensions may not be comparable across studies (Quay, 1979).

According to Achenbach (1978b), the value of classification systems for children should be assessed in terms of various criteria, including standardized descriptions of behavior and sufficient differentiation to include syndromes of particular subgroups. In addition, the classification systems should not depend on clinical inferences of people working with children and should reflect positive and adaptive skills as well as maladaptive behaviors or characteristics. They should simplify the grouping of children for research, epidemiological, etiological, and treatment effectiveness purposes and should facilitate quantitative measurement of change to enable clinicians to assess prognosis under different conditions (Achenbach, 1978b).

Individuals can be classified in several ways, and how one chooses to classify disorders depends on one's goals. Therefore, the purpose of the classification (whether clinical, research, or actuarial) is critical (Anthony, 1970). Achenbach (1974) cautions, however, that since no one system can take into account all of an individual's attributes, the clinician must remember that groups of children are classified according to only *some* characteristics (those which are related to the clinician's goals) and should resist the tendency to identify a whole person with the classified disorder.

Regardless of the classification system one uses, there are vexing problems surrounding the whole issue of classification and labeling of childhood disorders. First, some of the systems do not show consistently high reliability and validity. There appears to be considerable agreement regarding broad categories, but much less when more specific categories are included (Achenbach, 1974; Knopf, 1979; Schwartz and Johnson, 1981). For example, although there was high agreement in both DSM-II and DSM-III regarding psychosis, hyperactivity, conduct disorder, and mental retardation, with DSM-III slightly higher, there was disagreement in both systems regarding "anxiety" disorders, depression, and more complex cases (Mattison et al., 1979).

Secondly, the labeling of individuals can have a variety of negative effects for those individuals. There is evidence, for instance, of the strong influence that previous labels have on current diagnostic and classification practices, due in part to lack of clear criteria to distinguish healthy from ill (Achenbach, 1974); and the exactness and precision implied by many systems is more the exception than the rule in actual practice. Furthermore, many diagnostic terms imply prognosis and may unduly influence the therapy (Kessler, 1966). Moreover, the child must face or deal with the stigma of early labeling.

70

Such labeling may result in expectations of behaviors that fit the label (Achenbach, 1974), leading to self-fulfilling hypotheses (Ross, 1980).

Third, such classification schemes confer a status and validity on disorders, suggesting, for example, that specific categories are mutually exclusive, which they are not. They may also imply the existence of underlying diagnostic entities, an implication which may not be warranted and is not consistent with the views of behaviorally oriented clinicians who emphasize maladaptive behaviors as the central problem. The behavioral clinicians would further argue that such labels have little effect on the plans for intervention, as the task of changing behavior is the principal one, regardless of cause. Various classification schemes may also imply a discontinuity between abnormal and normal behavior which can be misleading, and classification into discontinuous categories also ignores processes and absorbs individual differences (Anthony, 1970).

Finally, as new editions of various diagnostic systems emerge, there are often shifts of symptom clusters or changed headings which reflect changes in the field but can further confuse students new to the field. For these reasons, *major* diagnostic categories are retained for discussion in this text. DSM-III diagnostic criteria are referred to in relation to some disorders, as are some of the factor analytic groupings consistent with the presentation of psychodynamic and behavioral approaches throughout. However, extended discussion of detailed classification schemes has been omitted to avoid unnecessary confusion or misinterpretation. Students interested in more detailed discussions of specific systems are referred to Achenbach (1974; 1978b), Anthony (1970), or the DSM-III (APA, 1980).

In summary, classification of some kind is necessary for identification and communication among professionals as a basis for diagnostic and treatment decisions as well as for continuing research into the nature of specific psychological disorders. In this text, both general types of classification are referred to throughout, with the understanding that all of the current systems have shortcomings and that the categorization and labeling of children has inherent dangers of which clinicians must be aware. A number of systems will probably always be necessary, as child psychopathology involves individuals in so many ways (Achenbach, 1974). However, the empirically derived, behavioral cluster approaches appear to hold the most promise for classification that is objective, clear, and can be consistently used.

Diagnostic Formulations

In view of the lack of agreement as to whether classification should be based on etiology and/or symptoms, the complexity and overlap in the area of diagnosis, as well as developmental considerations, Kessler (1966) has suggested that a diagnostic formulation might be more useful than labels and might maximize the accuracy of the information that is communicated. Such a diagnostic formulation describes a child's strengths as well as problems and therefore provides a more complete picture. There is also less chance of its sticking with a child and stigmatizing him or her indefinitely, or serving as a self-fulfilling hypothesis (Kessler, 1966). Finally, such a formulation is likely to facilitate clearer communication to other professionals working with the child. On the other hand, a diagnostic label means something slightly different to everyone who uses it and hence introduces distortions and misperceptions of a child which can affect both the prognosis and the treatment. Kessler further urges continually changing diagnoses and recommends more long-range studies to improve predictive ability and treatment decisions.

General Etiological Factors

There are many factors in the life and background of a child which might predispose that child to the development of a disorder, putting the child "at risk." The concept of risk is central, encompassing biological predisposition and vulnerability on the one hand and stress and adverse environmental influences on the other (Anthony, 1970). Many elements are common to the lives of all children in highly varied patterns and combinations. Others exist for some children and not for others. As the presence of these factors may or may not actually be associated with a disturbance, it is necessary to distinguish between *necessary* and *sufficient* conditions before embarking on a discussion of specific background variables.

A necessary condition is one that *must* exist in the child or the child's background in order for a disturbance to occur or develop, just as gasoline is necessary for a car engine to start (Achenbach, 1974). A sufficient condition, on the other hand, is one whose mere presence is enough; if it is present, a disorder will occur. If, for example, a specific neurological deficit has been found to be a sufficient condition in the etiology of hyperactivity, and it is present, no other factors are required for the hyperactivity to occur.

A condition can be necessary without being sufficient. To carry the gasoline analogy further, gasoline is necessary, but other conditions must be met also. The gasoline is a necessary condition but is not enough in itself (Achenbach, 1974); it is not a sufficient condition.

A condition can also be sufficient without being necessary. If the hypothetical neurological deficit were a sufficient condition and were present, it would inevitably lead to hyperactivity. But the presence of any other sufficient condition would likewise inevitably result in the disorder, whether or not the neurological deficit was present.

Thus a factor can be necessary or sufficient, or it can be both. If it is necessary but not sufficient, it must be there, but other factors or conditions or events must also occur or be present. If it is sufficient, its presence ensures that the disorder will occur. If it is both necessary and sufficient, it must be there, and nothing else is required. These are important concepts to keep in mind, especially later when controversial etiological issues are discussed. They may, in fact, help to clarify some of the apparently contradictory and confusing findings in the literature, and they can help to keep us from jumping to unwarranted, premature, or erroneous conclusions.

With these distinctions in mind, we can consider the various factors in a child's background that *may*, alone or in combination with other factors, predispose or lead to the development of disturbance. As has been mentioned, it must be remembered that these factors and characteristics exist in the lives of all children in an infinite variety of combinations and varying degrees. One of the diagnostic tasks is to learn how, for a particular child and family, the characteristics and variables, both physical and psychological, have interacted to produce the current behavioral and emotional picture.

A brief review of the many potential contributory causes follows, to introduce readers to the wide range of possible causal agents. The roles of these agents or factors and the ways in which they can interact and can be associated with the development of psychological problems are discussed at greater length in relation to specific disorders and in other contexts throughout the book.

Biological and Constitutional Factors

Biological and constitutional factors are all of the genetic, biological, neurological, and biochemical elements that, taken together, determine the child's physiological makeup. Included are constitutional

predisposition or weakness, genetic transmission of certain characteristics, chromosomal abnormalities, delays in biological maturation,
biochemical and hormonal or metabolic imbalances, and the child's
level of general health. Included also are basic temperamental characteristics such as the rhythmicity of biological functions, level of
activity, adaptability, and distractibility (Thomas et al., 1963). The serious and long-term effects on the child's physical and psychological
well-being of prenatal hazards such as exposure to radiation, drugs,
alcohol, nutritional deficits, rubella, maternal dysfunction or disease,
and other intrauterine events are well documented. Some biological
and genetic effects may not show up initially and only later cause
problems for the child.

Injuries, Traumas, or Disease

A child who has had a normal intrauterine environment, and therefore could be expected to develop normally, may experience a very
difficult birth or suffer birth-related injury or damage. As noted earlier, anoxia, or an insufficient supply of oxygen at birth and in the few
seconds after, can result in brain damage, the degree of which
depends on the extent and duration of oxygen insufficiency. Or children may incur brain damage later as a result of accidents, head injuries, or illnesses such as encephalitis or convulsions. When a child
experiences such a traumatic event, there may be direct damage from
the event itself, such as loss of speech or the use of certain parts of the
body after a serious head injury; there may also be psychological stress
and emotional upset after and because of the injury, which is super-
imposed on any direct loss.

Family Background

Many characteristics, communication patterns, and complex influences within the family affect the quality of the child's adjustment and
may contribute to the development of a disturbance. Family size, family makeup, and birth order obviously have a bearing on the kind of
parental attention and stimulation a child receives. The family's socioeconomic level has consistently been related to child-rearing practices,
intellectual and language development, attitudes toward education
and occupational aspirations, roles in the community, goals and ambi-

tions, and other aspects of the child's life. In addition, in homes where financial hardship is a constant problem, there is increased stress on the family and educational and social opportunities for the child are greatly decreased. The family members' cohesiveness, hobbies, routines (or lack thereof), friends, relatives, psychological atmosphere and adjustment, and general life-style all greatly affect the child and the child's developing attitudes, general competence, personality, and self-esteem. Thus it is clear that many factors may contribute to the creation of problems or inadequacies which can interact to produce a disorder.

Community at Large

Relevant factors which exist outside the family include educational and recreational facilities and programs, the quality of life in the community, and the general level of stress in society brought about by inflation, pollution, unemployment, crime, threats of war, and other problems. A number of people outside the family also have an important influence on the child. Teachers, friends, neighbors, and adult acquaintances form a network which affords the child a sense of belonging and may also provide support and counsel when such aid is not forthcoming from the child's family. Acceptance or rejection by peers is also a crucial variable in the child's development. As children mature, the influence of their peers becomes increasingly important as they gain independence and grow away from the family. The support and affection of friends—or the lack thereof—can significantly affect the level of the child's psychological adjustment.

Moreover, environmental and social events and characteristics are mediated by the child's perception, memory, problem-solving skills, capacity for abstract thought, and previous learning. In addition to such emotional characteristics as anxiety, fear, and hostility, a child's biological inheritance further affects the way in which the child perceives and responds to the events in his or her life.

Within the context of these diverse influences, the child's personality is developed with a unique patterning and interaction of abilities, interests, characteristics, attitudes, conflicts, and problems. Some of these patterns are more likely than others to be associated with specific disorders, and a child's vulnerability may be more or less pronounced at varying times in his or her life.

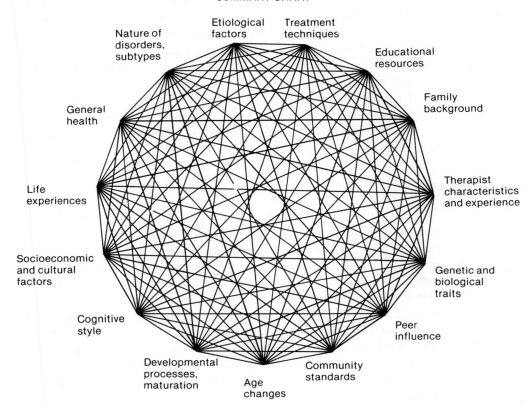

FIGURE 4.1   *Interactions among the complex influences on a child's development.*

Thus, the problem of diagnosis is a complex one. Ferreting out the possible physical and psychological characteristics and events which singly or in combination have led to a disorder is very challenging work; and a clinician should have as much information as possible about the child and the child's current and past environment. This is true whether one adopts a primarily psychodynamic, behavioral, cognitive, or biological stance toward the child's problems. In addition, there is a need to understand the intriguing and very challenging group of children who face many of the factors that are usually considered negative or destructive but who still somehow not only survive and grow up normally, but actually seem to thrive in spite of or because of them (Garmezy, 1979).

The summary chart in Figure 4.1 illustrates the highly complex and varied interaction of factors in a child's life which can contribute to the development of a disorder. Most research studies intersect the lines at specific points, addressing particular characteristics or factors. Until a broader understanding of all of the influences in a child's life is attained and more of the factors are addressed simultaneously, our ability to predict and control will remain inadequate, and contradictory findings will persist.

Careful assessment is thus an important and challenging undertaking indeed, the importance of which cannot be overemphasized. It is in the area of investigating and describing more fully the child's behavior, problems, strengths, and overall development that the specific tools and techniques discussed in the following chapter can be helpful.

Discussion Questions

1. How would you define normal behavior? What is the relationship of a child's behavior to his or her culture, past experience, models, and developmental problems?
2. Which criteria are of the greatest value in determining whether a child's behavior and adjustment are "normal"?
3. Discuss the need to find an underlying cause for the symptoms a child shows. Do you think that alleviating symptoms is a sufficient treatment intervention? Why or why not?

CHAPTER 5

Tools and Techniques of Assessment

The wide range of diagnostic tools and techniques from which a clinician can choose is presented herewith first, followed by a case study which illustrates how they might be selected differently by psychodynamic and behavioral diagnosticians.

In this chapter testing will be considered as one source of information in the assessment. It is not *the* answer, nor is it definitive, but it can be very helpful when used to supplement and clarify other information.

Purposes of Assessment

Not only does a thorough assessment allow the clinician to become thoroughly familiar with the client and the problems involved; it also provides a point of reference throughout the duration of contacts with the child. It allows comparisons of current behavior with past behavior, and current levels of functioning with previous levels. The assessment process should lead to a description of the problem, an estimation of its severity, identification of relevant factors suggesting interventions, and prognostic predictions (Sattler, 1982).

In addition to their frequent use as a tool by which the clinician can become acquainted with the problems of a referred child, assessments may also be utilized as part of broad screening programs, to determine educational placements, to aid in planning, to evaluate improvements in performance and the effectiveness of various remedial interventions (Reid and Hresko, 1981).

Sources of Diagnostic Information

The major sources of diagnostic information are interviews, medical and school reports, observation, and psychological testing. The kinds of information one gets from the various sources complement one another: interviews and medical reports provide important background information that cannot be obtained through testing or observation; through observation, the diagnostician learns first-hand how a child interacts with others and is able to evaluate the behavior of the child in situations which may not have been represented in the interview or which may have been distorted. School reports attest to a child's behavior in a more structured atmosphere and in response to specific demands, providing a record of achievement, although observation of other aspects of the child's behavior is an important part of the reports as well.

As various facets of a child's life yield differing kinds of information, the clinician can feel more confident about diagnostic statements and hypotheses if they are based on corroborative evidence from a number of areas rather than just one or two. By relying on an intelligence test score and observations from the testing session, for example, without the developmental background or any information about the child's behavior in the classroom or at home, a clinician increases the risk of misinterpretation. It is not realistic to assume that information from all areas will always be available; but, generally, the more sources one can draw from, the more accurate the assessment will be.

Interviews

The interview is one of the most important sources of diagnostic information. It may be conducted with the child alone, the parents alone, an entire family, or some combination of family members. It may be highly structured, in which case the clinician asks a series of special questions, or the clinician may allow the child or family member to talk about problems or concerns in a more open-ended, undirected way.

The interview provides an opportunity for the clinician to establish rapport with the client; to directly observe and assess the child's or the family's communication, language, and social skills; and to obtain independent background information regarding current problems and the conditions that sustain or exacerbate them. The establishment of a warm, accepting atmosphere will minimize anxiety and help both the child and the family to trust the clinician enough to be able to talk freely and develop a productive relationship. The competent and sensitive clinician accomplishes this by communicating acceptance, interest in the family's problems, and confidence in his or her ability to help.

The interview will provide, first, *introductory information*. This includes not only the child's vital statistics, such as name, age, birthdate, and family information, but the referring source and the referral problem. The referring source indicates who first took action about the problem; the referral problem chronicles the behaviors that were of concern to the referring source. If the problems for which the child is referred have existed for a fairly long time, finding out what prompted the person to seek help *now* can be very illuminating. What has, in fact, been the precipitating factor?

The diagnostician also needs to obtain *background information.* This will establish the context of the problem and the quality of the environment within which the child has been living. Questions should cover how the parents feel about the problem; whether there has been a recent crisis in the home, such as the death of a parent, a divorce, a serious illness, or any other upsetting event; and what family communication patterns are like. The clinician will also want to find out whether the family is generally happy and well functioning or whether there is considerable discord and friction; whether the marital relationship is harmonious or in continual difficulty; and whether there are problems with any of the other children in the family.

Some of this information can be gleaned through careful observation during family sessions: The clinician might note, for instance, whether all family members are allowed to express opinions or whether only adults are free to do so; whether one person speaks for everyone; and how the family handles disagreements and dissenting opinions. Positive and affectionate gestures—or their absence—are among the characteristics of the family that can be noted. Inconsistencies between such behavior and the content of the family's verbalizations can provide particularly helpful insights. Patterson (1977), for instance, found significant discrepancies between his direct observation of families and what parents actually reported during interviews.

For the purpose of prediction, interviews have less validity and reliability than testing, however, and there is always the risk of examiner bias (Cattell, 1965). Race, socioeconomic status, accent, and certain mannerisms on the part of the client may lead the examiner to form hypotheses, expectations, and attitudes that directly or indirectly affect work with that client. The examiner needs to be aware of his or her vulnerability to such bias and to guard against it.

The clinician also needs to know the child's *developmental history,* including information about the pregnancy and delivery, any problems at or shortly after birth, at what age various developmental milestones were reached, and how new situations have characteristically been handled. The child's general health history, including diseases and accidents and the reactions of the child and family to them, is important.

The clinician must also find out as much as possible about the child's *strengths and assets* in order to get as complete and balanced a picture as possible. All too frequently, the sole emphasis is on problems and weaknesses. Sometimes parents, for instance, are surprised at how difficult it is to think of things they like about their child or of strengths the child has. In the pain and frustration surrounding the problems that prompted them to seek professional help, the parents frequently lose sight of their child's good points. Moreover, performance is in part a function of the assessment conditions and the efforts of the diagnostician to elicit certain behaviors (Kazdin, Matson, and Esveldt-Dawson, 1981). These positive characteristics and skills are the very ones that need to be maintained and strengthened during treatment so that they can become bases on which other positive behaviors can be built.

Medical and School Reports

Medical records should be obtained from the family physician if there has been anything unusual or major in the child's history or if there have been any special medical problems. In addition, a thorough, up-to-date medical examination is essential to rule out the possibility of physical causes when there are such presenting symptoms as fatigue, stomachaches, and restlessness. Too frequently such symptoms are *assumed* to be psychological or to result from anxiety or depression when in fact they may well have a physiological basis. If they are not investigated medically first, one risks doing the child a gross disservice by proceeding without adequate information, using techniques and approaches that are highly inappropriate to the problem, and causing delay in obtaining the proper medical care for the child.

Information from the school about the child's functioning in school is also important, even when the referral was not made because of specific academic or behavioral problems in school. There is considerable interaction and consistency among the various arenas of a child's life, and problems in one area spill over into other areas and affect functioning there. Thus family problems or almost any other problems that are psychologically disturbing can affect the child's attitude, performance, or behavior at school. It is also important to know whether the child is acquiring the essential academic skills and forming good work habits. Although parents' opinions are useful in this regard, teachers' judgments can often provide invaluable insights into the nature of a problem. In addition, report cards, teachers' comments, and samples of schoolwork can be very useful to the diagnostician as representations of the child's actual life experience.

A full educational assessment, sometimes called a psychoeducational assessment, may involve such formal practices as testing but may also make use of a procedure known as diagnostic teaching which provides an informal assessment of basic skills through observation of a child's responses to a fairly standardized educational situation (Rhodes and Paul, 1978).

Observation

Behavioral observation is a very important source of information for the clinician. Although parents and others may give graphic descriptions of a child's behavior, there is no substitute for direct observation of that behavior. Behavioral observations can be made in the home, at school, on the playground, or in any other natural setting. They must be as objective, as possible, however.

First, specific behaviors must be very carefully identified and defined. Attempts to measure how "aggressive" a child is may result in conflicting reports from different independent observers because of varying opinions as to what constitutes aggression. On the other hand, if the observers agree to count the number of fights a child initiates, the observations and the criteria for including specific behaviors have been spelled out and can be reliably counted and objectively measured. This insistence that the behaviors be precisely defined helps to decrease the use of labels, which can hide the heterogeneity of the individual children included within a category (Quay, 1977).

Second, accurate recording of the observations must be made. Many rating scales, checklists, and recording codes have been developed for this purpose. Among them are Patterson's (1977) code for observing parent-child interactions; Cobb and Ray's (1976) code for observing classroom behaviors; Spivack and Swift's (1977) behavior rating scale for adolescents; and the Behavior Observation Scale, which objectively differentiates among mentally retarded, autistic, and normal individuals (Freeman et al., 1981).

Once the problem behaviors have been observed and recorded, a *functional analysis* is necessary in order to demonstrate how the various behaviors interact with and affect one another. One must determine what circumstances or events generally precede the occurrence of given behaviors, and what conditions or events reinforce and thus maintain such behaviors, in order to change some of the reinforcing conditions and thus decrease the undesirable behavior.

Finally, *careful monitoring* of the target behaviors and periods of continual observation are important to assess the effectiveness of any chosen intervention. Specific counting and charting procedures are well described by Ross (1980). In addition, Gelfand and Hartmann's (1975) book provides an extensive description of methods of data collection and data analysis for behavior therapy, including objectives, sample contracts, and the assessment of effectiveness.

Clinical observations of the child during an interview or testing can give very helpful clues to characteristic ways of functioning, anxiety level, coping mechanisms, and many other aspects of the child's personality. The way in which children attack a problem or respond to questions, for example, can indicate their level of organization, whether they are impulsive or reflective, whether or not they are confident of their abilities, and how flexible is their repertoire of behaviors for coping with the environment. The child who confidently approaches the task at hand in a highly organized way and who is justifiably pleased with the result presents a very different picture from the child who consistently complains that the job is too difficult, who starts before directions are finished, who asks for additional help, or who seems frustrated and upset during performance of the task. Such clinical observation can also lead to insights regarding the child's level of spontaneity; use of language; ability to relate to strangers, persons in authority, and other adults; and general coordination and physical health. Thus, sensitivity, sharp attention, and careful observation on the part of the clinician are vital diagnostic tools.

Psychological Tests

The psychological test is, in a sense, a highly structured behavioral observation. In this procedure, certain specified samples of behavior are elicited in a test (Lezak, 1976; Salvia and Ysseldyke, 1981) and then compared with norms for the child's age group. The accuracy of extrapolation from the test samples to real life, according to Lezak, depends in part on how precise the observations are and how similar the two situations are; but behavior is generally sufficiently stable and consistent over time to justify such extrapolation (Mash and Terdal, 1976). However, results from many of the tests in current usage should be considered tentative and should be confirmed and corroborated through more detailed assessment of the child's capacities (Sattler, 1982).

The examiner's relationship with the child is a crucial factor in the validity of the testing. Good rapport must be established with the child in order to elicit maximal performance. Apprehension may interfere with functioning and may result in a poorer performance than the child is capable of, although this situational anxiety in itself provides further important diagnostic information to the clinician.

Among the many kinds of psychological tests that can be used in various combinations to assess a child's behavior and functioning are intelligence, achievement, perceptual and visual-motor, personality, interest, and aptitude. The latter two categories, however, are rarely used in the assessment of children and adolescents with problems and thus will not be included in this discussion. Helpful information about them is contained in Anne Anastasi's (1976) excellent summary of various tests and inventories and their uses. Only a sample of the many tests available in each of the other categories is discussed here. For descriptions and evaluations of the myriad of tests available in all categories, students are referred to Buros's (1978) encyclopedic compendium.

INTELLIGENCE TESTS

The Wechsler Intelligence Scale for Children–Revised (WISC-R)

Probably the most widely used intelligence test for children is the WISC (Wechsler, 1949), or the revised version, the WISC-R (1974). This test is appropriate for children from ages six to sixteen and yields not only a total IQ score (Full Scale IQ) but also verbal and nonverbal IQ scores (Verbal and Performance Scales). The verbal section has five subtests (Information, Comprehension, Arithmetic, Similarities, and Vocabulary) which record the child's verbal skills, including ability to solve arithmetic word problems, capacity to think abstractly, fund of factual information, level of vocabulary, and common sense or social judgment. The nonverbal or performance tasks (Picture Completion, Picture Arrangement, Block Design, Object Assembly, and Coding) measure a number of aspects of the child's nonverbal functioning, including visual-motor coordination, integrative capacity, spatial skills, attention to detail, and ability to reproduce symbolic material rapidly. Optional subtests include Digit Span and Mazes.

Except for Coding, subtest items are given in the order of increasing difficulty, and the child proceeds until a specified number of failures for a given subtest is reached. Raw scores on each of the subtests are converted to standardized scaled scores, which then can be compared with standardized norms for the child's age group so IQ scores can be computed.

The full scale IQ thus obtained, however, can be highly misleading and can result in serious misinterpretations for several reasons. Not only is there the possibility that a child could proceed from one range of functioning to another on the basis of chance variation, but the single IQ score can obscure different problems and patterns of functioning. For example, one child may have achieved a Full Scale IQ score of 100 because both Verbal and Performance IQs were 100. This child's ability cannot be compared with that of the one whose Full Scale IQ score of 100 came about by averaging of a Verbal IQ of 80 and a Performance IQ of 120.

It is preferable to speak in terms of ranges of intellectual functioning such as low average, average, above average, superior, and so on. If an IQ score *must* be reported, at the very least all three scores (Full Scale, Verbal, and Performance) should be communicated in order to provide as much information as possible and thus minimize the risk of misinterpretation.

Moreover, children do not get the same scaled scores on all of the subtests, and the *patterning* of their scores is of great diagnostic importance. The particular combination of high and low subtest scores can help the clinician to pinpoint the nature of the child's problem and assess the areas of relative strength and weakness.

In addition to quantitative scores, the WISC-R also yields a considerable amount of qualitative data about a child both in the quality and in the particular content of a response. For example, the following three responses to the question "What would you do if a younger child started to fight with you" suggest very different personalities.

a. I'd walk away so he wouldn't get hurt.
b. I know I shouldn't hit him, but I'd probably let him have it anyway.
c. I'd punch him out so he'd know better next time.

Obviously, no one can make diagnostic inferences about a child's personality on the basis of one or two responses, but if a child's answer was "c" in the above example and if many other answers were in a similar vein, there would be reasonable grounds for a hypothesis of immaturity and considerable difficulty handling aggressive or angry feelings, and for the assumption that many fights or interpersonal conflicts had taken place at school and in the community. Thus, the substance of the child's responses, as well as their accuracy, can give important diagnostic information.

The *kinds* of errors children make can also reflect highly creative (positive) or very bizarre (negative) thought processes, depending on the nature of the responses and how unusual they are. Some children may give very unusual but highly creative responses to a question or take a very unorthodox but highly effective approach to a problem. Others' responses may also be statistically unusual but may appear instead to be bizarre, inept, and lacking a constructive quality that bespeaks mastery and competence.

Upward and downward age extensions of the WISC are also available (Wechsler, 1955; 1967). The Wechsler Preschool and Primary Scale of Intelligence (WPPSI) is for use with children ages four to six and a half, and the Wechsler Adult Intelligence Scale (WAIS) is for persons sixteen and over. Both have verbal and nonverbal sections similar to those of the WISC, and both yield IQs in those areas as well as a Full Scale IQ. The subtests are similar in the kinds of abilities and functions they measure, but the content is age-appropriate.

Wechsler's scales have spawned an enormous body of research literature. Extensive discussions of these scales as well as the Stanford Binet (to be discussed in the next section) can be found in Lutey (1977), Sattler (1974, 1982), and others.

The Stanford-Binet Intelligence Scale

The Stanford-Binet Intelligence test, which has evolved through many revisions and standardizations since early in this century, measures the child's performance on many different kinds of verbal and nonverbal tasks but yields a single IQ score. It is intended to measure a general intelligence factor, rather than measure intelligence as a composite of many component abilities, as the Wechsler scales do. It is highly correlated with academic performance, especially for subject matter with a verbal emphasis (Anastasi, 1976). It is designed for children two years old and over, and while it lists norms into early adulthood, it is more discriminatory at the lower ages and thus is less reliable at higher ages, especially at higher levels of functioning (Anastasi, 1976). It has frequently been used with retarded populations, where it yields, in addition to an IQ score, a test age which indicates the test level at which the individual is functioning, as distinguished from the chronological age. A child of ten, for instance, who performs on the test at the level of an average eight-year-old would be said to have a test age of eight.

The Stanford-Binet test is more cumbersome to administer than the Wechsler scales and consequently is used less frequently, particularly since the development of the WPPSI; but it is especially helpful with very young children, between the ages of two and four (Lutey, 1977).

The Peabody Picture Vocabulary Test (PPVT)

The PPVT (Dunn, 1965), revised as the PPVT-R in 1981 (Dunn and Dunn, 1981), is a measure of intelligence which, quite unlike the first two, requires no expressive language on the part of the child taking the test. Pictures of increasing complexity and abstraction are presented, and the child is asked to point to the picture that best describes the increasingly difficult words that are given. This is a helpful test for children who lack fluency or have some kind of expressive language problem, but it does require good interpretation of verbal input. It measures only vocabulary comprehension, however, rather than the multiple verbal and nonverbal functions measured by both the WISC and the Stanford-Binet. Because such tests measure only one function or aspect of intelligence, they should not be used to determine a child's placement (Salvia and Ysseldyke, 1981).

Raven's Progressive Matrices

Raven's Progressive Matrices, for children over six and adults, is a nonverbal test of reasoning which measures, for example, an individual's ability to make comparisons and to use analogies. It is a helpful screening tool for children with language difficulties and with physical or auditory problems. However, as its norms are dated, and it is less reliable and valid than the WISC-R or the Stanford-Binet, if used, it should be supplemented by other tests (Sattler, 1982).

Infant Scales

A number of scales have been developed to assess developmental progress in infants. These scales are not very predictive of later IQ scores because the latter are heavily dependent on verbal skills, which of course have not yet been developed in infancy. As they can be used to assess an infant's overall developmental progress in such areas as motor, perceptual, social, and early language skills, the score might better be considered a "developmental quotient" or DQ. Exceptionally low scores, however, may be predictive of later intelligence levels, as in the case of moderately or severely retarded children. These scales can also be used to screen for early signs of specific deficits or potential problem areas which need immediate monitoring or early remediation. There are scales to be administered to the newborn. An Apgar score (1960), for example, can be obtained for newborns one and five minutes after delivery to evaluate such physiological functions as heart rate, reflexes, muscle tone, respiratory function, and color, with very low scores indicating possible or potential difficulties (Sattler, 1982). Such scores are moderately predictive of future neurological status, but there is a need to evaluate also a wider range of responses (Brazelton, 1973). Brazelton's (1973) *Neonatal Behavioral Assessment Scale* for newborns is designed to assess abilities along dimensions related to such factors as development of social relations, state of consciousness, reactions to stimuli, and ability to organize, in an attempt to study subtle behavioral responses as the infant adapts to the new environment, as well as caretaker responses, to help predict caretaker-infant interactions.

Another infant scale is the revised *Denver Developmental Screening Test* (Frankenburg et al., 1975), which is designed as a screening instrument to help identify maturational delays in children up to age six. It yields data on a child's personal-social, motor, and language development (Sattler, 1982). The *Infant Psychological Development Scale* (Uzgiris and Hunt, 1975) is based on Piagetian tenets and assesses intellectual development from two weeks to two years, including such cognitive abilities as object permanence, schemata development, and

90

causality. Other examples of such scales are the Bayley scales (1969), Gesell and Amatruda scales (1947), and the Cattell Infant Scales (1960).

ACHIEVEMENT TESTS

The range of achievement tests is very broad and far beyond the scope of this chapter. These tests measure a child's general level of achievement as well as performance in specific areas. Although many of them are more familiar to and are more frequently used by educators, the results of such tests are also very important in the diagnostic work of psychologists. Two commonly used ones are mentioned here.

The Wide Range Achievement Test (WRAT)

The WRAT is one of the most popular and most efficient achievement tests for ages five to adulthood. It measures reading, spelling, and arithmetic functioning from nursery school through university levels. The reading part of the WRAT does not require comprehension, and the arithmetic section has computational problems only and not word problems. Because of these differences, some children may do well on reading on the WRAT but poorly on the WISC vocabulary subtest; or well on math on the WRAT and not so well on the WISC word problems, or vice versa. Such differences in performance on similar but different kinds of tests are of great help diagnostically to the clinician. For instance, if a child does well on the WRAT math problems but very poorly on the WISC word problems, the clinician might suspect a language problem in the child's arithmetic achievement difficulties rather than a lack of mathematical ability. The WRAT is brief and easy to administer and has been found to be highly correlated with other measures of academic achievement (Jastak and Jastak, 1965).

The Stanford Achievement Test (SAT)

The SAT is typical of the more extensive achievement tests available, which are made up of batteries of tests. The SAT includes six batteries, covering grades one to nine, and tests achievement in many different academic areas. Other such tests include the California Achievement Tests, which assess skill development from kindergarten to grade twelve, and the Iowa Tests of Basic Skills (Salvia and Ysseldyke, 1981). These batteries of achievement in both general and specific areas will not be described here; they are discussed in Anastasi (1976) and in Salvia and Ysseldyke (1981).

NEUROPSYCHOLOGICAL TESTS

Specific neuropsychological diagnostic tests are used to assess characteristics of or changes in brain functioning and their effect on behavioral and psychological processes (Feuerstein et al., 1979). Performance on a number of tests is measured, and inferences are made regarding possible neurological dysfunction (Feuerstein et al., 1979). The many tests are used to assess the quality of the child's perceptual and motor development and integration, and to compare it with that of other children of the same age. They can give helpful information about a child's integrative skills, degree of perseveration, ability to make conceptual shifts, concrete thought, and recall ability (Sattler, 1982). Only the most commonly used neuropsychological tests are included here.

The Bender Visual/Motor Gestalt Test for Children

In this test of visual-motor function, (Clawson, 1962), which is based on Bender's (1946) original test, the child is asked to reproduce geometric designs presented on cards. The accuracy of the reproduction, the kinds of errors made, the placement of the designs on the paper, and other performance aspects are noted, from which inferences are made about the child's problems. This test has developmental norms which indicate at which age children would normally be expected to execute the various designs and to which a child's performance can be compared. The Bender test, which has been in use for many years, has generated a significant amount of research. It has been of value in diagnosing brain damage and various psychological disorders as well as identifying certain kinds of personality and intellectual characteristics (Clawson, 1962). Again, the *kinds* of errors made are an integral part of the interpretation of the test and of the assessment of the child's problems.

The Frostig Developmental Test of Visual Perception

The Frostig measures five aspects of a child's visual-motor functioning: eye-hand coordination, figure-ground discrimination, shape constancy, position of objects in space, and spatial relations (Frostig et al.,

92

1964). Although its norms are based on three- to nine-year-olds, the authors suggest that it can be helpful clinically with older children, even those of high-school age, when serious learning problems are involved. Because it yields a perceptual age score for each of the five areas, as well as a total perceptual age score, the clinician can identify specific areas of strength or weakness in the child as compared with other children of the same age.

The Developmental Tests of Visual-Motor Integration (VMI)

The VMI (Beery, 1967) requires that a child reproduce on paper designs of increasing complexity and difficulty. It is appropriate for use with children up to age sixteen and has separate norms for boys and girls. It provides a fairly quick assessment of the child's percep-tual-motor functioning and yields a perceptual age score. As it is quite rigidly scored, so that a design missed can make a difference of as much as a year in a child's perceptual age score, a particular child's VMI score may be somewhat lower than one would expect in view of that child's performance in other areas. Like comparable tests, it also provides other important clinical information, such as the child's approach to problems, degree of self-confidence, and meticulousness.

The Illinois Test of Psycholinguistic Abilities (ITPA)

The ITPA, developed by Kirk and his colleagues (1968), is designed to more precisely define the nature of a child's learning difficulties by assessing very specific receptive, expressive, and integrative psycho-logical functions. There are twelve subtests which measure, for instance, such aspects of auditory and visual functioning as discrimi-nation, closure, sequencing, and memory, to name a few. The test is intended to indicate more definitively which cognitive components or skills are intact and which are lacking, in order to facilitate planning for a child (Lerner, 1981).

The ITPA is appropriate for children up to ten years of age and con-tains standardized norms against which to compare a given child. It is a fairly lengthy test to administer, but gives very detailed information about a child's functioning in many specific areas and at different lev-els. A more detailed discussion of the various levels and subtests and of its use with children can be found in Lerner (1976).

PERSONALITY TESTS

Personality tests are designed to elicit information about a child's psychological makeup, patterns of personality characteristics, behavioral response repertoire, constellation of problems, and, at least with some of the tests, unconscious motivation. Those most commonly used, along with various rating scales and personality inventories, will be discussed here. They are grouped into objective, subjective, and projective types for discussion purposes, although at times those distinctions are difficult to maintain.

Objective Tests

Objective tests are those which can be administered and scored easily, require a minimum of interpretation, and are most likely to yield scores or results on which clinicians can readily agree. Objective tests are common in medicine—blood pressure, height, and weight measures yield concrete information. In academic areas of psychological functioning there are objective achievement tests such as the WRAT whose scores are virtually unchallenged. However, in the area of personality testing, such objective and unarguable results are difficult to achieve and hence relatively rare.

Behavioral rating scales and checklists probably represent the most objective tools. Such rating scales as Quay's *Behavior Problem Checklist* can be used to identify deviant behavior and select intervention techniques as well as to measure the child's behavioral response to drugs and other therapy (Quay, 1977). The *Devereux Elementary School Behavior Rating Scale* developed by Spivack and Swift (1967), or their high school rating scale (1977), can be used to assess both academic and interpersonal behaviors. The *Adaptive Behavior Scale* described by Anastasi (1976) is based on observation of daily behavior of children with problems and has a developmental scale and a section to help assess specific behavior problems or disorders. It can be used by any adults in contact with the child or by an interviewer who is observing the child.

The *Child Behavior Profile* (Achenbach, 1978b; Achenbach and Edelbrock, 1979), for use with children from ages six to sixteen, yields information about a child's adaptive competencies as well as many behavior problems. When the information obtained from parents is

94

transferred from the *Child Behavior Checklist* to the profile, the clinician can get an overview of specific behaviors, how problems and competencies of the child cluster, and how the child compares with other children of the same age and sex. The test thus describes the child's behavior economically and meaningfully (Achenbach, 1978b).

One of the clear advantages of the behavior rating scales is that they can easily be administered by teachers and other concerned persons, whereas extensive training is required before tests such as those classed as projective can be conducted and interpreted properly.

Subjective Tests

Subjective tests are those on which individuals provide information about themselves in response to specific questions or on self-report inventories. Although they may be objectively scored, they are subject to distortion because of the individuals' limited self-knowledge, and/or the risk that the answers may be faked if the person being examined is trying to project a favorable or unfavorable image. For these reasons, the tests require somewhat greater interpretation on the part of the clinician, who must evaluate and assess the validity of the responses, their consistency, and the kind of motivation the subject was experiencing. They can, however, reveal differences in the way problems are perceived by the individual and by others. The individual's perception is of course critical, whether or not it is consistent with what is actually happening in the environment, because it is the determining factor in his or her behavior.

One of the most widely-used personality inventories is the *Minnesota Multiphasic Personality Inventory (MMPI)* (Hathaway and McKinley, 1967). Since it is standardized for ages sixteen and older, it has limited usefulness in a practice mainly concerned with children, but it can be given to older adolescents. It is a lengthy inventory of statements which subjects indicate are true or not true of themselves. Patterns of scores are depicted graphically for various scales which are assumed to reflect personality tendencies or characteristics. If scores are extreme enough or appear in certain constellations, pathology is suggested. The test can be machine scored, and lengthy computer printouts of elaborate personality descriptions based on the scales can be obtained.

Another scale is a *Fear Survey Schedule (FSS-III)* developed by Wolpe and Lang (1964) as a means of discovering areas of maladaptive anxiety. Subjects rate to what degree various experiences or situations disturb them, cause discomfort, or generate fear. As with other inventories, individuals can suppress expressions of certain characteristics in order to "fake good"; that is, present a healthier picture of themselves than is realistic—evidence that " . . . inventories and other aids are no substitute for the skill of the therapist" (Wolpe and Lange, 1964, p. 28).

Another helpful inventory is the *Vineland Social Maturity Scale* (Doll, 1947), which measures social independence. Responses are obtained from the parents about their child's performance in various self-help and social areas. Like any other inventory or self-report technique, this one has the potential for bias and distortion.

Projective Techniques

Projective tests involve the presentation of an ambiguous or neutral stimulus to which subjects must respond in some way, such as with the creation of a story about a stimulus picture. It is assumed that their responses will be determined by forces in their personalities, many of which are unconscious, and that they will thus "project" their personalities onto the stimulus presented. Such tests are unstructured, so that the persons taking them cannot rely on conventional responses and therefore must show their own individuality (Rapaport, Gill, and Schafer, 1968).

One frequently used projective technique is the *Thematic Apperception Test (TAT)*. Developed by Henry Murray in 1943, it consists of a series of pictures depicting people in various rather ambiguous situations, and the child is asked to tell a story about each picture. It is assumed that from an analysis of the child's identification with one of the characters—and the characteristics, conflicts, and problems ascribed to that character as well as to the others—the clinician will be able to infer certain things about the child. That is, the child "projects" his or her personality and perceptions into the story, and the clinician interprets the meaning and significance of those projections. The *Children's Apperception Test (CAT)* is similar but utilizes animal instead of human figures, on the assumption that children more readily identify with animals (Bellak and Adelman, 1960). It also shows scenes that are likely to elicit the problems and conflicts that are typical of many children. The *Blacky Pictures Test* (Blum, 1960), based on the same kind of assumptions, is a highly psychoanalytically-oriented test intended to reveal psychoanalytic problems and conflicts. The *Make-a-Picture Story (MAPS)* test (Shneidman, 1960) has the child choose characters to set up in a scene and then tell a story about the picture created. Thus, in addition to story content, the choice and arrangement of figures provide outlets through which a child can project his or her personality.

The Children's Form of the *Rotter's Incomplete Sentences Blank* (1950) is useful for discovering how children feel and how they perceive events in their environment. It consists of forty sentence stems which the child is asked to complete, such as "I like. . . ." or "A mother. . . ." or "I failed. . . ." Again, no single response is significant by itself, but *patterns* of responses, such as repeated references to failure or specific difficulties, can be helpful.

The *Rorschach Inkblot Test* is perhaps the best known of the projective tests. Developed by Herman Rorschach in the 1920s (Rorschach, 1942), it consists of ten cards imprinted with inkblots, of which five include color and five are black, white, and grey. The child is asked to tell what the inkblot looks like and what causes it to look that way. Depending on the content of the responses, the use of the various elements of the card, and other aspects of the responses, the clinician makes certain inferences about the child's personality characteristics and conflicts. The Rorschach test has generated much research and controversy, and there are many books available on its use and interpretation. More extended discussions can be found in Goldfried, Stricker, and Weiner (1971), Halpern (1960), Hertz (1960), and Rickers-Ovsiankina (1960).

There is not unanimous agreement as to the helpfulness of tests that purport to measure inner dynamics. Such tests have been heavily criticized on a number of fronts. Even among proponents, there is disagreement as to which specific tests are the most helpful, scientific, objective, misused, overused, or clinically productive.

This kind of testing requires a high degree of interpretation on the part of the clinician, which means that there is also greater room for disagreement about the inferences to be drawn from test results. Consequently, there is an even greater need to seek corroborative findings and confirming evidence from other areas. The test responses must be related to other data and be grounded in behavioral indices as much as possible to prevent the unfounded speculation for which projective tests have been so frequently and severely criticized.

The tests can be useful to the clinician in suggesting hypotheses which can then be followed up and investigated through other observations and sources of information, but they should not be used in isolation. The mandate for high levels of integrity, conscientiousness, and responsibility on the part of the clinician is clear.

There are other projective techniques, in addition to tests, which can be used in the assessment of a child. All are based on the same assumption: that children will project their personalities onto the stimulus or materials with which they are presented. Drawings, for instance, have been used extensively as a projective device (Buck, 1948; Burns and Kaufman, 1970; Machover, 1949) as well as an indicator of intellectual functioning (Goodenough, 1926; Harris, 1963). A child may be asked to draw a family or a person; based on the characteristics delineated or omitted, the kinds of distortion introduced, or the artistic quality of the drawing itself, certain inferences are made. Similarly, a child's play with such unstructured and ambiguous stimuli as clay, sand, and finger paints can elicit certain kinds of expressions which are then interpreted by the clinician. A child's play with puppets and dolls is also assumed to give the child an opportunity to project his or her personality into a situation.

Like the projective tests, these techniques require careful interpretation and should not serve as the sole source of diagnostic information about a child, no matter how helpful they may be in generating or suggesting hypotheses.

Good discussions of the use of projective techniques with children are to be found in Anderson and Anderson (1951), Rabin and Haworth (1960), and Rapaport, Gill, and Schafer (1968).

Test Selection

How does a clinician choose from among the many tests available? How can the range of potentially helpful tests be narrowed to a manageable and realistic number? The clinician has many variables to consider. Which tests are selected depends on the nature of the problems, the age of the clients, the theoretical perspective of the clinician, the reliability and validity of various tests, and the resources available.

First, one must consider the *reasons for a child's referral*, which in turn determine the questions that the assessment is to address. If the purpose is to evaluate problems that an individual is experiencing, one would select different tests than if one were engaged in broad screening programs or pursuing specific research questions. Assuming for the moment that the purpose of the assessment is to evaluate the problems of a child who has been referred, the clinician must still choose from a wide variety of tests. For example, if the child has been referred for school-related academic problems but has shown no serious behavioral difficulties, the clinician would likely emphasize intellectual, visual-motor, and perceptual functions in the testing. Some measure of the child's achievement level would also probably be included to determine the extent of any underachievement and to pinpoint deficits in specific skill areas. Some form of sentence-completion task might also be included to get more information about the child's self-perceptions and feelings about school, success, and family pressure.

If specific learning problems were not suspected, or if there was no evidence of any perceptual problems or confusion, the visual-motor tests might be eliminated from the battery of tests. Moreover, if a child had serious expressive language problems or limited verbalization ability or fluency because of a different cultural or language background, tests such as the Peabody Picture Vocabulary Test–Revised or Raven's Progressive Matrices would be more appropriate as assessments of general intellectual level than a test like the WISC-R, which relies more heavily on expressive language and might therefore underestimate a child's intellectual potential.

A child referred for behavioral as well as academic problems would likely be given similar tests. However, additional behavioral checklists or personality testing would be necessary to further assess the reasons for the behavioral problems and the conditions that were maintaining or exacerbating them.

Second, the *age of the child* affects the choice of tests to be used. Most tests have been designed and standardized for use with a specific age group. The standardization sample on which the test was developed should serve as an appropriate group against which to compare the child. If children who fall outside that range are given that test, the accompanying test norms are no longer appropriate and could be misleading.

Third, particular tests are selected according to the *theoretical orientation* of the diagnostician. Although clinicians of any of the major persuasions will show some commonality in their test selection, important differences in their fields of interest will dictate, in part, their choices. For instance, a behaviorally oriented clinician would not choose a Rorschach to assess underlying unconscious motivation. Conversely, psychodynamically oriented workers might use some behavioral checklists, for example, but would probably supplement them with various projective tests as well.

Fourth, a clinician should also select tests on the basis of their demonstrated *reliability and validity*. Although tests can also be used to generate hypotheses, as long as those hypotheses are confirmed through other data, generally tests chosen should have demonstrated or proven usefulness in consistently and reliably predicting other behaviors in which the clinician is interested. Detailed reliability and validity data for specific tests cannot be included in this chapter. However, more extended discussions of standardization samples and reliability and validity of all of the tests mentioned in this section, as well as descriptions and evaluations of many others, can be found in Buros's (1978) encyclopedic compendium of tests, or in Sattler's (1982) excellent book on assessment.

Children can become anxious during testing because of the nature of the material they are responding to or because of the content of their responses, and clinicians should be sensitive to the existence of such anxiety. Talking briefly with clients after testing and answering their questions gives clinicians an opportunity to reduce anxiety and to follow up certain issues or problems that have been suggested by the child's responses or comments during testing. Obviously, much depends on the examiner's sensitivity, skills, sense of responsibility, and integrity. Failure to reduce such test-induced anxiety before the client leaves the testing situation may jeopardize any future therapeutic relationship.

Integration

When clinicians have obtained as much relevant information as possible, they must assemble all of the pieces of the diagnostic puzzle. They must identify patterns and characteristics of the child and family and integrate them into a meaningful, consistent, coherent picture of the problems before them. Past training, theoretical stance, the personality of the clinician, and sensitivity to innumerable cues affect the

100

quality of this integrative diagnostic effort and the accuracy of the data analysis and interpretation.

A thorough and well-integrated assessment is crucial to providing meaningful help to a child and family, because it determines the course of action that the clinician will choose, the specific techniques of intervention to be used, and the measure of progress made in therapy. A less than comprehensive assessment can cause clinicians to enter blind alleys which bring no relief to the child and waste valuable time that could be spent on effective intervention. There is no substitute for information that is as extensive, broadly based, and objective as possible.

Models and Methods: A Comparative Analysis

Each clinical institution, school board, or private clinician uses a somewhat different combination of techniques and tests, depending on the nature of their client population, the theoretical perspective of the staff, the conceptual models that have been adopted, and the time and resources available. Although virtually all would agree on the need to get the most comprehensive information possible concerning the problems with which they have been presented, wide differences of opinion exist regarding what constitutes such useful information and the best methods to obtain it.

Although psychodynamically and behaviorally oriented clinicians might strongly disagree on the nature of the material to be included in interviews, the usefulness of the interview method is not usually disputed. Similarly, clinicians of each of the major models would likely agree on the importance of school reports as a source of significant information about the child's functional level and behavioral difficulties. Similarly, they would no doubt agree on the importance of medical records and the need to rule out significant medical, physiological, or biochemical disorders.

Major disagreements most frequently arise in the areas of observation and, particularly, psychological testing. Although both approaches consider observation to be very important, psychodynamic clinicians emphasize clinical observation during interviews and testing from which they draw inferences. They rely on reports of behaviors from others such as parents and teachers. Behaviorally oriented workers, on the other hand, emphasize direct behavioral observation in various settings; careful recording, counting, and charting of such observations are a key component of a behavioral approach to problems. The recording, along with the behavioral descriptions and definitions that precede it, provides the clinician with baseline data against which to compare future behavior and with supplementary information that may increase understanding of the current problem. Behavioral clinicians also use clinical observations, but the variety of settings in which they observe behavior, as well as the manner in which they record, monitor, and evaluate it, differs significantly from that of most psychodynamically oriented workers.

The most fundamental differences between the two approaches relate to the kind of psychological testing to be used. Behavioral diagnosticians rely primarily on the many objectively scored behavioral checklists, rating scales, and inventories that have been developed, a few of which have been discussed in this chapter. Psychodynamically oriented workers may use such techniques but may also use projective techniques, alone or in addition to the more objective indices. Because projective techniques are based on the assumption of unconscious motivation and unconscious processes, behavioral clinicians reject them as irrelevant and misleading. Behavioral clinicians are not interested in searching out underlying psychodynamic causes for the maladaptive behaviors they seek to change. They pay more attention to specific stimuli situations, although they do not totally exclude an individual's characteristics (Goldfried and Sprafkin, 1974). The behavioral clinicians, with their emphasis on observable and quantifiable behaviors, have frequently criticized the results of projective testing as too subjective, "fuzzy," ambiguous, untestable, and open to multiple interpretations. On the other hand, psychodynamic workers sometimes label the objective instruments as superficial, stating that the information they provide is not adequate for an understanding of the complexities of a child's personality.

Clinicians, of course, need not make a clear choice between one or the other avenue. There is obviously a tremendously wide range of techniques available to a practicing clinician. Which ones are selected depends on the nature of the problems, the age of the clients, the theoretical perspective of the clinician, and the resources available. A clinician needs to develop an awareness of the huge armamentarium available and choose from it those techniques which will be of most benefit to specific clients. A highly behavioral approach may be most

effective and efficient for some clients; for others, a more psychodynamic approach may be more appropriate; and for still others, a combination. Hypotheses arrived at on the basis of projective testing, however, must be related to interview, school, observational, or behavioral
indices in order to keep the diagnostic work as empirical as possible.
The following quote from Bellak expresses the principle well:

> *There is no slot machine diagnosis possible*—one cannot put in a coin and get
> out a diagnosis. . . . *Integration* of test results with other facets of the personality
> is an essential principle. (Bellak, 1971, p. 33)

Diagnostic considerations should not be limited to the first few contacts with the child, but should be seen as an ongoing function of the
clinician. As the child progresses with treatment, the therapist needs
to change the specific short-term goals for that child, a process that
requires reevaluation and reassessment. The absence of change also
requires reevaluation and reassessment in order to determine which
overlooked or newly developed factors may be precluding therapeutic
change and which techniques need to be altered (and in what way).
Because the child is still developing and therefore constantly changing, diagnosis must also be developmental (Stroh, 1960).

Finally, a diagnostic workup often has a therapeutic effect in itself.
The child and family frequently experience a measure of immediate
relief because steps are finally being taken to help them and to share
the responsibility for solving their problems, and because the clinician's authoritative and reassuring manner conveys confidence and
optimism about the outcome. In cases where prognosis is very guarded
and the outlook poor, clinicians still frequently provide relief for the
family through their recommendations of courses of action for the
parents, their participation in a mutual problem-solving venture, and
their support.

The following case study could be approached from a psychodynamic or behavioral perspective or from a more eclectic viewpoint,
with techniques drawn from both models. A split-page analysis comparing possible diagnostic procedures from each point of view follows
the case study in Table 5.1. There are also brief hypothetical but very
possible interpretive paragraphs on the respective data obtained. Differences in the content sought, the interpretation of the content, and
the general tone of the procedures can be seen even in such a brief
descriptive and diagnostic comparison.

CASE STUDY

John is an eleven-year-old boy who was referred because of behavior problems at school, aggressiveness on the playground, and underachievement in the classroom. He seemed unmotivated in school and demonstrated poor work habits. He had had problems as early as grade one, but they had increased in the last few years. Math was especially problematic for him. Parents described him as easily hurt, but self-reliant, independent, and prone to express aggression physically. They used both verbal and corporal punishment with John, and projected the blame for much of his difficulty onto the school.

The school reported that John had shown increasingly serious behavior problems on the playground. He had unpredictable outbursts as often as twice a day during which he punched other children or threw them down. The school did report, however, that these had decreased somewhat with John's recent interest in baseball. Although John was capable of doing the required work and sometimes did do it, at other times he refused and instead disturbed the class with noises and other disruptive behavior. Early report cards indicated that he had shown good early reading and math skills, but was aggressive when upset as early as kindergarten and showed increasing violent outbursts, distractibility, hastiness and disruption over the years. By grade five the teacher noted that his behavior problems were hampering his social development and interfering with his learning.

TABLE 5.1   *Diagnostic approaches*

	Psychodynamic	*Behavioral*
Interview	Obtain introductory and background information.	Obtain introductory and background information.
	Obtain a detailed developmental history.	Obtain a developmental history.
		Note such things as what usually precedes the occurrence of the problem behaviors and what reactions occur in response to John's behavior or demands.
	Assess family dynamics and communication patterns.	
	Make inferences about the psychological significance of various parent-child interactions, both past and present.	Determine which events or reactions in school or at home reinforce John's maladaptive behavior.
	Assess child's perception of the situation through his direct and indirect statements.	

104

	Psychodynamic	*Behavioral*
	Generate hypotheses about his inner psychological makeup and the kinds of conflicts he experiences.	
School and medical reports	Note the history of the child's school problems, any steps that were taken to correct them, and the success or failure of such interventions.	Note the levels of academic functioning and any behavioral problems described by the school personnel and reactions to them which might serve to reinforce them and maintain them.
	Assess interpersonal and academic interactions and difficulties of the child in school.	Obtain report cards and actual samples of the child's work in school.
	Generate hypotheses about how the child's psychological conflicts and problems interfere with his learning and social adjustments.	Note whether the child has any significant medical or neurological problems which might interfere with learning.
	Note whether the child has or has had significant medical problems, frequent accidents, or unusual diseases which could contribute to his current problem.	Note reactions of the child or his family to such medical difficulties which may have reinforced maladaptive behavior.
	Note his reaction to such diseases and the psychological significance they had for him.	
Observation	Note grimaces, gestures, verbalizations, and other behaviors of the child. Analyze them and their timing for possible clues to underlying attitudes or problems.	Observe the child's reactions to and during the interviews and testing.
	Observe the child's reactions to and during the interviews and testing.	Identify target behaviors which are the most problematic and which will constitute the main focus of therapy.
		Observe John in the classroom and with his family to note the interactions that occur, what precedes and follows them, and which events or circumstances are reinforcing to him. Record and chart such behaviors, using the coding system of Patterson, Cobb and Ray, or both in order to make these observations as objective as possible.
Testing	Administer the *WISC* for quantitative and qualitative data regarding his intellectual level, approach to problems, and	Administer a *WISC* to obtain data regarding John's intellectual level and behavioral characteristics which facilitate or hinder his performance.

TABLE 5.1 *Diagnostic approaches (continued)*

	Psychodynamic	Behavioral
	attentional and integrative skills. Analyze the content for possible clues to the child's conflicts and problems. Analyze the pattern of subtest scores.	Administer the *WRAT* to get an idea of any weak areas or significant discrepancies between his chronological age and grade placement or functional level.
	Administer the *WRAT* to get an idea of any weak areas or significant discrepancies between chronological age and grade placement or functional level.	Ask the teacher to complete the *Devereux Rating Scale* on John for an objective and quantitative report of his actual behavior. This will also provide baseline data.
	Adminster the *Bender-Gestalt* and *VMI* to investigate possible perceptual-motor or integrative difficulties.	Complete a problem checklist such as Quay's (1977) *Behavior Problem Checklist*.
	Administer the *Rotter Incomplete Sentences Blank* to get an idea of how John perceives various aspects of his life and how he feels about them. Note recurring themes and frequent concerns.	Administer the *Bender-Gestalt* and *VMI* to investigate possible perceptual-motor or integrative difficulties.
	Administer a *TAT* to try to get an idea of the child's ideals and aspirations, level of self-esteem, unconscious conflicts and impulses, and other psychological data.	Administer the *Children's Personality Questionnaire* or *Adaptive Behavior Scale*. Note patterns of maladaptive behavior and which behaviors are repeated most frequently. Compare John's scores on these behaviors with those of other children his age.
	Ask the child to *draw a family* and interpret the characteristics of his drawing in terms of his self-perception, intellectual level, and other personality characteristics.	
Impressions and recommendations	John is an eleven-year-old boy of average intelligence who has some long-standing perceptual problems which likely interfered with his early learning. Because of the consequent frustration and feelings of failure, he withdrew effort and began to act out his frustration in aggressive behavior. This behavior also brought him increased attention, albeit negative, and some status with peers which he could not get through more acceptable	John is an eleven-year-old boy of average intelligence who has some perceptual difficulty and is achieving at levels below those expected of a child his age. His problem-attack skills are poor, and he needs help to become more careful and more critical of his work. His aggressive behavior seems to occur in part as a result of his modeling of his father's aggressive

Psychodynamic	Behavioral
behavior or academic achievement. In addition, John is harboring considerable hostility toward his parents, who have used physical punishment frequently, and he may have displaced some of that anger onto his peers. His close identification with an aggressive father and his mother's projection of blame onto the school have resulted in John's projection of blame onto the school and in an avoidance of responsibility for his part in his problems. He has also probably received some subtle encouragement for his aggressive behavior from his father, who seems to experience some vicarious satisfaction from it. This family needs help clarifying some of these indirect and subtle communications so that John can begin to develop a better self-image and socially acceptable ways of expressing his anger and hostility.	behavior and his parents' reinforcement and encouragement of it. His aggressive and assaultive behavior brings him considerable attention at school, from both teachers and peers, and is thus reinforcing. In addition, verbal behavior and language skills are not strongly reinforced in his home environment. His lack of academic success and his repeated failures have reduced the amount of positive reinforcement for socially acceptable or competent, adaptive behavior. He needs training in and reinforcement for such behaviors.

If a psychodynamic approach were taken, although remedial academic work would also be recommended, most of the therapeutic emphasis would be on resolving the unclear communication and underlying conflict in the family. It would be expected that once those issues were clarified and John's self-esteem was built up, his academic and social functioning would improve.

If one took an exclusively behavioral approach, on the other hand, although specific remedial work might again be recommended, the major emphasis would be on devising a plan to change John's maladaptive behavior, with a program of reinforcers for specific behaviors in both academic and social areas, at home as well as in school.

An integrative-diagnostic approach and interpretation would incorporate some aspects of both approaches. For example, such an approach would utilize psychological tests, including projective tests, as well as behavior checklists or rating scales. Underlying pathological

107

processes and distorted patterns of communication might be discovered through such tests and might perhaps serve as the focus of later family therapy. At the same time, a program might be worked out to decrease the maladaptive behaviors and increase more acceptable and constructive ones through skills training and consistent reinforcement. Therapy would thus proceed simultaneously on both fronts.

Discussion Questions

1. Discuss the above case study and the diagnostic considerations in terms of the models presented in Chapter 2.
2. Discuss the case study above in terms of the child's needs. What steps would you recommend in order to ensure that those needs were met?
3. Choose one case study from the following chapters and develop the same diagnostic comparisons as were developed above.

PART III

Treatment and Remediation

Remedial Techniques and Interventions

The range of possible therapeutic interventions for use with children is very broad. Some are commonly utilized, whereas others are fairly esoteric or experimental and are being used only by a limited number of devotees. This discussion will focus on the specific kinds of intervention that are most frequently used and that therefore are most likely to be encountered in the literature. The types of treatment to be discussed are in no way mutually exclusive; in fact they are often used in various combinations.

The emphasis in this section is primarily descriptive, its purpose being to introduce the array of treatment approaches and techniques which are available. In the next chapter, problems encountered in trying to evaluate the effectiveness of various kinds of therapeutic intervention will be discussed, as well as methodological problems inherent in that evaluation.

Psychotherapy

The most widely used form of intervention has traditionally been some kind of psychotherapy. The many varieties of psychotherapeutic intervention have some characteristics in common. First, psychotherapy assumes a relationship between a therapist and a client which allows them to work together on the client's presenting symptoms. This relationship may be one-to-one, as in traditional psychotherapy; or it may be developed in the context of group or family therapy—or even conjoint therapy, where more than one therapist is involved. The therapy may be conducted in an office, hospital, school, or other setting.

The nature of the relationship and the way in which the therapist and client set about to work on the client's problems will depend on the theoretical orientation and skills of the therapist and on the age and characteristics of the client. Thus, there may be psychoanalysis (Freud, 1946; Klein, 1932), psychoanalytic psychotherapy (Chess and Hassibi, 1978), nondirective psychotherapy (Rogers, 1951; 1961), play therapy (Axline, 1947; Moustakas, 1959b), group therapy, activity therapy, or any number of others, some of which will be discussed in more detail later in this chapter.

Second, psychotherapy assumes the use of verbal exploration of difficulties as clients explain and discuss their problems, backgrounds, and feelings with a therapist. With children for whom verbalization

112

is not easy or who are too young to use language with great facility, play is used as the medium of communication. In play, many children can easily express their inner feelings and conflicts, and therapists who are sensitive to the kinds of messages children send through their play can respond to that language as they might to the more verbal language of older children or adults. With older children and adolescents, more conventional individual or group psychotherapy is appropriate; they may benefit greatly from being in a group of peers who are able to verbalize many of the same problems and conflicts that they themselves are experiencing. A closer look at some commonly used forms of psychotherapy follows.

Psychoanalysis

The use of psychoanalysis with children is best exemplified in the work of Melanie Klein (1932) and Anna Freud (1946). There is considerable emphasis in their therapy on an examination of the child's past, on the interpretation of the symbolic meanings of symptoms, and on uncovering unconscious dynamics and conflicts through careful study of the child's dreams and verbalizations. In analysis the therapist works to help the child resolve some of the classic analytic conflicts which arise during the various stages of psychosexual development, such as an Oedipal complex. The analyst may bring to light the child's disguised sexual and aggressive impulses, or may work to decrease the severity of the child's superego (Klein, 1932). Sometimes responses to the child's behavior have nothing to do with conflict or problems but are simply supportive to the child, as when the provision of food in the sessions reassures the child about the therapist's level of caring (Halpern and Kissel, 1976).

Traditional psychoanalysis is usually a long and expensive process; it may take as many as five sessions a week for four or five years (Chess and Hassibi, 1978). For the student interested in following a single, specific, detailed but not lengthy analysis of a child from start to finish (four months in this case), as well as the analyst's accompanying notes, Melanie Klein's *Narrative of a Child Analysis* (1961) is recommended. Sometimes "psychoanalytic psychotherapy" is used—a more limited form of psychoanalysis which is effective for mild disorders (Chess and Hassibi, 1978). Interpretations in such therapy are still analytic to a degree, but unconscious material is not so systematically explored

113

and uncovered, and the therapy is somewhat less frequent and requires a shorter period of time than classical analysis.

Nondirective Psychotherapy

In nondirective psychotherapy, a warm, accepting atmosphere in which the child can feel safe is considered essential for growth. An optimistic belief in the child's capacity for growth and self-development is apparent, and the therapist communicates unqualified acceptance, respect, and faith in the child. Supportive therapeutic techniques are based on the assumption that the child will grow if obstacles such as censure and criticism are removed. Focus is on the present, and the therapist listens in an understanding and empathic way and " . . . deals directly and immediately with his (the child's) feelings rather than with the problems or symptoms and their causes" (Moustakas, 1959b, p. 2). Nondirective psychotherapy is typically much briefer and less frequent than psychoanalysis, with the therapist and child meeting perhaps once or twice a week rather than daily.

Nondirective psychotherapy can be used with both children and adolescents, individually or in groups. It is generally conducted in a play context when used with younger children and in a more verbal form with older children and adolescents.

Play Therapy

The use of play therapy has become an important tool in the treatment of children because play is their natural mode of communication and expression. In play they can relive experiences, alter the world, and most important, control what happens. In the play sessions children can express hostility toward parents, siblings, or other figures with no fear of retribution; they can even construct families without specific troublesome members. Play figures can achieve great goals, allowing the child to experience feelings of mastery. Some children become less inhibited as they find complete acceptance in being permitted to express themselves and to enjoy various tactile and emotional experiences. Thus play therapy may be particularly suited to younger children, to older ones who have difficulty articulating their problems and conflicts, and to children who find it hard to express their feelings directly.

114

Play therapists may lean heavily toward psychoanalytic or nondirective techniques, which will influence how they respond to the child's play or how active they are in the sessions. Or they may be more eclectic in their approach; that is, they may draw from various theoretical orientations and use a variety of therapeutic tools, depending on the needs of the child. More emphasis is placed on the nondirective and eclectic approaches in this chapter, as they are more frequently used than classical psychoanalysis. Axline's (1947) description of a nondirective play therapy atmosphere is most graphic:

> The play-therapy room is good growing ground. In the security of this room where the *child* is the most important person, where he is in command of the situation and of himself, where no one tells him what to do, no one criticizes what he does, no one nags, or suggests, or goads him on, or pries into his private world, he suddenly feels that *here* he can unfold his wings; he can look squarely at himself, for he is accepted completely; he can test out his ideas; he can express himself fully, for this is *his* world, and he no longer has to compete with such other forces as adult authority or rival contemporaries or situations where he is a human pawn in a game between bickering parents, or where he is the butt of someone else's frustrations and aggressions. He is an individual in his own right. He is treated with dignity and respect. He can say anything that he feels like saying—and he is accepted completely. He can play with the toys in any way that he likes to—and he is accepted completely. He can hate and he can love and he can be as indifferent as the Great Stone Face—and he is still accepted completely. He can be as fast as a whirlwind or as slow as molasses in January—and he is neither restrained nor hurried. It is a unique experience for a child suddenly to find adult suggestions, mandates, rebukes, restraints, criticisms, disapprovals, support, intrusions gone. They are all replaced by complete acceptance and permissiveness to be himself. (Axline, 1947, pp. 16–17)

Because it is not intended to substitute or impose "good" behavior for "bad," according to adult standards, nondirective play therapy allows children to express themselves freely and by doing so to gain confidence.

The atmosphere of the playroom, the kinds of materials available, and the child's relationship with the therapist are central to any play therapy, regardless of the theoretical bent of the therapist. The playroom should be pleasant, colorful, and interesting to a child, but not overly stimulating. Some relatively unstructured materials should be available, such as clay, paint, and sand, to enable children to project their own world onto the material and to express their feelings and conflicts freely (Moustakas, 1959) without having the materials dictate or narrow their expression. The therapist may make specific toys or materials available to facilitate expression of certain problems or to elicit conflictful material. For example, the availability of dolls and dollhouses allows the child to re-create a family which may be a reflection of the child's actual family, a desired family constellation, or a perceived family grouping. The addition of such toys as guns, darts, and water pistols provides an easy opportunity for a child to express aggressive feelings or exhibit aggressive behavior, although such encouragement or props may not be necessary.

To bridge the gap in interests and abilities between younger children and adolescents, therapy with slightly older children may involve a combination of verbalization and such activities as walking, feeding ducks, and playing games. All of these activities help to relax the child, to develop rapport between the therapist and the child, to allow the child to express feelings and concerns more freely in a casual context, and to facilitate verbalization.

One very inhibited nine-year-old girl, for instance, rarely spoke and responded very tersely to questions. The bridge between her withdrawal and the therapist turned out to be the therapist's Old English sheepdog, which the girl adored. After of couple of sessions she was able to ask if she and the therapist could take him for a walk; and those walks became an integral part of each therapy session. Very gradually, during the walks, she was able to begin to initiate conversation and comments which then led to her increased ability to verbalize many of her fears.

Axline (1947), lists eight basic principles on which play therapy should be based, some of which have already been mentioned. They are a warm, friendly relationship; acceptance of the child; permissiveness; recognition of and reflection of feelings; respect for the child's problem-solving ability; letting the child lead; avoidance of hurrying; and establishing only the requisite limitations.

The early structuring of the play therapy sessions is important. Permissiveness should be conveyed, but limits must nevertheless be set. Limits are necessary regarding materials (destructiveness is not allowed), time allowed for the sessions, and the person of the therapist (abuse of the therapist is not tolerated). These limits keep the sessions tied to reality for a child (Axline, 1947). They make the child feel safe and secure, for he or she knows that if behavior or feelings get out of control, the therapist can and will enforce the limits and help the child reestablish control. Without such limits, the child may engage

116

in behavior that will serve to heighten anxiety or guilt, and the therapist may also become uncomfortable and anxious. Thus, the therapist must provide a boundary or structure within which growth can occur.

The following case study details the highlights of a period of play therapy with a nine-year-old girl. The series is described in some detail because it illustrates many of the above points, because it involves both analytic and nondirective components,—and because the client was such an interesting and expressive little girl.

CASE STUDY

Anne was a very small ten-year-old black-haired girl who was referred initially as an academic and behavior problem at school, with hyperactive and disruptive behavior, and as a behavior problem for the parents at home. The parents, particularly the mother, felt inadequate in their handling of her and felt guilty over largely negative responses to her, and were already worried that their problems would increase with adolescence.

Therapy with Anne was very interesting and rewarding in several ways. First, there were marked changes in her behavior throughout therapy and very definite changes in her areas of concern and ways of handling her problems. Second, she was a very expressive child and showed steady progress in her ability to articulate her feelings and conceptualize her problems and all of the possible solutions to them. Third, her behavior in therapy often complemented that of her parents in their therapy. When the entire family was seen together, she became increasingly verbal. Her therapy will be described in terms of these three aspects.

Although Anne was ten she looked more like a much younger child. She was not only short for her age, but very thin and poorly coordinated. When initially seen, she was extremely hyperactive and distractible, playing with one thing after another, talking rather superficially about herself and her family. She was much more eager to impress than to relate to the therapist. The playroom initially seemed too stimulating, but by the second session she had calmed down considerably and soon became very involved in coming to the clinic.

Early in therapy, Anne concentrated mainly on problems at school. She disliked it intensely, liked coming to the clinic because she could miss school, and thought of herself as "really dumb." The other children at school called her "a loser" which hurt and angered Anne but she had very little means for coping with this. The only real mention of her family in the early sessions was in her reconstruction of the physical layout of her own home using the doll furniture, without including people too much. Some of her drawings were at times rather bizarre with strange, cryptic messages written across the top which intrigued the therapist. Her emphasis on the time of the sessions and on the room number reflected her confused orientation, her attempts to structure the situation, and her efforts to decrease her apprehension.

Over the course of these early sessions, the therapists began to understand the kind of confusion that existed in the communications between the mother and Anne. For example, Anne's mother encouraged her to become involved in many after-school activities and lessons, but then reacted negatively when Anne became overtired or was unable to keep up with her schoolwork. Or the parents would urge Anne to invite her friends over on weekends and then complain about the noise or the messes they made. Anne was confused by these inconsistencies and became increasingly frustrated in her attempts to gain parental approval. During the initial therapy sessions, Anne responded very warmly to the therapist's accepting manner. She related a couple of incidents from school which seemed intended to shock or surprise the therapists and seemed relieved when the therapist's manner remained warm and accepting.

In the next few sessions, Anne showed a markedly wide range of behavior, including regressive, sometimes almost babyish mannerisms, considerable giggling and silliness, or whining on one hand and very aggressive, controlling, directing behavior on the other, which seemed to express her ambivalence toward the therapist as she became more involved in the relationship and also tested limits with her hostile behavior. She became increasingly able to verbalize what she wanted, but often used some of the play materials to express her hostility. For example, she sometimes used dolls to poke at the therapist or to throw things around the room. When she was confronted with the unacceptability of such behavior, she threw the dolls in a box and announced that they couldn't play anymore because of their roughness, and thereby projected her hostile behavior and feelings onto the dolls, so as not to endanger her relationship with the therapist.

After about four months of weekly sessions, Anne's behavior at one session was most unusual. She came in, sat in the corner on the floor, and rocked slowly back and forth. She finally picked up a mother doll and put its soft, quilted arms around a baby doll. As she did this, Anne glanced apprehensively at the

118

therapist as if to gauge her reaction. She seemed afraid to communicate such positive responses of the mother toward the child. The therapist simply commented, "The mother loves the baby." Anne was relieved at this reaction from her, as she had been afraid that the increased positive responses from her mother would mean that her mother was beginning to compete with the therapist in a sense. At the same time Anne voiced many somatic complaints, apparently to solicit attention and to test the therapist. After this session, Anne became increasingly able to express her feelings verbally but even more so in her play. She began to express her hostility toward her family in doll play, pretending they were ill, excluding various family members altogether, or contriving situations in which they suffered a variety of misfortunes or lived in trying circumstances.

As this aggressive phase began to decline, Anne became more positive during the therapy hours, for which she was consistently reinforced. She seemed to enjoy increased feelings of mastery and competence, symbolized in her play with some of the material. At the same time, progress was being made with her mother, whose attitude toward Anne became more positive and expectations more realistic. She began to reinforce Anne's positive behavior more frequently and began to react less negatively to behaviors she didn't like. Anne's performance in school began to improve, and she gradually began to develop more satisfactory relationships with peers, which provided further reinforcement for her positive behaviors.

Students who are interested in reading a detailed account of non-directive play therapy as it was actually conducted with a young boy are referred to Axline's (1964) *Dibs in Search of Self.*

A variant of play therapy known as *filial therapy* has been described by Guerney (1964) and Guerney (1979). Filial therapy involves training groups of parents in play therapy techniques for use at home with disturbed children, learning-disabled children, and those with other handicaps. Guerney (1979) reported significant improvement in behavior and in relations between parent and child, and generally more positive feelings. However, it is difficult to assess how much of the improvement noted was actually due to the parents' use of play therapy techniques and how much was due to such other factors as placebo effect and the parents' increased attention.

Group Therapy

Group therapy can also be used with children, as the sole treatment or in conjunction with other forms of treatment. With children of latency age or younger, it often involves play. With older children and adolescents, verbal discussions can be used, although there may be some limitations, as these children are not yet old enough for the self-motivation and introspective emphasis of psychotherapy with adults, yet are too old for play therapy involving activities that they have outgrown (Halpern and Kissel, 1976).

Like individual psychotherapy, group therapy can have various theoretical orientations. Nondirective play therapy can be applied to groups (Axline, 1947); behavioral techniques have also been used in group play therapy situations (Clement and Milne, 1967; Rose, 1972).

Groups can be set up in various ways. Heterosexual groups may be best for mid to late adolescence, and single-sex ones for latency-age children or young adolescents (Halpern and Kissel, 1976). Groups may represent one kind of problem or be more heterogeneous in their makeup. There are obvious drawbacks, however, in having a group made up of all inhibited children, where no one feels free to speak up and verbal modeling does not occur, or in having a group made up solely of acting-out children, where the possibilities of group contagion and difficult handling arise. A reasoned mix of problems and personalities appears to be most workable and effective.

Group therapy has been used with problems as diverse as inhibition/withdrawal and delinquency, where peer interactions and modeling are important. It has also been useful where the child or adolescent derives reassurance and support from being with others who have similar problems, such as a group of adolescents with common family problems.

There are definite advantages to the use of groups besides the obvious economy of reaching more children in the same amount of therapist time. Children in such groups get practice in relating to peers, and they discover how they are perceived by peers. They are also exposed to many different styles of relating, and important modeling behavior occurs. A shy child may become more assertive after observing specific expressive behaviors in another group member.

Children in a group situation have an opportunity to also "rest" for a while. As there are others on whom the therapist can focus, individ-

120

ual children can withdraw somewhat or consider some aspect of the discussion while others are interacting more directly with the therapist or with one another.

The dynamics of the group are important; the group develops certain qualities or characteristics which are, in fact, a function of the interactions of the whole group. The group therapist needs to be sensitive to the roles into which group members fall or place one another, such as scapegoat, leader, or bully, and must be ready to come to the assistance of children who are put into roles in which they are uncomfortable. Limits need to be set in group therapy as in individual therapy, and destructive behavior must be forbidden so that all of the children feel safe. Positive interactions and positive social behaviors occurring in the group need to be reinforced.

There are some disadvantages to group therapy. Each of the children in a group has less time with the therapist and perhaps, in that respect, a less intensive psychotherapeutic experience. The therapist has less control over the therapy both because of the makeup of the group and because of the influences on any given child from other members of the group.

When a child is seen in a group, the parents are usually seen also, as they are when a child is in individual psychotherapy. The parents can be involved in a group with other parents or in individual sessions with a therapist, who may be their child's therapist or who may maintain close contact with the child's therapist.

The relative effectiveness of group therapy, however, has not been any more clearly demonstrated than that of individual psychotherapy. Abramowitz (1976), for instance, in her recent review of outcome research on various forms of group therapy with children—including activity therapy, behavior modification, and verbal and play therapy groups—found little solid evidence for the effectiveness of groups. A third showed improvement, a third showed a mixed response to treatment, and a third showed no improvement. She did conclude, however, that the groups using a behavioral approach more often showed a positive or at least a mixed outcome.

The following rather detailed case study illustrates some of the aspects of group therapy that have been discussed in this section as well as other aspects of nondirective psychotherapy. Brief individual descriptions of the boys precede a discussion of the group's interactions.

CASE STUDY

Dale, Robert, Allan and Michael, ages nine to twelve, who had been referred for varied reasons, were included in a boys' therapy group which met over a period of five months. Allan and Michael were behavior problems in school and at home, with much acting out and controlling behavior, and Allan had been put on half days at school. Dale was overinhibited and immature for his age, and Bob was very withdrawn and constricted. It was felt that social interaction and socialization experiences in a group setting would be of benefit to all of the boys. Both a male and a female therapist were involved.

The initial approach of the therapists was primarily exploratory and was as permissive and nondirective as possible. The therapists tried to foster an atmosphere in which the boys felt free to experiment, to express themselves, and to develop satisfying relationships with both peers and adults, setting limits only when necessary.

Dale initially engaged primarily in solitary activity and was very compulsive (e.g., counting dots on the ceiling). He often engaged in activity separate from the others or took up the others' activity by himself after they had done it together. Much later, when he did invite competition in a game he had practiced, he frequently lost, after which he usually remained somewhat more aloof and condescending. Except for occasional involvement in vigorous play, he was typically involved verbally either making quips, snide comments, or jeering remarks or instigating aggressive and/or competitive activity between other boys, while at the same time staying out of it himself as a somewhat amused observer.

As soon as he was introduced, *Michael* assumed the role of the bully in the group and seemed able to relate only in an aggressive, bullying way. Verbal behavior was minimal on his part, and if aggressive behavior seemed to be subsiding, Michael usually provoked some, as this seemed to be the only area in which he felt competent or capable of competing with the others. At times he became rough, and the therapists had to intervene to prevent the others from being hurt.

Allan initially served as the catalyst which started most group interactions. Although he had seemed to be the social, polite "host" of the group very briefly at the start, his aggression and thinly-veiled hostility soon became apparent, and he became more interested in winning, made accusations of cheating, and changed games when he was losing. He showed almost frenzied activity at times and soon elicited considerable competition and then hostility.

122

The introduction of Michael, a latecomer to the group, brought a striking change in Allan's coping mechanisms; Allan changed from a controlled child to a frightened-looking child. He began taunting behavior for the first time, directed at Michael, and stressed the "we" aspects of the group. He told Michael how things were done in "our" group, in order to preserve some of his status and control and to warn Michael not to intrude too fully or rapidly. He also approached the female therapist for the first time, asking her to play a game with him when the activity with Michael got rougher. This was a brief interlude and seemed to be a means by which he could seek out protection while saving face and catching his breath. He initiated considerable aggressive activity at the end of the hour because he knew the therapists would be ending the session promptly when the time was up.

Bob joined activities cautiously and tentatively at first and followed Allan's lead for a long time. Once he asserted himself in making some rules that disagreed with Allan's, there was increasing expression of aggression, which went from harmless play to throwing objects at the others, requiring the therapist to intervene. Ticlike facial grimaces appeared simultaneously with the increased aggression and seemed to reflect a combination of fear, anticipation, and excitement. Gradually Bob became more appropriately assertive, and when only he and Michael were present, he became the leader in initiating activities.

During the initial sessions of the group, the boys played and behaved in an essentially parallel way, doing what they wanted to individually while at the same time sizing up the others. There was relatively little relating to one another or to the therapists as they felt their way around the new situation.

With the introduction of Allan, activity became more intense, with increased competition and testing of limits with aggressive behavior. The general tenor was—and remained— active. Some pairing off of the boys occurred, with Allan and Bob engaging in activities together either without or against Dale. Increasingly strong competition and greater hostility followed.

With the introduction of Michael to the group, there was an abrupt change in coping mechanisms. All three of the others united against him as he immediately assumed the "bully" role. The boys for one session were more sedate, working on models and using more verbal than physical communication and aggression, but this did not carry over, and the hours changed relatively little. They involved strongly competitive and very aggressive behavior. Frequently there were somewhat perfunctory remarks made by the boys to discourage negative behavior such as fighting, but these became almost ritualistic and were rarely adhered to.

It did not seem to matter that there were two adults present, nor did the sex of the therapists seem to make a difference. Behavior vis-a-vis peers was paramount. The therapists had, in fact, created a unique situation for interaction. It was one of free interaction with few limits, where the boys were forced to participate, both because they were not allowed to leave the room and because the other boys would not let ones who normally withdrew do so. The adults seemed to serve primarily as creators of the situation and as implicit protection, as they would set limits if necessary. In this setting the boys began exploring methods of coping and had to develop new defenses, as they were prevented from always responding with the usual ones such as withdrawal or bullying.

At the time of termination, Bob showed the most change of all the boys. He had gone from a withdrawn, overinhibited boy to an active one who had taken on some of the leadership functions. Mike remained physically aggressive, provoking fights, and seemed unable to use verbal modes of communication effectively. Allan had learned to compromise and had learned that he could be well liked even when he was not controlling. Dale became somewhat less constricted and more mature. His increased maturity seemed to make him aware of the fact that he was older than the others and may help to explain his greater aloofness and condescension in later sessions.

Family Therapy

As was mentioned briefly in Chapter 2, another approach to the problems of children and adolescents is a family systems approach. This one is predicated on the assumption that the referral problem is not that of the child only but is a result of the way in which family members interact with one another and with the child. According to this view, behavior develops from modeling and reinforcement contingencies within the family, not just individual characteristics; and the interaction of family members maintains the behavior of other members (Weathers and Liberman, 1978). Thus, family therapy represents an orientation to problems rather than a therapeutic method; that is, the diagnosis and treatment unit is interactional processes rather than individuals, and disorders are considered relationship problems

124

(Haley, 1971). Problem resolution, then, depends on changing those interactions. There is no universal form of family therapy; its distinctiveness lies mainly in its view of the family as " . . . a small, interdependent, dynamic social system" (Werry, 1979b, p. 91).

Many clinicians have observed that families of all sorts tend to establish very strong rules and a special equilibrium within the family to which all members contribute. One member may have the role of a scapegoat, for example, and be blamed for virtually everything that goes wrong. Another person may be the "family achiever"—the one who does many things well and collects accolades for the family, giving the family a "good name." Another may be the "sickly one" who is overprotected and catered to far more than objective reality requires. Moreover, the physiological characteristics of young children can influence the family's interactions (Hetherington and Martin, 1979). If one member of the family receives therapy and changes certain behaviors and the others do not, that individual may no longer fit the established role in the family, and the delicate balance may be upset. Other family members may then become anxious and disturbed, and may even attempt to minimize or undermine the therapy or nullify the changes that have been made. Families are arranged along hierarchial lines, with definite rules, and family members behave in such a way as to keep specific sequences of interactions operating; the therapeutic task is to change those sequences (Haley, 1976).

Thus it has become increasingly clear that involvement of the entire family is not only helpful but necessary—that is, the family system must change to accommodate beneficial changes in individuals (Weathers and Liberman, 1978). When a child is referred, then, the problems are seen as family problems, and the treatment goals involve other family members as well. When a young child is the subject of treatment, the therapist may focus on the parents because of the quick responsiveness of young children to changes in parental handling (Weinberger, 1971).

One of the most common goals, and probably the most critical to any family, is to explore and improve patterns of communication among family members. Expectations of and attitudes toward one another, and the ways in which these are communicated within a family, are issues of central importance with which the therapist must deal. More open expression of conflicts and feelings may occur as a result of family therapy (Weeks and Mack, 1978), and the family members will need guidance in putting new and effective patterns of communication into practice.

The means by which the therapist tries to effect change in a family varies according to the therapist's theoretical perspective; there may be a psychodynamic (Ackerman, 1958), interactional, or behavioral emphasis.

One communication-based approach to families was developed by Satir (1967). Her model is process-oriented, stressing relationships, especially within families, and the inadequate and conflicting verbal and nonverbal messages that are sent by dysfunctional family members. Satir maintains that if there is a functional and gratifying marital relationship, the children will thrive. The therapist's task is to improve methods of communication or interaction among family members; the therapist serves both as a communication model and as a resource person to the family.

Behavioral approaches are relatively new to the notion of the family as a system and have so far been concentrated on particular two- or three-way interactions (Werry, 1979b). A behavioral emphasis involves a behavioral analysis of the problem and the use of reinforcement and modeling in the context of family interactions (Liberman, 1970). The maladaptive behavior must be identified, specific goals must be set, and an analysis of the environment must be done to determine what environmental conditions support or maintain the problem behavior and what patterns of social reinforcement exist among family members (Liberman, 1970). In this model, the therapist is an educator, working with the family, and "sick" labels are not necessary (Liberman, 1970). It is felt that a system of intervention that determines the reinforcement exchanges between different combinations of individuals is more effective and faster than one that is directed solely at individuals (Weathers and Liberman, 1978a; Liberman, 1970).

Family members can be seen all together or in various combinations or subgroups of members (Halpern and Kissel, 1976). In his brief therapy, Weinberger (1971) found that parallel visits in which the child and parents were seen separately by the therapist were the most effective for children between seven and eleven years of age. With older children, especially adolescents, he advocated family sessions, with all members seen at the same time. Another possibility is to see the adolescents alone for part of the therapeutic hour and then ask them to bring their parents into the session (Adams, 1974).

126

For thorough coverage of several aspects of family therapy as well as exposure to many innovative variants, the reader is referred to Guerin's (1976) encyclopedic volume; Halpern and Kissel (1976), Chapter 7; or Ackerman (1970). Familial correlates of various disorders have been described by Hetherington and Martin (1979). For students interested in reading detailed accounts of actual families in therapy, Papp's (1977) book of full-length case studies is recommended, as well as Haley and Hoffman's (1967) text in which they present interviews with therapists who explain their specific handling of family therapy sessions.

Behavior Therapy

A second broad kind of intervention which is also widely used is behavior modification or behavior therapy. Although the two terms are often used interchangeably, behavior therapy is actually a subset of behavior modification—an application of behavior modification to clinical problems (Graziano, 1978). Graziano summarizes behavior therapy as follows:

> Behavior therapy . . . assumes that a person's psychological problems are largely determined by current environmental factors; that the most effective intervention for many clinical problems is the careful, systematic manipulation of specified environmental variables; that such manipulation will result in predictable improvement; and that self-control is the general goal of behavior therapy. (Graziano, 1978, p. 29)

This type of therapeutic intervention, which is usually relatively brief, is based on learning-theory principles. Its emphasis is on overt, observable behavior and environmental events, rather than underlying intrapsychic causes of problems which are explored in many forms of psychotherapy. The main goal is to identify target (problem) behaviors, and then set up programs to eliminate those behaviors and substitute more acceptable or satisfying ones. A behavior therapy program can be used to decrease a problem behavior and/or to increase a positive or prosocial behavior (Gelfand and Hartmann, 1971). It most frequently involves the client in relearning specific behaviors and attitudes through a program of primarily operant (instrumental) or classical (respondent) conditioning; the program itself can take many forms.

Systematic Desensitization

One fairly commonly used behavioral technique based on classical conditioning is *systematic desensitization*. This is a procedure in which a hierarchy of anxiety-producing situations or events is elicited from a client, who is then trained in specific relaxation techniques. These techniques are then used in the face of events in the hierarchy, beginning with the least anxiety-provoking situation or event. When the client is able to relax in the presence of (or with the thought of or discussion of) the least anxiety-provoking event, the therapist presents the next one. This procedure continues until the client has become "desensitized," that is, can induce relaxed feelings even in conjunction with the most anxiety-producing event.

Workers have used relaxation and desensitization in the treatment of a wide range of disorders, including asthma (Alexander, 1972; Moore, 1965), phobias (Wolpe, 1969; Wolpe and Lazarus, 1966), and others to be discussed later.

Operant Conditioning

Most commonly used is an operant or instrumental type of conditioning program, which reportedly is used twice as often as cognitive and social learning models combined (Phillips and Ray, 1980). The main goal in operant conditioning is to improve a child's behavior by changing the reward value of specific behaviors. An attempt is made to decrease the amount of reinforcement that a child receives for undesirable behavior and to elicit desired, usually incompatible behaviors, which are then rewarded. In order to rid a child of tantrums, for example, there must be a change in their reinforcing properties, one of which is the mother's attention. The mother must withdraw her attention when her child has a tantrum: she must ignore it and reward other, more desirable "nontantrum" behavior, such as asking politely for something. Since learning theory predicts that reinforced behavior is more likely to recur than nonreinforced behavior, the desired behavior should increase in frequency if it is rewarded, and the undesirable behavior (in this case tantrums) should decrease if it is not reinforced. Reinforcement contingent on the desired behavior is significant not only in facilitating learning but also in maintain-

128

ing gains (Lovaas et al., 1976). Sometimes therapists have used classical and operant conditioning techniques together effectively by changing from one to another at various points in therapy (Lazarus, Davison, and Polefka, 1971).

With behavorial interventions, baseline data on the target behavior are typically obtained before a course of therapy is begun. That is, the frequency of the problem behavior is carefully and objectively noted at the start. Specific behavioral and therapeutic goals are then set, based on the data. Careful records are kept of the occurrence of specific target behaviors in order to chart progress toward those goals. Acceptable or desired behavior is rewarded, whereas maladaptive or undesirable behavior is not. Although adult and peer attention is a very potent reinforcer for a child, use of tokens and other concrete reinforcers to reward behaviors that one wants to encourage, will further increase the likelihood that those behaviors will be repeated.

The nature and timing of the rewards is essential to the treatment's success. One must be certain that the "reward" that has been chosen truly has reinforcement or reward value for the child. If it is not something the child cares about, there is no relevant or effective reinforcement. In addition, the timing or *schedule of reinforcements* is important. Partial reinforcement, for instance—rewarding certain behaviors only some of the time—makes those behaviors more resistant to extinction. If the mother in the previous example resolves to ignore the child's tantrums in a supermarket but gives in once in a while because of her own fatigue or preoccupation, the tantrums will persist much longer than if she consistently ignores them every time they occur. Similarly, delaying reinforcement for behaviors until after they have appeared in several settings may encourage generalization of the behavior (Fowler and Baer, 1981).

Behavioral techniques have been found to be especially effective with autistic and other psychotic children (Lovaas et al., 1965; Bucher and Lovaas, 1968; Lovaas et al., 1967; Lovaas, Schreibman, and Koegel, 1976) whose verbal capacities have been seriously impaired. They have also been used particularly successfully with very young children and with retarded children, with whom verbal psychotherapy is not usually considered to be very helpful. The behavioral techniques can be useful in effecting behavioral change in acting-out, delinquent adolescents, with whom a psychotherapeutic relationship is difficult if not impossible to develop and insight is neither sought nor achieved. Behavioral techniques allow one to substitute actions (such as reinforcement, rehearsal, relaxation) for symbols (words, dreams, ideas) or to combine them (Lazarus, 1971).

Modeling

Modeling has been used successfully in many instances to effect behavior change in both normal and disturbed children. It is a much more efficient means of developing social skills than trial and error because it conveys necessary information more graphically and faster (Rosenthal and Bandura, 1978). Moreover, appropriate behavior needs to be elicited to be reinforced, and modeling of that behavior may be a necessary first step (Rosenthal and Bandura, 1978).

Modeling is often used in conjunction with other techniques, such as systematic desensitization. In one study, for example (Ritter, 1968), a group of five- to eleven-year-old phobic children observed models in increasingly bold interactions with feared snakes. Another group had actual physical contact with the snakes as well. Although the group with the actual contact showed greater reduction in their avoidance behavior, both groups showed less avoidance behavior than an untreated group.

Modeling procedures have been used with a wide range of problems, including children's fears, antisocial behavior, inadequate social skills, withdrawal, aggression, attentional difficulties, autism, and retardation (Kirkland and Thelen, 1977; Rosenthal and Bandura, 1978). They may also be combined with *role-playing* or behavioral rehearsal. Role-playing as a kind of rehearsal of behaviors to be learned has been particularly useful in training children in social skills. Kelly (1981), for example, used puppets to role-play peer interactions; he found the device especially helpful in situations where social skills training was needed by a child being seen individually. However, *in vivo* or real-life practice is also needed, along with modeling, feedback, and reinforcement. Role-playing has led to decreases in disturbing behavior and has helped children to develop new skills, at least short-term, although more information is required regarding the maintenance of the treatment effect (Kirkland and Thelen, 1977). All of these procedures are referred to again in later chapters in relation to specific disorders.

130

Implosive Therapy (Flooding)

Implosive therapy, developed by T. G. Stampfl, relies on the learning-theory tenets of desensitization and extinction. The basic idea is to expose an individual to significant levels of conditioned stimuli (that is, flooding) which are anxiety-provoking, as in phobias. The treatment is based on the assumption that symptoms develop as a result of fear and avoidance of aversive stimuli. When one's worst expectations regarding outcome are not realized and there are no concomitant aversive effects, fear of that stimulus will decrease and become extinguished (Levis and Hare, 1977). This exposure can be *in vivo* (actual exposure) or *in vitro* (symbolic or imaginal exposure), but Ultee, Griffioen, and Schellekens (1982) have found that the former led to better results than either the latter or the control situation, with no significant difference between the *in vitro* and control groups.

The procedure emphasizes emotional arousal (Levis and Hare, 1977). The technique can integrate psychodynamic concepts also by including symbolic, analytic, anxiety-provoking material or themes, which are worked through before the next higher themes on the anxiety-arousing hierarchy are addressed (Stampfl and Levis, 1967).

Devotees of this method claim effectiveness with a wide range of problems, including depression, phobias, anxiety, and obsessive-compulsive reactions as well as psychotic reactions; they also claim a reduced treatment time, with marked change occurring in one to fifteen sessions (Stampfl and Levis, 1967).

There have been many criticisms of the method, however, on ethical, methodological, and clinical grounds. It has been argued, for example, that there has been much confounding of results; that no evidence exists for implosive therapy's superiority over systematic desensitization; and that it is not ethical to expose individuals to such traumatic treatment, especially when systematic desensitization may be just as effective (Morganstern, 1973). Moreover, others (de Silva and Rachman, 1981) have argued that exposure is simply not a necessary condition for fear reduction.

Multimodal Therapy

Lazarus (1973) has argued that patients usually have a number of specific problems which should be dealt with by a number of specific treatments, across at least six or seven dimensions. He recommends that imagery and cognitive processes be invoked, as imagery in rehearsing future stressful areas ("psychological 'fire drills'") can play an important role in preventing problems. He feels that psychotherapeutic interaction involves seven modalities all of which should be used. The seven modalities are behavior, affect, sensation, imagery, cognition, interpersonal, and drugs (acronym: BASIC ID). According to Lazarus, if therapy is not working or is stalled, each modality should be examined to see if one area is being neglected.

All of these forms of behavior therapy with children and adolescents are discussed later in relation to specific disorders and are described well elsewhere (Achenbach, 1974; Graziano, 1978; Rutter, 1975). In addition, a good summary of these and other behavioral techniques and methods may be found in Wolpe (1969) or Wolpe and Lazarus (1966). The use of a variety of behavioral techniques to change a multitude of specific behaviors is described and documented in Daniels's (1974) impressive collection of studies concerning management of behavior problems, as well as in Schaefer and Millman (1978), Craighead, Kazdin, and Mahoney (1976), Graziano (1971), Lazarus (1971), and others.

There is controversy, however, over the permanence of behavior change achieved through the use of these techniques. Some have suggested that the *maintenance* of new, adaptive behavior does not seem as well assured as behavior *change* and requires more work (Graziano, 1978). In addition, the substitution of adaptive behavior for maladaptive behavior in no way guarantees that new stimuli will not elicit new maladaptive behavior (Chess and Hassibi, 1978). Others have reported maintenance of gains for nearly a year after treatment (Lazarus, Davison, and Polefka, 1971) and have suggested that one must extend the therapeutic environment in order to maintain gains in treatment (Lovaas, Schreibman, and Koegel, 1976). Such an extension exists, for instance, when parents have been taught behavior modification principles which they can continue when the child is returned home. Lazarus (1973) argues that the more different modalities that are involved in any therapeutic system, the more lasting the results will be.

Others, worried about *symptom substitution*, claim that if a symptom is alleviated and the underlying cause is not removed, another symptom will appear in its place. Many behavioral therapists, however, believe that such substitution is rare after behavior modification and can be dealt with as any other behavior would be dealt with (Rose, 1972). If it is true that symptom substitution may occur when a child's maladaptive behavior is decreased but the child has few positive alternatives to use to secure reinforcement (Gelfand and Hartmann, 1971), the obvious solution is to ensure that the child learns desirable or prosocial responses to replace the undesirable ones.

Disagreement and controversy notwithstanding, there is no doubt that the behavioral workers' greater emphasis on the child's environment and its influence on behavior has added a significant dimension to the study of childhood disorders. Their techniques have often brought about changes in behavior when other methods have failed (Rutter, 1975), and they can be easily taught to parents and teachers for use within the family or at school.

Finally, unlike the situation that existed during the 1960s, when separation of behavior approaches from psychotherapy was the norm and the influences of each on the other were ignored, the 1970s saw more frequent attempts to integrate them (Harrison, 1977). Therapists can, for instance, facilitate changes in specific behaviors while at the same time implementing verbal, "psychotherapeutic" discussions about those changes. Or subtle psychological changes may occur in parents as they chart and discuss problems with a therapist. Such approaches as that of Clement and Milne (1967) and Weinberger's (1971) brief therapy illustrate how therapists can incorporate the positive aspects of both. Weinberger, for example, advocates concentrating on current behavior and the difficulties it causes and recommends drawing up an initial contract with parents concerning both their expectations and those of the therapist. However, the therapist also takes an active psychotherapeutic role in confronting the child about specific behaviors, discussing problems, finding out how the parents are contributing to the problems through their behaviors and expectations, suggesting alternatives, and discussing changes with the child. Maximum therapeutic time is six weeks and twelve sessions. Finally, Lazarus (1971) suggests that a comprehensive approach with behavioral, humanistic, and personalistic aspects may contribute significantly to the development of more effective psychotherapy.

The following case study, which illustrates both the application of behavioral techniques and the involvement of an entire family as was outlined in the section on family therapy, is taken from Schaefer and Millman's (1978) book describing many kinds of therapy for use with a wide range of problems in children.

133

CASE STUDY

A six-year-old boy was referred as being uncontrollable. He refused to follow any instructions, had temper tantrums, was aggressive, and swore. In addition to his extreme disobedience, he often provoked others. The father spent very little time at home and interacted with his children in an irritated, punitive manner. The mother felt totally inadequate with her family.

Family therapy was carried out weekly for eleven months by three therapists: One saw the mother, one saw the boy, and one visited the father. The mother was interviewed in order to assess home reinforcement contingencies. A brief written description and discussions with her were used to help her understand operant conditioning to be used with the child. In play therapy, compliance shown by obeying adult commands was chosen as a significant behavior. Eye contact and correct responses to brief commands (for example, "Put the blocks on the table") were recorded and reinforced with candy and social approval. The boy's inattention or lack of compliance resulted in the therapist not responding for sixty seconds. Later, eye contact and following commands were reinforced only if both occurred together.

The mother and her therapist observed and discussed effective techniques used in the play therapy and then entered the playroom. The mother made several commands and ineffectively used the arranged contingencies. With discussion and practice, the mother improved and became effective in controlling her son's behavior. At home, a reward system using stars was designed and extinction of the undesirable behavior was employed.

As the boy's behavior improved, his older brother became disobedient and aggressive and fought with him. Both boys were seen together in the playroom, where working together on command and spontaneous cooperation were reinforced. Independent rewards were more effective than rewards for both working together. Two large cardboard counters were used. When both were cooperative, they each gained three points. If only one was cooperative, he would earn one point. Aggression resulted in the loss of five points. Points were used to purchase ice cream or visit an animal laboratory. The number of points required was raised each session. . . .

Improvement was sporadic and uneven, with time out being quite effective. The boy had to learn that unacceptable behavior would not influence the therapist's refusal to respond. Cooperation between the brothers was quickly fostered by the contingencies used, and obedience and cooperation were greatly increased. With peers, the boy was rarely provocative. The mother reported that an improved relationship with her

134

husband resulted from their working together on their children's problems. (Schaefer and Millman, 1978, pp. 448–449)

Cognitive-Behavioral Interventions

A broadening of behavioral techniques to include the alteration of cognitive processes was mentioned in Chapter 2. Cognitive-behavioral interventions use behavior modification techniques but also involve an individual's cognitive activities, including attitudes, beliefs, and attribution, in an attempt to effect change. Therefore, they lie between the behavioral and cognitive approaches, using many behavioral procedures based on performance but focusing on both behavioral and cognitive problems (Kendall and Hollon, 1979). A comparison of the two approaches and the differences in treatment that result is shown in Table 6.1

The cognitive behavior therapy techniques which began in the 1960s involve teaching cognitive strategies by using a variety of train-

TABLE 6.1 *General characteristics of cognitive-behavioral interventions*

	Treatment target	Treatment approach	Treatment evaluation
BEHAVIORAL	Behavioral excesses or deficits	Behavioral "learning theory" interventions. Environmental manipulations (e.g., token economies, contingency management)	Observed changes in behavior with rigorous evaluation
	Behavioral excesses or deficits	Behavioral interventions. Skills training, information provision (e.g., modeling, role-playing)	Observed changes in behavior with rigorous evaluation
COGNITIVE-BEHAVIORAL	Behavioral and cognitive excesses and deficits	Broadly conceived behavioral and cognitive methods	Observed changes in behavior and in cognition with methodological rigor
	Cognitive excesses or deficits	Cognitive interventions with adjunctive behavioral procedures	Examination of cognitive and, to a lesser extent, of behavioral changes
COGNITIVE	Cognitive excesses or deficits	Semantic interventions	Changes in cognitions, "integrative changes"; often, but not always, nonempirically evaluated

Source: P. C. Kendall and S. D. Hollon, eds., *Cognitive-Behavioral Interventions: Theory, Research, and Procedures* (New York: Academic Press, 1979). Reprinted by permission.

ing methods (Hobbs et al., 1980). According to Hobbs and his colleagues, these methods generally fall into three classes: (1) direct instruction in problem-solving, as when a child is presented directly with a coping strategy (for example, "Look and think before you do it"); (2) self-instructional procedures, where a child rehearses verbal statements to use in a problem-solving situation, a "private monologue" (for instance, "If I keep going, I'll do fine"); and (3) cognitive modeling, where a child is exposed to a model who is using the coping strategies and who may also verbalize the strategy. We will take a brief look at some samples from the broad array of such techniques.

Many of the cognitive-behavioral approaches rely on training children in various *verbal mediation techniques*. For example, Kanfer and his colleagues (1975) trained five- and six-year-old children to use verbal mediation to emphasize their competence and control in a dark situation, and thereafter the children tolerated the dark better than a comparison group.

Self-instructional training with modeling has also been used successfully to modify impulsive behavior in children (Kendall and Finch, 1978; Meichenbaum and Goodman, 1971). Although six weeks' training in verbal mediation through modeling and verbalizing cognitive activity did not result in reduced aggressive behavior in one study of six- to eight-year-old aggressive boys, it did result in more prosocial behaviors and in improved performance on cognitive tests (Camp et al., 1977). Moreover, the boys were more like normals than a control group of aggressive children who did not receive training. In another study, when the effects of a token reinforcement system were compared with those of a self-regulation system, both decreased disruptive behavior and improved task behavior, but changes were greater with self-regulation and were better maintained after teacher controls were withdrawn (Neilans and Israel, 1981). Bornstein and Quevillon (1976) also found that self-instruction facilitated on-task behavior, with generalization of gains from laboratory to classroom and maintenance of gains nearly six months later.

Many workers have used *attentional training* procedures to remedy specific problems. For example, in one study (Ribordy, Tracy, and Bernotas, 1981), attentional training, in which nine- to twelve-year-old children were rewarded for successfully inhibiting irrelevancies and for good attending behavior, led to the ability of high-test-anxious children to perform as well as the low-anxious ones. Those in the placebo and control group made more errors than those in the low-anxious group. The finding did not hold for older children in the study (sixth graders); the effect was the highest on the fourth graders and marginal on the fifth graders.

Cognitive behavioral approaches have been used for a wide range of problems, including such diverse ones as impulsivity, aggression, fear of the dark, and delinquency, but there is a lack of consistent findings in that no one dependent variable has improved consistently (Hobbs et al., 1980). Moreover, there are methodological problems in that much of the work has been done in laboratory situations rather than in a natural environment, and much work has been done with nonclinical cases (Hobbs et al., 1980). In addition, it is not clear whether mediational processes from the training are the ones responsible for behavior change, although that is often assumed; and many studies use test performance as a criterion rather than changes in the target behavior itself (Hobbs et al., 1980). Also, as interpersonal behavior is reciprocal, or bidirectional, there is a need to evaluate the context and the significant others in the environment before implementing a program to train self-control in children (Meichenbaum, 1979).

Extensive descriptions of the use of cognitive-behavioral techniques to treat a wide range of problems, including alcohol and eating disturbances, depression, anxiety, delinquency, pain, and lack of assertiveness, can be found in Kendall and Hollon (1979). The authors note that although this area of intervention is still incomplete, it allows for greater flexibility regarding models and approaches and also provides experimental rigor regarding its assessment and evaluation.

Medical Therapies

Chemotherapy, or the use of medication, is the type of medical therapy now most commonly used with children, such radical therapies as shock therapy, insulin therapy, and psychosurgery having become a thing of the past in the treatment of children. Medication can be seen as one aspect of a multifaceted attack on a problem. It cannot be used on a continuous basis to try to "adjust" relationships (Kanner, 1972), but it may be used as an adjunct intervention, either in addition to or followed by other kinds of intervention, or to make a child more amenable to other kinds of therapy. Medication may, for instance, be used to calm down and help organize the thought of a psychotic child, before other kinds of intervention are tried. Or it may be used to improve the concentration and decrease the hyperactivity of a very distractible, learning-disabled child; but that child still needs remedial, academic assistance as well.

Gualtieri and Hawk (1981) offer four criteria for evaluating the use of drugs: the severity of the disorder, the specificity of the drug effects, the chances of success with other interventions, and the likelihood of enhancing other therapies with the use of the drug. They further suggest that drugs be used very carefully and only after other, behavioral techniques have first been tried wherever possible, especially with milder disorders, or after counseling and psychotherapy have failed with anxious, dependent, withdrawn, or oppositional children.

Drugs are used to directly alter physiological functioning (Schwartz, 1978). Their function is to eliminate target behaviors or symptoms, not to "cure" a syndrome or disorder. That is, drugs are not available to treat specific diagnostic categories, but rather to minimize such symptoms as insomnia, hyperactivity, impulsivity, psychotic thought disorders, and some aggressive behaviors (Campbell, 1976) which are associated with specific disorders.

For a description of some of the drugs used for specific symptoms or behaviors, the reader is referred to Campbell (1976), Campbell and Small (1978), Minde (1977), or Gualtieri and Hawk (1981). The use of medication with hyperactive children is discussed in more detail in Chapter 10.

As many children and parents worry about the possibility of dependence or addiction when medication is used with children, full explanations should be given to them, including information about the drug's addictive qualities as well as its possible side effects. Children receiving medication should also be reevaluated frequently; the therapist should evaluate the effectiveness of the drug with thought to changing the dosage if necessary, changing the type of medication, or taking the child off the medication altogether. Gualtieri and Hawk (1981), for instance, report that "drug holidays" at six-months to two-year intervals will often show that the child no longer needs the medication.

There are important differences between the effects of drugs on children and on adults which must be taken into account. For example, there is some evidence that children suffer less than adults from the side effects of some drugs, that they are " . . . biologically more

138

sturdy" (Campbell, 1976, page 247). Moreover, the same type of medication can have different effects on different children. For example, phenobarbital can lead to both hyperactive and depressive behavior, and antihistamines can act as either a stimulant or a sedative (Gualtieri and Hawk, 1981). The age of the child is very important; children under ten seem to react differently to drugs than those over ten (Minde, 1977).

The use of drugs has the potential for more pervasive or encompassing effects with children than with adults because the child is developing at a rapid rate in many areas. Campbell (1976), for one, urges more research into the important effect of drugs on children's cognitive functioning, as some drugs may even be contraindicated for children because of their powerful and often adverse effects. Drugs may interfere with such cognitive functions as attention, perception, information processing, or organization and integration of perceptions and may cause deterioration in behavior (Gualtieri and Hawk, 1981). As there is a problem of generalized impairment of cognitive functioning with high dosages, the lowest possible dosage is best (Gualtieri and Hawk, 1981).

It appears that medications can play an important role as an adjunct therapeutic aid, but they must be used with reason and caution and parents and children should be well informed about them. Further research into their benefits and risks, as well as their differential effects on children at different ages, is needed.

Biological interventions besides drugs, such as biofeedback, can also be used to facilitate self-regulation (Schwartz, 1978). Such others as megavitamin therapy are not currently considered to be appropriate treatments (Gualtieri and Hawk, 1981). Gualtieri and Hawk suggest that a controlled diet may be helpful for some hyperactives, but report that there is no evidence that a poor one will cause hyperactivity or learning problems in normal children. The role of diet in hyperactive children is discussed in more detail in Chapter 10.

Residential Treatment

Residential treatment or milieu therapy is another fairly common form of intervention. Milieu therapy is actually a broader term than residential treatment and refers to any environment in which everything is arranged for its therapeutic benefit. In practice, however, such a milieu is usually found only in a residential treatment center where all facets of a child's living situation are planned to be of therapeutic benefit and all staff members, from therapists to director to maintenance people, are chosen for their ability to contribute to and aid the therapeutic process. In such a context, "therapeutic" could mean anything from proper basic care to education that is a realistic preparation for life (Redl, 1966).

Residential treatment has distinct advantages and can be a very effective form of intervention. First, a child can be separated from a destructive or even dangerous milieu, which often brings an immediate improvement in the child's behavior (Kleiser, 1973). Removal of the child from the home, for instance, provides relief not only for parents, who are thus given a break from the constant pressure and anxiety of dealing with serious problems, but also for the child, who is separated from the nagging, blaming, accusations or other negative behaviors to which he or she has been subjected. The vicious circle in which parents and child may have become embroiled is broken. For this reason the child who arrives at the treatment center may hardly resemble the one pictured in the reports that preceded him or her. Second, there is the possibility of more total control of a child's life in a residential treatment center than in an outpatient therapy situation. Routines, problems, encounters with others, expression of feeling and relationships with authority figures all occur in the context of a treatment setting and, usually, in the presence of various staff members who are able to note patterns of behavior, stimuli to which a child is especially sensitive, precipitants of negative behavior, and other aspects of the problem. Third, because work in the treatment center *is* a job or vocation for the staff, dedicated as they may be, and they still have a life outside of the treatment center, staff members are better able than parents to maintain some psychological balance and equilibrium (Kleiser, 1973). Unlike parents, who suffer increasing frustration, stress, and fatigue, they are able to get away from the strains and pressures of dealing with problem children, even though the need for the child to deal with many different people in the center may in some ways be a disadvantage. Fourth, the residential treatment center offers the child a much higher degree of acceptance and tolerance than was found outside, and this in itself may produce positive effects (Kleiser, 1973).

These advantages are balanced somewhat by important disadvantages or problems. First, residential treatment is very expensive, and there are increasing demands for accountability and evidence to show that the cost brings benefits that cannot be obtained through the use of other less costly interventions. Second, residential treatment removes children from the normal mainstream of society and places them in a rather artificial situation where there is more attention, tolerance, nurturance, and special programming than they will find outside the institution. Therefore, return to the community nearly always requires special care and planning and often means adjustment difficulties and some regression. One follow-up study (Van Evra, Louis, and Kays, 1979) showed a consistent dip in functioning between discharge and a three-month follow-up period, which highlighted the difficulties with reentry into the community and the need for careful after-care programs. Third, unless families are also involved during the child's stay, there may be a tendency for them to withdraw, shifting to the treatment center the responsibility for "fixing" their child. In an interesting effort to combat this problem Critchley and Berlin (1981) involved the parents of psychotic children in every aspect of the child's program in a milieu treatment center. The authors found that such involvement eased the disturbance, facilitated nurturant and limit-setting behavior of the parents, and improved the prognosis.

In summary, residential placement is an expensive and rather extreme measure which should be resorted to only after other, less radical kinds of intervention have been tried. It should be restricted to those for whom such intensive care is absolutely essential (Crisis, 1970). However, when such placement becomes necessary because other programs are insufficient or no longer viable, it is a therapeutic alternative that offers certain definite treatment advantages.

Educational Interventions

For some disorders the therapist may not choose to use any of the interventions discussed so far. Rather, the emphasis may be on intervening educationally. For example, with mentally retarded or learning disabled children, the main therapeutic task may be seen to be one of changing the educational setting or academic curriculum of the child to facilitate academic progress and the learning of specific skills, and perhaps also to reduce stress. Thus, the child may be transferred from a regular classroom to a special class, or may spend part of a day in a resource room receiving specific remedial help. A child may need material broken down into smaller units. Or a child may require a more structured environment, although the evidence does not favor having children in isolation, such as in study cubicles (Reid and Hresko, 1981).

Educational interventions may include specific remedial programs in reading or math or may involve more broadly defined education or training in social skills and interpersonal relationships, in self-care, or in self-control. The major difference from other therapeutic approaches is that educational interventions do not emphasize the need to understand causal factors in the child's disorder. Rather, the emphasis is on working out remedial educational strategies which will enable the child to learn and function more effectively, whatever the cause of the problems.

These interventions are discussed in more detail in later chapters, especially Chapter 9 on mental retardation and Chapter 10 on learning disabilities.

Other Interventions

Environmental Therapy

Environmental manipulation, sometimes known as environmental or situational therapy, focuses attention on the child's total social-psychological environment and tries to provide a humane, sensitive, and supportive environment, whether in school, in church groups, or in other areas (Crisis, 1970). As children are more dependent on their environments than adults, they may be less able to deal with the stresses of a pathogenic situation without outside intervention (Mushin, 1977). Environmental manipulation may mean, for example, transferring a child or changing an unproductive and perhaps destructive school placement. It may involve educational programs aimed at altering parents' behavior and attitudes and helping them to become more effective parents (Adams, 1974; Van Evra, 1974), in order to create a healthier environment for the child. Any kind of manipulation or intervention that is aimed at changing the context within which the child behaves, rather than the child's behavior, could be included under this broad category. Unlike behavior therapy, which

142

also changes environmental contingencies and other aspects of the environment, this kind of intervention does not aim to change specific behaviors within the child but rather to make the total environment healthier and more conducive to growth and change.

Home Care

Home care, or assistance in the home draws heavily on the services of paraprofessionals such as tutors, homemakers, public health nurses, and others to significantly increase the range of help available. It is especially good when basic stimulation and care in the home are poor (Crisis, 1970) and has the distinct advantage of keeping the child at home while at the same time improving the quality of care there. It may include helping with the family budget, giving nutritional and meal-planning information, advising parents on child care and child development, arranging immunization for the children, helping with housework, or even providing the mother with some relief by baby-sitting for an afternoon. The improved quality of care that results also has beneficial effects on other children in the family and thus serves an important preventive function. It is more economical than removing children from the home and placing them in expensive residential or specialized day-treatment programs, and at the same time it keeps them in as normal a situation as possible.

Crisis Intervention

Crisis intervention must, by definition, be immediate, action-oriented, and decisive. Crises such as a suicide attempt do not allow for the luxury of taking time to form a therapeutic relationship. Immediate help may mean removal from a noxious situation, as in cases of abuse, and placement in a foster home or secure or semisecure institution or treatment center. Or it may involve medication, restraint, or some other form of intervention. Children in a crisis situation, frightened by the intensity of their own and others' feelings, need the security of external intervention and control. Later they can be helped to work on the underlying problems, using one or more of the other interventions discussed in this chapter.

Selection of Intervention Techniques

The therapist's choice of a technique or combination of techniques from this array depends on many factors.

First a therapist's *theoretical orientation* influences to a large extent, and limits, the kinds of treatment that will be considered. For example, a behaviorally-oriented worker would hardly choose a lengthy psychoanalysis for a client, nor would a psychodynamically-oriented therapist rely solely on a program of operant conditioning to alleviate a child's symptoms. On the other hand, a therapist with a cognitive-developmental approach would use techniques that involved changing the cognitive processes related to the maladaptive behavior.

The therapist's *experience* also affects the kind of treatment selected. Therapists may have discovered, on the basis of their own clinical experience, that certain techniques or combinations of techniques are particularly helpful with specific problems and they will therefore tend to rely on those. There should also be, however, continued openness to change in the interventions used as new findings appear in the literature regarding the *demonstrated effectiveness* of various techniques with specific problems.

The *age of the child*, the *nature of the problem*, and the *appropriateness of a technique* are also important and interrelated determinants of the treatment selected. For example, play therapy would be much less appropriate and less likely a choice for a depressed adolescent girl than for a depressed eight-year-old, as the former is rather old for play therapy. On the other hand, if circumstances warrant (e.g., a severe expressive language problem makes verbal psychotherapy untenable), a variant of play therapy might be tried in order to facilitate communication of problems and feelings. Similarly, a ten-year-old child with a severe dyslexic problem would not need—or be a candidate for—extensive psychodynamic psychotherapy. Rather, a therapist would likely find a combination of specific educational interventions, as well as some supportive counseling, to be considerably more appropriate and effective.

Finally, the *resources available* may be yet another determinant of the choice of treatment. A therapist may, for instance, ideally prefer certain educational placements for a child, or may wish for a combination of educational and remedial programs. However, such realistic factors as geographic limitations, limited school personnel, funding cutbacks, overcrowding, or other factors beyond the therapist's control may limit somewhat the actual program that can be implemented. Similarly, a therapist may view family therapy as the best and most effective way to intervene for a child who has been referred. If, however, the parents steadfastly refuse to get involved, the therapist's choice of a program must be tempered by the reality of the situation, and other interventions must be sought and implemented.

The choice of treatment is a very important one and depends on a number of factors, some of which are beyond the therapist's control. Methods for evaluating the effectiveness of these many kinds of treatment, as well as problems involved in such research, will be discussed in the next chapter. The application of the various therapeutic strategies and approaches with specific disorders as well as some of their limitations, will be demonstrated more clearly in Part IV.

Discussion Questions

1. Evaluate the apparent strengths and weaknesses or benefits and problems associated with each of the specific therapeutic interventions discussed in this chapter.
2. Search the literature for material confirming or refuting the apparent strengths and weaknesses of each approach.
3. Discuss which principles and characteristics of therapy are illustrated by the case studies presented in this chapter.

CHAPTER 7   # Treatment Effectiveness

The evaluation of treatment effectiveness is of central importance. However, given the wide range of therapeutic techniques, the various theoretical perspectives, the personal biases of individual clinicians, as well as serious methodological problems and shortcomings, the evaluations of treatment have not so far yielded satisfactory or definitive results; direct comparisons of studies in the area are difficult if not impossible.

There are studies that claim superior results for one particular technique or intervention; that find certain techniques particularly helpful for certain age groups or with specific disorders; that suggest that the theoretical perspective or particular technique used is less important than the personality of the therapist; and that indicate that comparable rates of improvement occur whether or not an individual receives treatment.

Although this is clearly a very difficult area in which to find clear and unequivocal answers, clinicians must try to determine which factors are crucial to effective intervention in order to understand the relative effectiveness of various approaches. That understanding is important to theoreticians as well as to the clinician who deals daily with probabilities of success and has to make informed choices and judgements about treatment procedures.

This chapter provides a look at some of the methodological difficulties involved in the evaluation of treatment effectiveness, various kinds of research designs that have been used to study it, some criteria for effectiveness, and reports of some of the many apparently controversial findings. The emphasis in this chapter is on methodological issues, with further discussions and reports of the effectiveness of specific techniques included in later chapters on specific disorders.

Methodological Problems

Many significant problems confront attempts to evaluate treatment effectiveness, among which are the following:

Causation cannot be inferred from correlational relationships. While it may be tempting for the clinician to assume, given obvious evidence of improvement in a child's behavior after exposure to a given technique, that the technique itself was the effective variable, one must be cautious about drawing such a conclusion. Unless a controlled study can be done, involving the usual experimental safeguards, it is impos-

148

sible to infer causation from an association between use of a technique and improvement. Moreover, even if children have been randomly assigned to treatment and control groups, conclusions concerning the effectiveness of the particular treatment may still be erroneous for reasons to be discussed later in this chapter. Finally, even when a treatment has had demonstrated success, that success cannot be used to confirm or "prove" one's theoretical position about the etiology of the disorder (Burbeck, 1979; Ross, 1980; Sherman and Baer, 1969).

Definitions of terms used to characterize treatment effectiveness may be vague or ambiguous. Words such as "improved" or "good" are notoriously unclear (Ullman and Krasner, 1969), as are notions of what actually constitutes therapy itself. Levitt and his co-workers (1959), for instance, pointed out that the number of hours constituting psychotherapy could range from one to seven hundred, depending on one's views. Obviously, greater definitional precision is needed before treatment effectiveness can be assessed.

Isolation of treatment effects is difficult. Sampling problems, situational variables, and life experiences make comparisons between treated and untreated subjects problematic, and placebo effects and varying experience among therapists can confound the data (Paul, 1966). In addition, it may be difficult to isolate different kinds of therapy as independent variables (Miller et al., 1972). Highly controlled experimental situations, careful study of individual cases, adequate control groups, long-term follow-up, and other kinds of empirical support, all advocated by Beck (1976), are rarely available. Where longer-term follow-up studies and outcome evaluation studies are available, they are often methodologically weak (Eysenck, 1961; Paul, 1966; 1967a; 1967b; Ullman and Krasner, 1969).

Client characteristics as well as therapist characteristics affect the evaluation of treatment effectiveness. The age, sex, and background of both client and therapist affect treatment effectiveness. In addition, therapeutic technique, therapeutic environment (home, office, institution), and time factors (number of treatment contacts and the length of the follow-up periods) are all relevant in the evaluation process, as are the criteria used to evaluate the treatment's effectiveness (Paul, 1969).

Research with children presents special problems for the assessment of treatment effectiveness. "Symptom" behaviors may occur in basically normal children and then spontaneously decrease over time in the normal course of development (Levitt, 1971). Therefore, a "baseline recovery rate" (Levitt, Beiser, and Robertson, 1959, p. 338)—that is, an estimate of how such spontaneous improvement will occur—must be established. Obviously, treatment-related improvement must be distinguished from spontaneous improvement. In addition, symptoms may change with a child's age, a phenomenon that Levitt referred to as "developmental symptom substitution" (Levitt, 1971, p. 477), further confounding attempts to relate therapeutic intervention to specific behavioral changes.

Finally, in therapy with children the focus of treatment is not on the child alone. Hence, improvements in the child's behavior may be due to the therapy the child received, that which the parents received, or some combination or interaction of factors (Levitt, 1971).

One needs to find out which techniques are effective for what kinds of problems, as no one technique will likely show itself to be best for every problem (Ross, 1972). Paul (1969) summarized nicely the methodological problems facing researchers when he stated that the ultimate questions are "What treatment, by whom, is most effective for this individual with that specific problem, under which set of circumstances, and how does it come about?" (p. 44). These are questions no single study can answer, although there have been methodological improvements (Phillips and Ray, 1980).

There are many *kinds* of studies that can be done to demonstrate or evaluate treatment effectiveness. A discussion of some of the many kinds of experimental designs that can be used, as well as some of the methodological difficulties inherent in them follows.

Experimental Designs

The kinds of research the clinician is involved in and the answers he or she is seeking will determine which of the wide variety of available experimental designs should be chosen.

Pretest/Posttest Design

Many studies involve a pretest evaluation or assessment, followed by a specific intervention, then a posttest evaluation. The assumption is that if the posttest evaluation indicates improvement over the pretest, the therapeutic intervention was successful. It is important to include a control group that receives no treatment to help to clarify developmental changes and/or spontaneous improvement. In addition, the inclusion of a placebo group also allows one to determine whether any changes that occurred were due to such factors as extra attention, rather than a specific technique.

Reversal Experimental Design (ABAB)

In the ABAB design the effectiveness of a given treatment is assessed by withdrawing the treatment and noting whether the problem returns. A, in this case, refers to baseline measures, B to measurement during the experimental procedure (Risley, 1969). Subjects demonstrate certain symptoms (A), and a specific treatment is begun (B). If they show improvement, the treatment is then stopped to see if problem behaviors or symptoms return (A). If they do, the treatment is started again (B); and if the symptoms disappear again, it is assumed that the treatment is causing the effect that is being observed. Such procedures can be used with groups or individuals, but sometimes may not be possible for methodological and ethical reasons (Kratochwill, Brody, and Piersel, 1979), as follows.

Multiple Baseline Design

A multiple baseline design may be more useful in evaluating the effectiveness of an intervention technique when therapeutic results persist even after the experimental procedure or treatment is stopped, or when ethical considerations preclude withdrawal of a treatment. A child whose attentional problems have decreased because of a specific intervention technique, for example, may continue to show improved attention even after that technique has been stopped or withdrawn. In a multiple baseline design, baselines are obtained for a behavior in more than one situation, and therapeutic procedures are first introduced in one situation. If there is change, the procedure is introduced in another situation, and the results are compared with the rate of behaviors in situations where the experimental procedure has *not* been introduced. In the example given above, for instance, attentional problems might be noted in the classroom, at home during homework or study periods, and in a Sunday School class. If a multiple baseline design is used, data would first be obtained in all three areas, and then a specific technique aimed at the attentional problems would be introduced into one area such as the classroom. If attention improved there but remained the same at home and in Sunday School, the technique would then be introduced into a home study period and the effect noted. If improvement followed there as well but did not occur in the Sunday School class, one might conclude that the technique was in fact having the desired effect. This procedure could be used for different behaviors of one person, for a single behavior of one person in various situations, or for the same behavior of different children measured simultaneously in the same situation (Risley, 1969).

Factorial Designs

Factorial designs are used to evaluate different kinds of treatment or intervention simultaneously and in interaction with other variables such as age, sex, and type of problem. Such designs can clearly show the error in trying to use a single technique with many kinds of children (Achenbach, 1974). Miller and his colleagues (1972), for instance, used such a design to investigate several variables simultaneously. They randomly assigned sixty-seven phobic children, ages six to fifteen, to various treatment groups, including reciprocal inhibition, psychotherapy, and a waiting list control group. The children were then independently assessed after twenty-four sessions or three months on the waiting list, and again six weeks after. The data indicated that therapeutic effectiveness was a function of the age of the child. Treatment was most effective for the younger children (six to ten), regardless of therapist experience or technique, but neither treatment worked with eleven- to fifteen-year-olds.

Single n Design

Many studies involve a single subject. This type of study, referred to as a single *n* design or a case study approach, may be presented in relation to either psychodynamic or behavioral techniques. An important concern with such studies is how to determine whether observed changes occurred as a function of the intervention or would have occurred without it (Kratochwill, Brody, and Piersel, 1979). If evaluated rigorously and varied systemically, studies of such single cases, or small groups without controls, can be useful in illustrating new techniques (Achenbach, 1974). However, they are not sufficient to evaluate effectiveness, as there is no way to determine how typical they are or what proportion of an author's cases have had such outcomes (Achenbach, 1974).

Some of the methodological problems inherent in a case study approach can be circumvented through the use of various other experimental designs, some of which have been discussed in this section. Kratochwill and his colleagues (1979) discuss these techniques as well as others in more detail and recommend more controlled comparison studies.

Criteria for Effectiveness

Closely related to methodological considerations are the criteria the researcher uses to evaluate treatment effectiveness, criteria that depend on the purpose of the therapy. Most therapists, regardless of theoretical stance, would agree on the need to change behaviors that interfere with a child's adaptive behavior or self-esteem and would consider failure to do so a treatment failure (Achenbach, 1974). Ross (1972) suggests that treatment can be considered to have been successful when maladaptive behavior has become adaptive and deficiencies in behavior are no longer present. However, measurement can only tell us when therapy is *not* effective; it cannot, in itself, indicate the cause of any evident improvement (Risley, 1969).

Of the many evaluation criteria that have been used, including ratings and objective criteria, psychological assessment, and clinical evaluation or opinion, none seems to be superior to the others either theoretically or empirically (Levitt, Beiser, and Robertson, 1959). Some writers (Eysenck, 1965; Risley, 1969) have attempted to clarify the issues by distinguishing between clinician and experimenter, or between clinical criteria such as symptomatic improvement and experimental criteria such as methodological precision. Risley (1969) has suggested that both therapeutic and experimental criteria be used in the evaluation of behavior modification. The experimental criteria determine whether a specific therapeutic endeavor, of whatever type, actually *caused* a behavior change. The therapeutic criteria, on the other hand, indicate whether changes that have occurred are of significance to the person or are considered important by society. Perhaps behavior therapy can serve as the meeting ground for the different emphases (Clarizio and McCoy, 1976), with experimental

153

techniques being applied successfully to clinical situations (Franks, 1965).

As behavior analysis extends into more complex behavior, social validation—or the assessment of the social acceptability and importance of any changes (Kazdin, 1978)—may help researchers to avoid focusing on behaviors that are not relevant, and may be one way to establish a relationship between objective behavioral components and more complex behavioral classes (Minkin et al., 1976).

Kazdin (1978) has suggested that criteria for evaluating effectiveness of treatment may well expand to include consumer acceptance of treatment, cost effectiveness, and ease of service delivery. There are problems with including such consumer satisfaction ratings as criteria, however. Parents may indicate improvement when their child has been in any treatment (Miller et al., 1972). Furthermore, given the frequency of spontaneous improvement as well as the possible therapeutic effects of suggestion, to be discussed at greater length later in this chapter, testimonials are inadequate indications of the value of certain techniques (Beck, 1976).

Other criteria that might be used to evaluate various intervention strategies are aspects related to their effectiveness, such as total amount of time spent in therapy, utilization of the child's natural environment, dependence on family or paraprofessionals, and size of population that might be served by them, as well as factors related to implementation and cost (Sajwaj, McNees, and Schnelle, 1979).

Werry (1966) offered three simple criteria to be used in the evaluation of a treatment: whether it is safe, effective, and practicable. Finally, some (Robins, 1972; Ullman and Krasner, 1969) maintain that effectiveness should depend not on whether the child has improved, but on whether behavior has changed more effectively with therapeutic intervention than without.

Studies of Effectiveness

Studies have been done both to demonstrate separately the relative effectiveness of psychotherapy and behavior therapy with various subjects and differing problems and to compare the two directly in an effort to show the superiority of one over the other. Although some trends are clearer than others, there is considerable controversy and many contradictory findings.

154

Psychotherapy

Psychotherapy has historically been the most frequently used treatment. Although clinicians have attested to its usefulness and effectiveness with a wide variety of problems, empirical confirmation for this conviction has been lacking. Recently more and more studies have attempted to rigorously examine the effects of psychotherapy. Many of these have suggested that psychotherapy appears to be no more effective than such nonspecific factors as attention, reassurance, support, and suggestion, which people might normally be expected to encounter in the course of their daily experiences. In one study (Strupp and Hadley, 1979) college professors chosen for their ability to form good relationships with students saw as much improvement on the average in troubled patients as did trained psychotherapists, and both groups of patients were slightly better than controls. However, if neither the therapist nor the technique makes a significant difference, then the factors that actually effect change are not known (Miller et al., 1972). Love and his colleagues (1972) also found psychotherapy to be consistently ineffective across socioeconomic levels, at least regarding improved grade averages.

Some of the studies most critical of psychotherapy have been those of Levitt (1957, 1959, 1971) and his colleagues. In a review of dozens of studies of psychotherapy with children over a thirty-five-year span up to about 1960, Levitt found that there had been improvement in an average of two-thirds of all of the subjects at the end of treatment and in three-quarters of the subjects in later follow-up studies. However, he found the same percentage for his control group, which consisted of children who had been accepted for treatment but who had "defected." That is, they had failed to follow through to obtain treatment, but still showed improvement rates similar to those of the treated group. Although the children ranged in age from preschool to twenty-one, most were under seventeen; the median age was ten (Levitt, 1957).

Levitt's findings set off a predictable storm of controversy which still continues a quarter of a century later. His controls were criticized by Eysenck on the grounds that defectors do not constitute an ideal control group because those who quit while on the waiting list may have been less disturbed and would be expected, therefore, to show more spontaneous improvement (Eysenck, 1965). In addition, the long follow-up periods may have obscured differences between the treated and untreated groups (Achenbach, 1974).

However, there have been many other reports of a two-thirds improvement rate in treated and untreated groups (Eysenck, 1961, 1965; Shepherd, Oppenheim, and Mitchell, 1971), and the controversy begun by Eysenck in 1952 and fueled by Levitt's studies continues (Garfield, 1981). In an effort to reconcile this consistently negative finding with the clinicians' belief that psychotherapy is truly effective, Eysenck (1961) suggested that perhaps the natural improvement that occurs without psychotherapy reinforces the therapists' ideas regarding the value of their methods. Such clinical convictions of effectiveness may even preclude acceptance of findings that question the efficiency of some treatments (Eysenck, 1952).

Negative findings concerning psychotherapy are not confirmed by everyone, however, Shore and Massimo (1969; 1973) found that when psychotherapy was combined with job placement and remedial education in the treatment of delinquents, subjects showed better overall adjustment than did an untreated control group. However, the weighting of each of those factors or conditions was not discussed, so the contribution of psychotherapy to the better adjustment is not at all clear. After ten years the treated group was still showing adequate adjustment, whereas the control group continued to deteriorate; but again, the influence of initial differences in resources and abilities was not clear.

Others (Bergin, 1971; Smith and Glass, 1977) have also concluded from their reviews of outcome studies that there is at least modest evidence of psychotherapy's effectiveness. The number of studies yielding such evidence is greater than could be expected by chance, although an average, moderately positive effect may obscure multiple processes, some of which may have no effect, or, worse, may be detrimental (Bergin, 1971). Bergin did conclude, however, that traditional therapies may be relevant for only a few disturbances.

Behavioral Therapy

Many workers (Baker, 1969; Clement, Fazzone, and Goldstein, 1970; DeLeon and Mandell, 1966; Eysenck, 1961, 1965; Kent and O'Leary, 1976; Lovibond and Coote, 1970; Paul, 1966, 1976b; Rachman, 1973; Ross, 1972) have found learning theory and behavioral approaches such as conditioning and desensitization to be more effective with a wide range of problems than either psychotherapy or no treatment. In spite of such enthusiastic endorsements for behavioral techniques, it is important to remember Sherman and Baer's (1969) cautions about the need to demonstrate that the operant procedures used were in fact responsible for the changes noted; the need to exert the maximum control possible with clinically significant questions; and the need to refrain from going beyond the data or logic in explaining why behavioral techniques work. More data are required regarding the generalization of treatment effects (Clarizio and McCoy, 1976) and the permanence of such effects, as some findings recorded at the end of treatment have changed by the time of follow-up studies (Clement, Fazzone, and Goldstein, 1970; Kent and O'Leary, 1976). Matarazzo (1980) claims that there is little substantive evidence for the effectiveness of behavioral techniques in either treatment or prevention, and that where change does occur there is still a problem with maintenance of change. On the other hand, Wallick (1979) reports that two years after the use of desensitization with specific fears in a two-year-old, gains were still being maintained, with decreased intensity of other fears as well.

Phillips and Ray (1980), in a recent review of outcome studies and reviews of the child behavior therapy literature, concluded that such therapy is not developmental enough, that it needs more complex functional analyses, that it should place more emphasis on description and assessment, and, that it should use adequate designs on a more consistent basis.

Spontaneous Remission and Nonspecific Effects

The "spontaneous remission" that has often been reported may be due to informal therapy that occurs through contacts with clergy, friends, physicians, or teachers who provide some attention, reassurance, and support (Bergin, 1966). Thus, it may be virtually impossible, according to Bergin, to arrange a no-treatment control group except in institutions, because subjects seek such other therapeutic contacts in the community. Moreover, developmental changes may result in improvement and shifts in symptom patterns. If then, it could be shown that certain types of problems (or children) have a higher likelihood of spontaneous improvement or that certain problems are likely to disappear with age, parents could be given appropriate advice and support, and better use of their sometimes limited resources could be made (Shepherd, Oppenheim, and Mitchell, 1966).

Smith and Glass (1977), in their review and statistical integration of almost four hundred controlled evaluations of counseling and psychotherapy, concluded that a typical treated client was better off than 75 percent of those not treated, but few important differences existed among the types of therapy. That is, their statistically controlled comparison of psychodynamic, systematic desensitization, and behavior modification therapeutic effects revealed no difference in effectiveness between a group of all behavioral therapies and a group of nonbehavioral therapies. This finding emphatically underscores the need for careful evaluation of nonspecific effects such as attention, which may confound data on treatment effectiveness. Moreover, if treatment effectiveness depends in part on the type of disorder, attempts to study the relative effectiveness of one technique over another without regard for specific disorders might obscure differential effects (Eisenberg and Gruenberg, 1961). Finally, the effects of therapy on prosocial behavior should also be assessed (Abramowitz, 1976).

Therapist Characteristics

It has been suggested that the type of therapy is less important than the therapist. Kanner (1972) insisted that the basic aspect of psychotherapy is not the technique or school but rather the therapist himself or herself, and progress has been related to therapist characteristics such as warmth, empathy, and experience (Bergin, 1971).

Worsening with Treatment

Some writers (Bergin, 1966, 1971; Craighead, Kazdin, and Mahoney, 1976; McCord, 1978) have even suggested that at times treatment may lead to worsening or negative effects, although the evidence has been criticized as being too weak to support the claim that psychotherapy *caused* such worsening (Sobel, 1978). Furthermore, the condition of subjects may worsen without treatment (Rachman, 1973; Shore and Massimo, 1969, 1973). In some cases, lack of evidence for deterioration may be due to a concentration on less disturbed and hence more resilient children or to the use of measures that are not designed to detect such worsening (Abramowitz, 1976).

Conclusions

The area of evaluation of effectiveness is clearly clouded by controversy, methodological difficulties, and ambiguous or equivocal findings. However, based on the research findings reported, some preliminary observations can be made.

First, the fact of a client's involvement or prospective involvement in treatment can have beneficial effects on that individual's problems. Second, there are suggestions that behavior therapy has some advantage in terms of effectiveness when compared with other therapies on various kinds of measurable results, although more data are necessary. Third, psychotherapy frequently results in little advantage as compared with no-treatment conditions, despite the conviction of many clinicians that it is highly effective. Fourth, apparent spontaneous improvement is a significant phenomenon which makes the use of nontreatment control groups imperative but methodologically difficult. There is a need for more research to ascertain the variables involved in such "spontaneous" improvement. Finally, the significant effects of such nonspecific factors as attention, support, reassurance, and frequent contact need to be more rigorously investigated. Since numerous studies have shown that age, duration of problems, type of disorder, length of follow-up period, and other factors seem to make a difference in how effective a given treatment technique is shown to be, more complex research designs need to be developed to take more variables into account simultaneously. Factorial designs seem to show the most promise in this regard.

Discussion Questions

1. Which variables do you feel are most crucial in evaluating the effectiveness of a course of treatment? How many of those variables do you think could be studied simultaneously?
2. Discuss possible reasons for a child's "spontaneous" improvement.
3. Design a study to investigate which of three interventions is most helpful for anorexic girls, delinquent adolescents, or learning-disabled children.

PART IV

Types of
Disorders

CHAPTER 8   # Developmental Disturbances

The symptoms usually included in a discussion of developmental disorders are described and conceptualized differently by different authors. Some discuss them in relation to specific syndromes, some incorporate them in a "catchall" category for problems that don't fit neatly anywhere else, and some do not include them in their discussions at all. Authors with a psychodynamic stance perceive them to be symptomatic of underlying neurotic disorders and therefore prescribe psychotherapeutic intervention. Workers with a behavioral stance, on the other hand, tend to perceive them as maladaptive behaviors or habits which are not necessarily associated with other symptoms but which have resulted from faulty learning; they prescribe the relearning of new, more adaptive behaviors.

However they may be classified, clearly many symptoms and behavior problems arise in the course of a child's developmental progress. In this book the term developmental disorders will include two broad categories of behavior. The first group, to be discussed briefly, will comprise behaviors that, although frequently problematic, are common at particular developmental stages. The second group will refer to disordered behavior that deviates from normal developmental patterns and reflects a child's failure to master certain developmental tasks, as in habit disorders, maturational lags, and other developmental disturbances. Behaviors in either grouping may or may not be associated with other conflicts, disturbances, or signs of maladjustment. The bulk of the discussion in this chapter relates to the second category.

Age-Related Problem Behaviors

Although age-related behavior disorders are seen in many if not most children at specific ages and are relatively "normal," they nonetheless cause problems for the child and family. They emerge at certain developmental periods more frequently than at others, as the child confronts the demands and expectations of those periods. Problems in this category are usually relatively transient; can be managed by the family, albeit sometimes with difficulty; and do not generally require professional intervention. If they are not handled wisely, however, they can become more severe or extensive and may then require professional treatment.

For example, normally developing children show stress reactions in the presence of strangers at about six months of age, and signs of separation anxiety when their mother leaves toward the end of their first year or when they enter nursery school. These "disordered" behaviors indicate that the child's socialization is developing normally. How the mother handles these *normal disturbances*, however, is very important. If her behavior confirms their idea that separation is dangerous, she may increase their dependent behavior. If, on the other hand, she conveys her confidence in their ability to handle a new situation, the likelihood of their developing confidence in their own ability is greatly increased. Thus, while the "disordered" behavior is entirely normal and predictable and is in fact a sign of the child's growth, the environmental reaction to it can influence greatly whether it turns out to be a healthy, growth-producing experience or develops into one that is not.

Many different behavior problems occur in nonclinic or normal children. For example, childhood fears often take characteristic forms. They are likely to have specific content at particular ages—that is, they tend to be "stage-specific" (Schwartz and Johnson, 1981). Younger children often fear concrete stimuli such as loud noises, dogs, and darkness; whereas older children fear more abstract events such as kidnapping, death, and getting lost (Miller, Barrett, and Hampe, 1974; Schwartz and Johnson, 1981).

LaPouse and Monk (1964) studied the incidence of problem behaviors in normal children between 6 and 12 years of age and found that age was inversely related to behavior problems—that is, the incidence of problems was higher in younger children than in older. The problems they found most commonly were bed-wetting, fears, nightmares, loss of temper, overactivity and restlessness, and nail-biting. As these are also frequently seen in clinic populations, they have often been assumed to be "symptoms," or abnormal behavior. However, unless the incidence in clinic populations is compared with the incidence among normal children, their importance as a sign of disordered behavior may be overemphasized. In other words, they may in fact be temporary "normal disturbances" seen in a significant proportion of children in the course of their development.

Suddenly increased environmental demands, then, may lead to exaggerated responses to developmental stress; and although these are usually resolved without major difficulty, they can lead to serious parent-child conflicts or problems (Warme, 1977). It is not necessary to reiterate here all of the normal problem behaviors that children show as they confront the various developmental challenges during each age period. Such discussions can be found in any developmental textbook. However, a brief discussion of some of the *special problems of adolescence* is in order.

During adolescence there are frequent conflicts between the adolescent's wishes and those of the parents. There are also differences between parent and child in the perceived developmental tasks during adolescence (Erickson, 1978). Part of the special difficulty during this period is due to the occurrence of internal changes in psychological and biological drives with which the child has difficulty coping (Warme, 1977). Adolescents are faced with the task of separating themselves from their families and becoming independent adults. At the same time, they are still dependent in many ways, however much they would like not to be. There are very strong—and often conflicting—communal, environmental, and peer pressures to behave in certain ways. Adolescents need to develop their own sense of values but may have difficulty when options presented to them by the media, by their family, by their friends, and by their school environment are very different and often directly contradictory. Faced with conflicting loyalties, they may have to engage in frequent confrontations with their parents as they try to forge their own identity.

While these pressures are being exerted on them, they are still expected to achieve at a satisfactory level at school and to embark on a program that will eventually lead them into some worthwhile occupational pursuit. They may be expected to help finance their education and other needs through part-time employment. They may also be expected to be active in school clubs or church groups. All of the energy needed for this busy life is required at the same time that physiological changes are using up large amounts of energy. As a result adolescents may be tired much of the time and irritable or depressed. Their developing sexuality is a new area with which they must cope. Again, there are conflicting messages and expectations regarding how they should handle their feelings and how they should behave.

It is not necessary to reiterate the many developmental tasks that the adolescent faces; they are well described in the available books on

166

adolescence. What is essential here is to emphasize the importance of the environmental reaction to "normal disordered behavior." If, for example, adolescents are not taken seriously, or are ignored, ridiculed, or rejected, they are thrown back on their own resources to cope with demands in many areas simultaneously. They are not likely to have the energy, the capability, or the experience to handle such a situation. They must then turn to possible solutions or resources that they do know about. These may involve undesirable activities with friends, use or abuse of drugs or alcohol, acting-out behavior, or even self-destructive behavior. Although these behaviors may be engaged in experimentally by any adolescent, and are in fact fairly common examples of "normal disordered behavior" during this period, they may be relied on to a greater extent and as a more permanent solution if the child does not experience the appropriate parental or environmental responses to his or her concerns. If the parents can convey their understanding of the problems faced by their adolescent children, offering guidance and suggestions but allowing independent decision-making appropriate to the children's age and setting firm limits only when they appear to be necessary, the adolescents feel more secure. They are then better able to develop mature and independent coping mechanisms. Such handling of age-related problems will go a long way toward preventing those common behaviors from becoming more serious and longer-lasting "developmental disorders."

The next section deals with problems arising out of a child's failure to master developmental tasks that are ordinarily managed without major difficulty. Such problems frequently involve the continuation of behaviors that are normal at one age into an age period when their occurrence is not normal.

Developmental Disorders

Habit Disorders

Basic developmental routines and behavioral control are mastered without great difficulty by the majority of normal children. For some children, however, that mastery and control become problematic and can result in the following behavioral disturbances.

EATING DISTURBANCES

Pica

Pica is a disorder in which young children eat inedible substances; it can lead to serious health problems, depending on the substance. The name comes from the Latin word for magpie, or "scavenger bird" (Millican and Lourie, 1970). Children with this disorder may eat such varied substances as crayons, starch, plaster, wood, and cigarette butts, often preferring them to food (Millican and Lourie, 1970). Most cases of lead poisoning, for example, which is alleged to be the most common urban disease excluding infections (Greenberg, 1970), are related to pica (Rudolph, 1977).

A number of factors have been implicated as causes of pica. One hypothesis is that it occurs because of a nutritional deficiency in the child. However, there is little support for such a deficiency as a causal factor. In one study (Gutelius et al., 1962), although low levels of hemoglobin and ascorbic acid as well as poor diets were found to be associated with pica, the researchers could not conclude that nutritional deficits had caused the pica. Administration of iron was no more effective than a placebo saline solution in breaking the habit. In addition, the researchers made a rather surprising observation that most of the subjects were heavy and liked to eat, so there was an adequate intake of food.

Pica has consistently been found more often in families of low socioeconomic levels, although it does appear in all social classes (Millican and Lourie, 1970). There is a high incidence among blacks; as many as one-third of the black children in Washington, D.C., between ages one and six may be affected (Gutelius et al., 1962). It has been linked to unsatisfactory home situations with inadequate play facilities, minimal care and supervision, many emotional problems, and incompetent parenting (Kanner, 1972; Millican and Lourie, 1970). However, despite the many organic, nutritional, socioeconomic, psychological, and cultural factors that have been implicated, their relative importance is not known and the etiology is not well established (Millican and Lourie, 1970). Pica is rarely seen in children whose needs are being met (Kanner, 1972), however, and educational and supportive interventions have been found to be most effective (Millican and Lourie, 1970). Approaches aimed at educating the mothers regarding the dangers of the child's behavior and specific techniques for handling the behavior, along with supportive help from social workers regarding financing, housing, and marital problems, were effective in most cases (Millican and Lourie, 1970).

Anorexia Nervosa

The term anorexia refers to appetite loss, but anorexia nervosa refers to a serious form of eating disorder in which the child embarks on a program of self-starvation which can become life-threatening. Typically, the child either refuses to eat or induces vomiting so that food will not be digested and metabolized. There is increasing isolation and self-absorption (Bruch, 1978). Such children are usually thin by any objective standard but consider themselves to be fat. Most frequently seen among adolescent girls, it is one of the few disorders that affect girls more than boys, with a ratio of about ten to one (Tolstrup, 1970). The child may literally become skin and bones and may require intravenous feeding as a life-sustaining measure. Death occurs in 15 to 21 percent of these individuals (APA, 1980).

Models to explain this perplexing disorder have included psychodynamic, family interactional, behavioral, and medical ones (Bemis, 1978). Explanations have involved such diverse factors as a denial of sexuality, a fear of growing up, incorrect identification of hunger sensations (Bruch, 1961, 1970), specific patterns of parent-child interactions and expectations (Bruch, 1978; Tolstrup, 1970), cultural reinforcement for slimness (Bemis, 1978), and others. The families are often outwardly normal and very polite and frequently deny any problems except the child's weight loss (Bruch, 1970; 1978). This normality, according to Bruch, masks a serious underlying disorder on the part of the child, in which there are many inner doubts, feelings of unworthiness, and thought disturbances (Bruch, 1978).

Excerpts from a report by Bruch of an anorexic girl are reproduced below to provide a glimpse into the disordered life of an anorexic. The patient was twenty years old and had been sick for five years.

At fifteen Alma had been healthy and well-developed, had menstruated at age twelve, was five feet tall, and weighed one hundred twenty pounds. At that time her mother urged her to change to a school with higher academic standing, a change she resisted; her father suggested that she should watch her weight, an idea that she took up with great eagerness, and she began a rigid diet. She lost rapidly and her menses ceased. That she could be thin gave her a sense of pride, power, and accomplishment. She also began a frantic exercise program, would swim by the mile, play tennis for hours, or do calisthenics to the point of exhaustion. Whatever low point her weight reached, Alma feared that she might become "too fat" if she regained as little as an ounce. There were many efforts to make her gain weight, which she would lose immediately, and she had been below seventy pounds most of the time. There was also a marked change in her character and behavior. Formerly sweet, obedient, and considerate, she became more and more demanding, obstinate, irritable, and arrogant. There was constant arguing, not only about what she should eat but about all other activities as well.

When she came for consultation she looked like a walking skeleton, scantily dressed in shorts and a halter, with her legs sticking out like broomsticks, every rib showing, and her shoulder blades standing up like little wings. Her mother mentioned, "When I put my arms around her I feel nothing but bones, like a frightened little bird." Alma's arms and legs were covered with soft hair, her complexion had a yellowish tint, and her dry hair hung down in strings. Most striking was the face—hollow like that of a shriveled-up old woman with a wasting disease, sunken eyes, a sharply pointed nose on which the juncture between bone and cartilage was visible. When she spoke or smiled—and she was quite cheerful—one could see every movement of the muscles around her mouth and eyes, like an animated anatomical representation of the skull. Alma insisted that she looked fine and that there was nothing wrong with her being so skinny. "I enjoy having this disease and I want it. I cannot convince myself that I am sick and that there is anything from which I have to recover." (Bruch, 1978, pp. 1–2)

Medical attention is required immediately, but psychotherapy, family therapy, drugs, and operant behavioral methods have also been used singly or in combination.

A variety of family therapy techniques have been used with anorexic patients and their families. The most successful appear to be those with a family systems approach in which the eating disorder is seen as a family problem and/or a means by which confrontation of other family problems is avoided.

The question of autonomy and independence is central to many approaches (Bruch, 1978; Reinhart, Kenna, and Succop, 1972; Rosman, Minuchin, and Liebman, 1975). The issue of whether or not the child eats has often turned into a strong power struggle between parents and child; the therapeutic tack is to defuse or undermine that issue or that struggle. For example, Reinhart and his colleagues (1972) arranged for two different therapists to see the parents and the child, and both independently made the eating issue the child's responsibility. They found that outpatient treatment using that approach was as effective as inpatient treatment. They used hospitalization only as a last resort, and only briefly, when the parents were not able to tolerate the symptoms. The brief hospitalization was then followed by outpatient psychotherapy.

Another family systems approach is the "family lunch" technique of Rosman and his colleagues (1975). In this approach, the therapist eats lunch with the family, at which time the family's interactions about eating can be observed directly and interventions made immediately. The therapist uses different methods depending on the age of the child and the rigidity of the family. For example, with more rigid families in which the child is clearly resisting, the therapist may precipitate a crisis or a change by having each parent in turn try to get the child to eat (that is, take responsibility). Maladaptive methods which emerge can then be changed, or the therapist may disengage the parents altogether. In less rigid families, where there is not a power struggle, attention to eating behavior may be discouraged altogether and discussion of family background, roles, interactions, and problems encouraged. The goals with this approach are to broaden the problem to make it a family problem, to change the focus from an eating problem to a problem of interpersonal interactions, and to stop the parents from using eating behavior to avoid conflict (Rosman et al., 1975).

Once again, there is disagreement on the relative merits of behavioral methods and more psychodynamically oriented techniques. Fair success has been reported with the use of operant techniques. Blinder and his colleagues (1970), for example, using physical activity as a reinforcement contingent on gaining weight, achieved rapid weight gain in hospital treatment of four to six weeks' duration. Patients were allowed six hours outside the hospital on any day their weight was up half a pound from the previous day and there was no confrontation about eating. The procedure employed resulted in a rate of improvement comparable to that obtained with other methods, although good follow-up studies are needed to assess whether such weight gain during hospitalization is temporary (Bemis, 1978).

Behavior therapy has been criticized on several grounds. The efficiency with which behavioral methods bring about weight gain may actually *increase* the child's conflict and preempt the last bit of control the anorexic has (Bruch, 1978). Much of the reported success may be due to the selection of patients and the voluntary admission of anorexics who will contract for weight gain (Bruch, 1978). In addition, if weight loss is a *symptom*, then simple weight gain may leave the person with the very personality problems that led to the disorder (Bliss and Branch, 1960).

Kellerman (1977), however, in a review of published reports of behavioral therapy, found that the evidence did not support Bruch's criticisms. Rather, he found that there was not only a decrease in maladaptive behavior with relatively good gains, but a positive change in other behaviors as well. Kellerman concluded that behavior therapy was the treatment of choice for anorexia because it was the most successful in bringing about weight gain and in maintaining such gains. In any case, prognosis is better for young patients and for those who get treatment soon after onset (Bruch, 1978), and there is a move toward a more eclectic approach to this disorder (Bemis, 1978).

Obesity

Eating beyond the satiation level is aversive and will not occur unless there are strong reinforcers for eating beyond that level (Ross, 1980); obesity on a psychogenic basis is relatively infrequently seen in psychiatric practice (Tolstrup, 1970). Bruch (1961, 1970) suggested that in both anorexia and obesity the person ingests abnormal quantities of food because of an inability to correctly identify sensations of hunger and other bodily sensations. She attributes this inability to faulty early learning in an environment that was not responsive to early signs and signals from the child. However, the idea that people of normal weight respond to internal cues whereas obese individuals respond instead to external ones such as the appearance of food or time elapsed has been criticized as an oversimplification (Rodin, 1981). External and internal cues cannot be separated so clearly because external cues can affect internal ones. According to Rodin (1981), obesity is determined by the interaction of genetic, psychological, metabolic, and environmental factors and events, with no single cause and probably no single cure.

Operant techniques have been used in the treatment of obesity. Aragona and his colleagues (1975), for example, found a method of contracting for weight loss goals quite effective. When the children, ages five to ten, failed to meet the predetermined criteria for weight loss, the parents were penalized through the loss of a monetary deposit made at the beginning of treatment. Mahoney and Mahoney (1976) also found behavioral techniques to be more effective than others, although not consistently so across individuals.

ELIMINATION DISORDERS

In most children the task of acquiring mastery over sphincter and bladder muscles and attaining self-control in toileting proceeds more or less smoothly. Once such control is achieved, it tends to be permanent except during rather unusual disturbances or illnesses. However, such control is inadequately managed by some children and remains intermittent or weak over an inordinately long period of time. Or children may at a later age revert to earlier, less mature functioning and relinquish control for varying periods of time. The following problems are examples of elimination disorders.

Enuresis

Enuresis is a term used to refer to a child's persistent, frequent, involuntary urination past the age of three or four in the absence of clear organic pathology (APA, 1980; Lovibond and Coote, 1970). Sometimes a distinction is made between primary enuresis, in which a child has never been dry, and secondary enuresis, in which a child has been continent for a period but returns to a period of involuntary urination (APA, 1980; Lovibond and Coote, 1970). Incidence estimates range from 3 to 13 percent of children (APA, 1980; Kales and Berger, 1970), depending in part on their ages; the disorder is seen twice as frequently in boys as in girls (Warme, 1977).

Enuresis not only concerns parents but also interferes with many aspects of the child's life. It may result in ridicule from peers, exclusion from invitations for overnight visits, inability to attend camp, and other social difficulties.

Many causal explanations have been given for the appearance of enuresis. It has been seen as a symptom of an underlying disorder or, more simply, as an independent maladaptive behavior or habit which does not necessarily indicate an underlying disturbance (Baker, 1969; Lovibond and Coote, 1970; MacKeith, 1968; Mowrer and Mowrer, 1938) and can be attacked directly. It has been related to immaturity

(Kanner, 1972); inadequate cortical control over reflexive functions—that is, deficient neural maturation (Lovibond and Coote, 1970); anxiety and stress (APA, 1980; MacKeith, 1968; Young and Morgan, 1968); faulty training in proper habits (Mowrer and Mowrer, 1938); family disturbance (Young and Morgan, 1968); and other factors. Whatever the cause, the symptom may result in anxiety, maladjustment, and other problems.

Many different techniques have been tried with the enuretic child, with varying rates of success. Psychodynamically oriented clinicians, who assume that the enuresis is a symptom of underlying problems or conflicts, may involve psychotherapy or play therapy or whatever other technique they would use to treat any other neurotic disorder. Both classical and operant conditioning techniques have been used by behaviorally oriented clinicians. Perhaps the best-known technique using classical conditioning is the bell and pad technique introduced by Mowrer and Mowrer in 1938. It consists of a special pad which is wired to set off a buzzer when contact with urine is made. The aim is to condition the child to associate the bladder distension with the buzzer and thus train the child to wake up in response to that sensation without the buzzer.

A review of studies using this procedure suggested that it is effective (Werry, 1966) and is superior to traditional psychotherapy (De Leon and Mandell, 1966). Kimmel and Kimmel (1970) attempted to gradually increase the child's tolerance for bladder distension cues so that he or she would neither wet the bed nor wake up to go to the bathroom. Using operant rather than classical conditioning and rewarding the child's control for increasing lengths of time during the day, they had rapid success in removing this symptom even in cases where the child continued to experience other serious problems.

Conditioning techniques have been reported to work in as many as 85 to 90 percent of cases (De Leon and Mandell, 1966; Lovibond and Coote, 1970), and symptom substitution has apparently not been a problem (Mowrer and Mowrer, 1938; Werry, 1966). On the contrary, the child usually experiences considerable relief when such an embarrassing symptom is removed (Werry, 1966). Although fairly high relapse rates have been found in conditioning groups, the symptoms in such relapses tend to be less severe and retraining is rapid (De Leon and Mandell, 1966).

Drugs have been used in the treatment of children over six (Warme,

1977). However, they are not clearly beneficial and, where effective, may have to be withdrawn gradually to prevent a relapse (Lovibond and Coote, 1970).

By adolescence, most children have become continent (APA, 1980). In view of the possibility of spontaneous remission in more than 50 percent of the cases occurring before age six or seven, treatment before that time may not be justified for a number of reasons, including lack of motivation, poor understanding of the treatment, and the possibility that the treatment will frighten the child (Werry, 1966).

Encopresis

Encopresis, which is rarer than enuresis, involves inadequate control of bowel movements past the age when such control is usually mastered and in the absence of physical disorders. More common in the lower socioeconomic classes and in boys, it occurs in approximately 1 percent of the population (APA, 1980). Some see it as a neurotic manifestation which requires psychiatric treatment of underlying conflicts rather than direct treatment of the bowel function (Kanner, 1972), whereas others have used operant conditioning successfully (Neal, 1963).

SLEEP DISTURBANCES

Most normal children have occasional periods of difficulty with sleeping patterns because of illness, overexcitement, anxiety, or other conditions. However, their problems are relatively transient and mild. A few children have more persistent and more serious sleeping disorders which affect the quality of their sleep, their general health, and their psychological disposition. These sleep disorders can take a variety of forms.

Insomnia

A child with insomnia may have considerable difficulty falling asleep night after night. Or the child may get to sleep fairly quickly but wake up periodically during the night and be unable to get back to sleep. Either situation is very frustrating; and the more upset the child becomes, the more difficulty there is getting to sleep. Parents may be unable to sleep themselves because of the child's wanderings, complaints, noisemaking, or restless moving about. The level of frustration and exasperation that may result can easily carry over into daytime hours, with increased fatigue, irritability, and other problems.

Nightmares and Night Terrors

Both nightmares and night terrors may be indications of problems with a child. An estimated 1 to 4 percent of children experience terror disorders at some time, but they vary greatly in their occurrence, usually disappear by adolescence, and are not consistently associated with psychopathology (APA, 1980). According to some, dreams reflect processes that develop concurrently with waking mental processes (Foulkes, 1979).

There are important differences between nightmares and night terrors, however. Night terrors are more severe than nightmares, usually last longer, and are not remembered by the child (APA, 1980; Kanner, 1972). Night terrors typically occur earlier in the night, during the phase of deep sleep, and involve more intense autonomic reactions (Hartmann, 1981). They may be more a problem of nervous system arousal than a dream disturbance and may be due to an immature nervous system, though they can worsen with stress or emotional problems (Hartmann, 1981). Nightmares, on the other hand, appear to be anxiety dreams, after which the individual goes back to sleep more easily; they occur at all ages, whereas night terrors are most common in childhood (Fiss, 1979).

A good comparison between nightmares and night terrors, or *pavor nocturnus*, is found in the following excerpt from Kanner (1972). Night terrors are described first through reports from several mothers.

"About one half hour after retiring he cries and raves in his sleep for about ten minutes. He cries that the children are after him."

"He has had night terrors since the age of two years, cries about two hours after being put to bed. The cry sounds like he is terribly afraid. He does not remember the affair afterwards. When he was younger he used to get them four to five at night, now only when he runs around an awful lot or if he has a temperature. Last winter when he had the flu he had three attacks in one night. When he has the attacks he jumps out of bed. He grabs me around my neck, puts his feet around my body, and keeps crying for me, not realizing that I am right there."

176

"He has had night terrors for about two years. He has them from one every night to once in two or three weeks. He sits up in bed, looks very scared, tries to get out of bed, perspires heavily, and cries or screams. I sleep in the same bed and try to wake him as soon as he moves. When I try to quiet him he seems to want to get away but after a while he would calm down and go back to sleep." (p. 479)

Kanner contrasted those descriptions with the following account of nightmares.

A thirteen-year-old boy with astigmatism, dental caries, enlarged cervical glands, and a functional systolic murmur, slightly retarded in intelligence, of a fairly stable family, the only child of overambitious parents, had many fears, cried easily, had been fidgety all his life and especially since he began to go to school. He often woke up at night complaining of being afraid and reporting that he had just had a bad dream which frightened him. Something was coming after him; cats grew larger and larger until they seemed like elephants, or a huge ball was rolling toward him increasing in size as it became nearer. He could give a vivid picture of what had happened in the dream and was easily reassured. It took, however, some time before he went to sleep again. The incident roused his interest, and he kept discussing it with his mother, asking questions about the nature and prophetic meaning of dreams. (p. 479)

Use of reciprocal inhibition and operant reinforcement has led to improvement and maintenance of gains, after three or four sessions in which stimuli associated with anxiety were specified and reality factors maintaining it (including protectiveness of parents) were changed (Kellerman, 1980). Mild tranquilizers may also reduce the occurrence of night terror by decreasing the amount of stage-four sleep (Hartmann, 1981).

Somnambulism

Sleepwalking usually occurs during the first half-hour to three hours of sleep, which is a period of deep sleep and nonrapid eye movement (APA, 1980; Kales and Berger, 1970). (REM refers to the rapid eye movement stage of sleep, which is a later stage and often associated with dreaming.) Somnambulism is usually not clinically significant (Warme, 1977); isolated episodes are experienced by as many as 15 percent of all children (APA, 1980). Characteristics of sleepwalkers that were not found in the control group, such as low motor ability and low awareness, suggest the possibility of central nervous system immaturity (Kales et al., 1966a, 1966b), although the authors did not find differences between controls and sleepwalkers in total time spent in sleeping or in REM sleep (Kales et al., 1966a). Interestingly, the experimenters were able to start the sleepwalkers walking by standing them up during their slow-wave stage of sleep, but could not do so with normals. Individuals who have this problem also have a higher incidence than normals of other problems associated with NREM sleep, such as enuresis and sleep terrors (APA, 1980). There were strong family histories of somnambulism, and the authors concluded that organic and functional factors were involved (Kales et al., 1966b).

MOTOR AND RHYTHMIC DISORDERS

Thumb-sucking

Thumb-sucking, sometimes labeled nonnutritive sucking, is normal in infants but usually disappears by twelve to eighteen months (Davidson, 1970). Reasons given for persistence beyond that age in many children depend on one's theoretical perspective and are controversial. There is some consensus that the habit is not necessarily dangerous, from either a dental or a psychological point of view, before age three or four; but when it continues beyond age five, there may be consequences. The dental evidence is unclear—malocclusion may or may not result—but the habit is most problematic in children over five (Davidson, 1970). It has sometimes been taken as a sign of underlying problems if it continued into elementary school, but in one study no important differences were found between thumb-sucking and non-thumb-sucking children, and no clear evidence was uncovered to support the notion that it may be dangerous to stop it abruptly in older children (Davidson, 1970).

Tics

Tics are quick, repetitive, purposeless involuntary motor movements of a particular part of a person's body (APA, 1980; Kanner, 1972). They can be tonic tics, which consist of longer contractions and almost continuous movement, or clonic tics, which are more abrupt and briefer (Yates, 1970b).

Tics have been related to movement restraint or inadequate play material (Levy, 1944) and to unhappiness, conflict, and emotional

178

stress (Kanner, 1972). They appear to be outside of the person's control, persisting in an autonomous fashion, and have usually been found to be very difficult to treat (Yates, 1970b). However, they can be voluntarily suppressed for minutes or hours (APA, 1980; Yates 1970b), and behavioral techniques have been used successfully in their treatment. For example, by making such environmental events as white noise (negative) and music (positive) contingent on tic control, Barrett (1962) reduced multiple tics of a patient who had not previously been helped by drugs or psychotherapy.

Kanner (1972) noted that tics sometimes arise from habitual or customary gestures. The reduction of stress may be a means to alleviate the problem, and appears to have played a fairly large role in resolving the following case.

The last point is illustrated by a seven-year-old moderately retarded girl who, in addition to an affective upheaval caused by the discovery that she was a foster child, developed a horror of school, where she could not comply with the requirements. She had always presented a feeding problem, which was tremendously exaggerated on the mornings of school days. She had long been in the habit of pushing away with her right arm the food and bribes proffered by her foster mother during breakfast and the clothes with which her foster father tried to dress her so that she should not be late in her class; upon leaving the house, it was noticed that she continued jerking her right arm (which carried the book bag). She did not jerk it on her way back from school or at any other time of the day. When she was legally adopted by her fond foster parents and placed in an ungraded class, her jerking disappeared, together with her feeding difficulties. (p. 406)

A specific tic syndrome was described in 1885 by Gilles de la Tourette, after whom it was named. The disorder involves progressive motor incoordination, especially in the face and upper limbs, which also affects speech. Kelman's (1965) review of studies of forty-four cases over the past sixty years revealed that victims were generally males of average intelligence and had typically been afflicted with the disease since the age of ten or before. Although no organic cause has yet been identified, drugs appear to be helpful for symptomatic treatment, particularly haloperidol, or Haldol (Chapel, Brown, and Jenkins, 1964). When drugs are administered, the complete deterioration predicted by Gilles de la Tourette does not occur, and the disease can be controlled somewhat (Kelman, 1965).

179

Stuttering

Stuttering usually begins before age twelve; peak periods of onset are between two and three and a half and between five and seven years of age (APA, 1980). Its characteristics in the early stages are very similar to the irregularities and dysfluency of speech normally seen in young children. There is disagreement as to what is normal dysfluency and what is abnormal, since many repetitions occur normally (Dalton and Hardcastle, 1977). Stages in the development of stuttering typically involve a sequence of repetitions, delay and blocking, and, later, avoidance or substitutions (Froeschels, 1943; Jones, 1970). There may be frequent periods of spontaneous improvement or recovery in the early stages (Jones, 1970) or in mild cases (APA, 1980). There may also be "concealed stuttering" in which a person stares blankly. Stuttering usually does not occur with whispering or singing (Froeschels, 1943), leading Van Riper (1978) to suggest that it may be more a disorder of communication than of speech.

There is disagreement as to whether stuttering is due to conflicts, learned behavior, or organic or constitutional factors (Van Riper, 1978). Among the factors that have been found to be associated with or used to explain the appearance of stuttering have been laterality and lack of clear dominance (Jones, 1970), faulty speech training, underlying psychological problems (Moncur, 1955), and a high incidence of family disorders (Despert, 1946). Many have taken a more eclectic view of causation, suggesting that there may be different causes in different individuals and that the causes themselves are less important than the conditions which maintain the problem (Van Riper, 1978). Although research to find an organic base has led to conflicting results, a prominent view points to an impairment in the auditory feedback mechanism (Dalton and Hardcastle, 1977).

Most stutterers, despite their stressful condition, are quite normal (Van Riper, 1978). The anxiety and avoidance behavior they sometimes exhibit may be seen as secondary reactions to the stuttering rather than primary causes, and situations that cause the child to feel self-conscious can intensify the problem (Jones, 1970).

There is disagreement concerning the most effective form of treatment, the choice depending, of course, on one's viewpoint regarding causation. With children the treatment is developmental, and changing according to the stage of the child (Dalton and Hardcastle, 1977). In the 1940s researchers (Despert, 1946; Froeschels, 1943) advocated various breathing, articulation, and chewing exercises, alone or in combination with psychotherapy. More recently Jones (1970) stressed the need for psychotherapy aimed at the person's anxiety and self-concept as well as specific modification techniques such as desensitization. Moreover, stutterers often have very supportive relationships with speech pathologists (Van Riper, 1978).

In general, the aim is to elicit and reinforce fluent speech or to modify the stutter so that there is less need for avoidance, either of which involves learning (Van Riper, 1978). Most methods fall between a singular emphasis on a presumed underlying cause or on the speech itself, involving attention to the dysfluency and to the psychological aspects (Dalton and Hardcastle, 1977). Counseling with parents or groups of parents, play therapy, and creative drama may also be helpful (Van Riper, 1978).

Elective or Selective Mutism

Elective or selective mutism is a rare condition with no organic basis in which the child does not speak except with a very few intimates (Reed, 1963). Although there is occasionally some spontaneous remission, it tends to be persistent and hard to treat. Reed noted that although it has been seen as a specific disorder, it seems actually to be a learned psychological reaction which various factors precipitate. Of the children he studied, some used it to gain attention, some to reduce fear. There was nothing very unusual or traumatic in their backgrounds, and he attributed improvement to work done to help them relearn and improve their social behavior.

Kratochwill (1981) concluded that behavioral approaches are just as effective, and usually more so, than psychodynamic ones, although there are methodoligical problems involved. He maintains that behavior therapy is the treatment of choice for selective mutism. He also urges a focus on behavioral manifestations, including social withdrawal and social skills deficits.

An extensive review, including both psychodynamic and behavioral perspectives, is to be found in a book by Kratochwill and his colleagues (1978).

Maturational Lags and Deficits

For some children the normal sequence of development in motor, language, cognitive, affective, and social areas is disturbed or delayed. These children may demonstrate satisfactory developmental competence in some areas while at the same time showing delayed development in others. A child might, for instance, be competent in language and cognitive and social areas but very poor in motor coordination tasks. Children may show lags in one or more areas at the same time and to varying degrees.

MOTOR DEVELOPMENT AND PERFORMANCE

Problems with gross motor coordination may cause clumsiness and frequent falls or poor skill development. Delays in fine motor coordination may result in inability to use pencils and crayons efficiently or to engage in proper left-to-right tracking of the eyes across a printed page, a skill essential to learning to read. Speech peculiarities may be a consequence of the inability to coordinate the fine motor musculature required in speech. Or delays in ability to control and organize motor behavior may result in hyperactive behavior.

LANGUAGE DEVELOPMENT

Children may experience lags in receptive or expressive language, in the complexity or fluency of language, in the use of oral or written language, or in other aspects of language development. These and other language problems and delays are discussed more fully in Chapter 10.

COGNITIVE FUNCTIONING

A child with a maturational lag may be slow to acquire concepts or have difficulty with other aspects of abstract thought. Such delays are also associated with delays in language development because of the close interaction of the two areas. These delays, which may be relatively slight or very serious, are discussed more fully in Chapter 9 on mental retardation and Chapter 10 on learning disabilities.

AFFECTIVE AND SOCIAL AREAS

Children suffering a lag in affective and social areas may behave in socially immature ways—acting silly, brusque, demanding, dependent, or impulsive—longer than would normally be expected. They may be less able than normal children to cope with stress or to handle play activities with other children. They may show delays in learning to share, in learning to abide by rules, in identifying with and imitating adult behavior, and in their general socialization. Such lags in the attainment of independent functioning have been attributed to maternal overprotection (Levy, 1943), maternal rejection (Clarizio and McCoy, 1976), parental mishandling of dependency during stress (Stendler, 1954), disturbances in the attachment process (Ferguson, 1970), and parental inconsistency in showing nurturant behavior or handling dependent behavior (Ferguson, 1970). While dependence is necessary for proper socialization, excessive dependency may cause problems for children and disturbances in their socialization (Clarizio and McCoy, 1976).

In all cases of maturational lag, the child is behind parental expectations in one or more areas. How such delays are handled can have far-reaching effects. A child who is experiencing a slight language delay, for example, may benefit from patient, extra help from parents who are interested, affectionate, and caring and who view the problem in a calm manner that conveys reassurance. Such a reaction to the child's situation will greatly increase the likelihood of preventing other, more serious difficulties. If the parents panic or become highly exasperated or critical of the child who is experiencing difficulty, they may create other problems, such as decreased motivation. They may exacerbate the original problem, causing a further reduction in language use and fluency because the child will become very self-conscious about speech; they will almost certainly precipitate some damage to the child's developing self-esteem by adding to his or her feelings of failure.

This is not to say that parents should ignore the problem or refuse to help. They should encourage the child by offering positive reinforcement for efforts expended and progress made. They should also investigate the possibility of physical problems which, if found, should be dealt with promptly. They must be careful not to expect more than their children are capable of achieving, as unrealizable expectations cause undue anxiety and frustration. And of course such reactions to delayed functioning as shame, ridicule, and anger can have very negative effects.

Other Developmental Disturbances

The habit disorders and maturational lags described on the preceding pages vary greatly in their severity and in the duration of their effects. Although some of them can be quite persistent, others respond fairly quickly to specific kinds of intervention. There are other more profound developmental disturbances, however, which may have more pervasive effects on the person's development over a very long period of time, if not a lifetime. Mental retardation and severe cognitive-affective disorders such as autism and symbiotic infantile psychosis are examples of long-lasting "developmental disturbances." Since they are given detailed consideration in other chapters, several of the other serious problems of infancy will be considered briefly here.

Greenberg (1970) speaks of *atypical behavior* in infancy. In addition to various feeding, elimination, and sleep disorders, there may be motoric disorders, such as head-banging or rocking, and disturbances in arousal level, with consequent hyper- or hypo-responsiveness (Greenberg, 1970). If such atypical behaviors emerge in infancy, they should not be treated lightly; intervention is necessary to prevent increasingly deviant development (Greenberg, 1970).

Failure-to-thrive is a serious disorder of infancy in which the child's growth is retarded despite adequate food. Although this condition occurs mainly in institutions, it can also occur at home, where it is associated with neglect, depression, and rejection on the part of the parents (Greenberg, 1970). Gains are generally made quickly with good care (Greenberg, 1970).

Severe disorders of infancy may occur in the affective sphere. The classic work of Spitz (1945) and Spitz and Wolf (1946) pointed to the effects of separation from the mother and inadequate stimulation, found most frequently in institutional settings such as hospitals and foundling homes. The authors described *anaclitic depression* in infants, a severe disturbance which involves such depressive symptoms as lethargy, poor appetite, and sadness. In studies of very young children, Spitz identified *hospitalism,* in which physical and mental deterioration follow prolonged hospitalization. Spitz attributed a great part of the children's problem to lack of stimulation and stressed the irreparable damage that is done if mother-child interactions are restricted too much. Spitz's work has been criticized on methodological grounds (Pinneau, 1955), but many others, including Bowlby (1960) and Rutter (1972b), have also emphasized the importance of the early mother-child relationship.

Conclusions

It is evident that a solid grounding in developmental psychology and normal processes and patterns of development is essential to a study of psychological disorders in children and adolescents.

Environmental response to the occurrence of "normal disordered behavior" is crucial in determining whether the child masters the developmental tasks of that period (in which case growth is facilitated) or fails to master those tasks (in which case more serious disorders requiring professional intervention may develop). The weight of the evidence suggests that when intervention is required, behavioral techniques are generally more effective in decreasing maladaptive behaviors than are more psychodynamically oriented therapies alone. However, much more clarification is needed in this area.

Discussion Questions

1. What are some possible reasons for the apparent lack of success or effectiveness of psychotherapy in the treatment of habit disorders?
2. What are some of the means by which maturational lags can be distinguished from other disorders—for example, in the language area? What criteria might be used to make such a distinction?
3. Consider the relative effectiveness of various approaches to the handling of the "normal disturbances" discussed in this chapter. What advice would you offer parents who are faced with some of these common "disturbances" of behavior in their children?

Mental Retardation

The term *mental retardation* embraces all children who are functioning at a retarded level, but causal factors, as well as life experiences, progress, independence, and functional capacity, vary greatly. In this section various subgroups of retarded children will be discussed, along with more general issues and problems related to their care and remediation.

Theoretical/Descriptive Background

Definition

The definition of retardation given by the American Association on Mental Deficiency is as follows: "Mental retardation refers to significantly subaverage general intellectual functioning existing concurrently with deficits in adaptive behavior, and manifested during the developmental period" (Grossman, 1977, p. 11). This definition stresses clearly the important role of subaverage intellectual functioning but also, very importantly, the role of impaired adaptive capacity. Adaptive behavior here is defined as " . . . the effectiveness or degree with which the individual meets the standards of personal independence and social responsibility expected of his age and cultural group" (Grossman, 1973, p. 11). These include sensory-motor, communication, self-help, socialization, academic, and vocational skills (Seim, 1980). As these expectations vary for different ages, deficits of infancy and early childhood likely differ from those of early or late adolescence.

Significantly, the above definition is very behavioral. That is, it refers to the current behavior and status of a child rather than to etiology. It does not imply prognostic statements, as prognosis is more highly correlated with motivation, associated conditions, and opportunity (Grossman, 1973). Low IQ is no longer a sufficient condition for classification as a retarded child. Rather, impaired adaptive capacity must also be present, as is indicated in Figure 9.1.

Although adaptive behavior and intelligence are positively correlated, there is enough individual variation to warrant using separate measures and to require the presence of deficits in both before a label of "retardation" is applied (Grossman, 1973). Thus, a child may be considered retarded at one time and not another; such a classification is always relative to social norms and expectations for the child's chronological age. Social adequacy may be the most basic test, because

INTELLECTUAL FUNCTIONING

	Retarded	Not Retarded
Retarded	Mentally Retarded	Not Mentally Retarded
Not Retarded	Not Mentally Retarded	Not Mentally Retarded

ADAPTIVE BEHAVIOR

FIGURE 9.1   *Adaptive behavior and intellectual functioning. Source:* H. J. Grossman, ed., *Manual on Terminology and Classification in Mental Retardation* (Washington, D.C.: American Association on Mental Deficiency, 1977), p. 14. Reprinted by permission.

many children who have adequate social skills would be identified as retarded if the psychometric definition (IQ below 70) alone were used (Telford and Sawrey, 1977).

The AAMD definition excludes the "borderline retarded" category, substituting "borderline intelligence" as the preferred term. Borderline intellectual functioning refers to a child with an IQ between 71 and 84 and associated adaptive deficits (APA, 1980).

According to the Diagnostic and Statistical Manual of Mental Disorders (APA, 1980), or the DSM-111, other disorders such as hyperactivity and attentional deficits are three or four times more common in retarded than in normal children, although they are not always present. There may be other behavioral problems or neurological disorders as well.

Classification

The labels people use tend to depend on their professional vantage point and remedial emphasis. For example, educators have traditionally used the terms "educable" and "trainable" mentally retarded in describing retarded children because such terms are descriptive of the teachers' educational goals for specific children or groups of children. Psychologists and psychiatrists, on the other hand, more frequently classify retarded children according to IQ level. They may speak of mildly, moderately, or severely retarded children, for example, terms which have replaced the much older and fortunately obsolete terms of moron, imbecile, and idiot. Many would now like to eliminate the term retardation altogether and refer to these children as mildly, moderately, or severely developmentally handicapped. A comparison of the labels and classifications is reproduced in Figure 9.2.

Classification of retarded children according to the AAMD definition requires an assessment of their level of functioning in both intellectual and adaptive areas. The WISC-R and Stanford-Binet are standard measures used to assess IQ, and their intellectual criterion for retardation is an IQ of 70 or below, which is two or more standard deviations below the mean. The child's adaptive behavior can also be categorized in four major levels, from I to IV. If specific norms were available, Level I would also be comparable to two standard deviation units below the mean (Grossman, 1973). According to Grossman, the AAMD Adaptive Behavior Scale (Nihira et al., 1974), the Vineland Social Maturity Scale, and other assessment devices can be used to measure various behaviors that contribute to the individual's overall adaptation. Patterns of adaptive behavior and associated age-expectations should be noted in order to estimate the extent of an individual's deficits. Such patterns can also be used to plan the individual's remediation program.

Mentally retarded children are sometimes classified according to etiology, but such classification is not recommended because it is of no value in planning an educational program and because neurological tests lack the sophistication necessary to detect damage in every case (Hallahan and Kauffman, 1978).

Children who are classified as *mildly retarded* have IQs between 50 and 70; they comprise 80 percent of the mentally retarded population (APA, 1980). These are the children sometimes referred to as "educable." They are not noticeably different from normals in their physical characteristics and general health. According to the DSM-III, children in this category are often indistinguishable from normal children. During the preschool years they can develop language and social skills, and they have little sensorimotor impairment. They are capable of about grade six academic skills. As adults they can adequately pursue many occupations (Telford and Sawrey, 1977), although they may need outside assistance when they face stressful situations.

Children classified as *moderately retarded* have IQs between 35 and 49, and their adaptive capacity is more seriously impaired. Sometimes referred to as "trainable," they represent approximately 12 percent of

Educational terms	Intelligence measure	Obsolete terms	Adaptive behavior	Rate of development & learning	% Incidence
	Normal 85–115			Normal or standard rate	68.26
Slow learner 75–89	Borderline 70–84	Moron 50–84	Level I	$\frac{4}{5}$ to $\frac{9}{10}$ normal rate	13.59
Educable 50–74	Mild retardation 55–69		Level II	$\frac{1}{2}$ to $\frac{3}{4}$ normal rate	2.14	83
	Moderate retardation 40–54	Imbecile 20–49	Level III		
Trainable 25–49	Severe retardation 40 (Wechsler) 20–35 (Binet)		Level IV	$\frac{1}{4}$ to $\frac{1}{2}$ normal rate	0.13	13
Custodial 25	Profound retardation 20 (Binet)	Idiot 0–19	Level V	0 to $\frac{1}{4}$ normal rate	.01	4

FIGURE 9.2 *Comparison of developmental characteristics and classification categories of mentally retarded children.*
Source: Robert D. Seim, "Development Characteristics of Mentally Retarded Children: Classification Categories Compared," from a lecture presented at the Institute for the Study of Learning Disabilities, St. Jerome's College, University of Waterloo, Ontario, 1980. Used by permission.

the retarded population (APA, 1980). According to the DSM-III, they can learn to talk or communicate during the preschool years, but are only minimally aware of social conventions. They can benefit from vocational or occupational and social training and with supervision can care for themselves. They are not likely, however, to exceed a grade two level of academic achievement. As adults they may be partially self-supporting in semiskilled or unskilled settings but need close supervision and require guidance when faced with even mild stress.

Children classified as *severely retarded* have IQs between 20 and 34 (APA, 1980); they are sometimes referred to as the "dependent retarded" (Grossman, 1973). They account for about 7 percent of the retarded population (APA, 1980). According to the DSM-III, children in this category manifest poor motor development during the preschool years and develop little or no speech. They may learn to talk during their later school years and can learn basic hygienic skills. They profit little from vocational training, but as adults they may be able to do simple work tasks with close supervision. Unlike mildly retarded children, who are found more frequently in the lower socioeconomic level, the severely retarded are randomly distributed across socioeconomic levels and do not have higher numbers of siblings and parents who are retarded (Birch et al., 1970). They are more likely to have clear or demonstrable organic problems.

Children classified as *profoundly retarded* have IQs of less than 20 (APA, 1980); they are sometimes referred to as "life-support" individuals (Grossman, 1973). They account for only about 1 percent of the retarded (APA, 1980). According to the DSM-III, they manifest only minimal sensorimotor functioning during their preschool years. They may show some motor development during the later school years, and many benefit from minimal self-care training. Although when they reach adulthood some speech and greater motor development may occur and they may be capable of very limited self-care, they require constant supervision in a very structured environment.

The DSM-III also includes an "unspecified" category in which retardation is presumed but the child cannot be tested because impairment is too severe, because the child is too uncooperative, or because the child is an infant.

Although these categories can serve as guidelines, they do not dictate intervention programs. Individual children may sometimes be best served in programs designated for other categories (Grossman, 1973).

As helpful and behavioral as the AAMD classification system is, Taylor (1980) found it used surprisingly rarely in the literature. His review of research in the AAMD and mental retardation journals revealed the following: 28 percent of the authors used the definition; 20 percent of all of the articles reviewed had made small errors in terminological use; and accuracy could not be determined in an additional 23 percent of the articles. Forty percent used only the terms "mental retardation" and "retardation," with no information regarding level of retardation or classification.

Diagnostic Considerations

As classification can significantly influence the kind of help a child receives and the plans that are made, careful diagnostic assessment is imperative. The definition of the intellectual criterion includes the proviso that the IQ rating be attained through individually administered tests rather than brief or group tests (Grossman, 1973). In addition, because adaptive functioning is one of the major criteria and adaptive scales are not sufficiently valid or reliable to be used alone, good clinical judgment in the assessment of adaptive behavior is essential (APA, 1980). Parents can be involved in diagnostic procedures, because the laboratory-type assessment situation has diagnostic value in itself (Brown, 1975). Some clinicians prefer to do "psycho-situational assessments" within more normal contexts and situations, such as classrooms, where children's actual abilities, functioning, and intelligent behavior can be assessed and observed as the children interact with the environment (Bersoff, 1973).

Although such observation is not likely to replace IQ scores in the very near future, it is certainly an important source of additional information about children and their functional and adaptive capacity. IQ scores as usually measured can give helpful information when they are seen in the context of a child's functioning in a wide variety of situations, including real-life ones (Brown, 1980). Generally, the younger the child is, the more difficult it is to diagnose mental retardation, except in the case of profoundly impaired children (APA, 1980).

Another problem in accurately diagnosing retarded children is distinguishing between retardation as a primary classification and retardation as a secondary symptom in other disorders. Some children who are very disturbed may function at a retarded level during the course of their disorder but not after effective intervention. For example, a child who is severely depressed may, on a measure of intelligence such as an IQ test, obtain a very low score and simultaneously show very poor adaptive skills. Although that child could be classified as mentally retarded according to the AAMD definition, he or she may actually be manifesting retarded functioning only as a symptom secondary to the depression. Conversely, a child with Down's syndrome would be classified as mentally retarded as a primary classification. The types of retardation being dealt with in this chapter are examples of the primary classification.

Finally, other problems—deafness, for example—can result in a mistaken or inaccurate diagnosis of retardation unless the central problem is discovered. Hence the need for careful, thorough diagnostic procedures must again be underscored.

Personality and Learning Characteristics

Considerable study has been devoted to the areas of attention and memory, which are crucial to the understanding of retarded children. Deficits in memory, especially of abstract material (Suran and Rizzo, 1979), and attentional problems (Robinson and Robinson, 1970; Suran and Rizzo, 1979) have been reported. There is some evidence to indicate that retarded children demonstrate short-term but not long-term memory deficits when compared with nonretarded children. That is, there are differences in immediate recall and hence what gets into the memory system, but no differences once the material is in that system (Brown, 1980). The short-term memories may be poor because such children do not use good learning strategies such as grouping items and rehearsal, although they can be taught to use such rehearsal (Hallahan and Kauffman, 1978).

Mentally retarded children are sometimes characterized as more rigid than those who are at the same mental age level but who are chronologically younger. Zigler (1971) reported data to support the notion that such rigidity is in part a result of social deprivation and increased motivation for social reinforcement rather than intellectual retardation. He found, for instance, that noninstitutionalized retarded

194

(and hence less socially deprived) and normal children did not differ significantly on his experimental task, but both differed significantly from institutionalized retarded.

A higher number of personality and behavior disorders have been attributed to mentally retarded over normal children, but there is disagreement regarding the extent and the cause of such disorders (Brown, 1980). Among children who do not have clear physiological deficits, there is much evidence against the existence of unique personality characteristics (Brown, 1980). In other words, retarded and nonretarded of the same *mental* age are similar, although retarded and nonretarded of the same chronological age do differ. Therefore, perhaps personality develops more slowly in retarded than in normal children but does not involve unique characteristics. In addition, low social acceptance may lead to a low self-concept (Suran and Rizzo, 1979).

Mentally retarded children have been described as more other-directed and dependent than normal children, perhaps as a result of their frequent past failures and their tendency to mistrust their own solutions (Zigler, 1969). On the other hand, some retarded children may actually experience less failure than normal children because their environment rewards success and ignores failure; their learning might even improve if they were more realistically made aware of their failures as well as their successes (Brown, 1980).

Cognitive Deficits or Delay

Retarded children show deficits in basic cognitive processes such as perception, reasoning, and memory when they are compared with normal children of the same chronological age, but the distinctions are less clear when they are compared with nonretarded children of the same mental age (Brown, 1980).

An ongoing controversy between deficit and difference hypotheses concerns the type of learning problems experienced by mildly retarded children without obvious physiological damage or disorders. According to Zigler (1969, 1971), who holds a developmental view, cognitive development in such mildly retarded children progresses through the same sequence of stages as that of normals but at a slower *rate* and to a lower upper *limit*. Zigler suggests that this relationship between rate and limit of retarded and normal children is similar to the one between normal and superior children, and maintains that cognitive achievement or performance is determined by the cognitive level of the person, regardless of how long it took to get to that level.

The cognitive development and associated cognitive processes affect the quality of information-processing, which in turn profoundly affects behavior; but the tendency to view retarded children as a homogeneous subgroup with specific personality deficits arises in part from categorization and labeling (Zigler, 1971). Zigler advocates looking not only at how retarded children differ from normals but also at how they are similar.

The defect or difference theorists, according to Zigler, would argue that the levels are not the same in persons with different IQs. That is, if a person with an IQ of 66 and one with an IQ of 100 are both at one cognitive level (but at different chronological ages), their functioning is not the same. The defect or difference theorists would maintain that such scores reflect more than just *rate* of cognitive development and include how the child processes information. As different rates of development and different IQs reflect differences in the rate of processing information and learning, at every level children with low IQs will handle tasks requiring information processing and learning differently from those with high IQs (Weir, 1967).

Causation

There are three hundred known or suspected causal factors in mental retardation, but such factors account for fewer than 25 percent of the retarded population (Love, 1973). For the other three-quarters, mostly children with IQs of 50 or higher, the etiology of the disorder is unclear (Birch et al., 1970). Some of the causes are well known, and some children can be treated early enough to prevent retardation from developing. Others are less clearly discernible but correlate highly in the backgrounds of retarded children. Terms that were previously used to separate mental retardation into cases of *endogenous* (genetic and constitutional, or "inner") and *exogenous* (biological, physical, and social influence, or "external") origin are now obsolete (Grossman, 1973). They have been replaced by the newer "cultural-familial retardation" and "organic/brain-damage" respectively (Hallahan and Kauffman, 1978).

196

ORGANIC/PHYSIOLOGICAL CAUSES

Hereditary Factors

Arthur Jensen (1969) created a predictable uproar when he rekindled the nature-nurture controversy during the 1960s. He maintained that most racial and social class differences in intellectual level are a function of inherited differences and that environmental factors and events play a minor role. Of those environmental factors that do exist, he suggested that prenatal ones have the greatest influence (Jensen, 1970). Jensen's views led him to question the assumptions of some specific educational and enrichment programs regarding the important influence of environmental and cultural differences on IQ scores; he stressed instead the development of specific skills.

Earlier work of Skodak and Skeels (1949), however, in their study of one hundred adopted children, revealed that adopted children had a consistently higher intellectual level than what might have been predicted from the educational, socioeconomic, and intellectual level of their natural parents. They had apparently responded to security, intellectual stimulation, and an emotionally healthy relationship. The higher intellectual level of those adopted in early infancy was maintained into adolescence. In another study Skeels (1966) reported attainment of normal intelligence levels by retarded children after a program of early nurturance and stimulation.

Such evidence directly contradicts that of Jensen and supports the much more widely held view that environmental influence is of critical importance. Individuals may vary, however, according to their genetic constitution, in their susceptibility to possible harmful factors (Robinson and Robinson, 1970). And although the environment is likely to be maximally important during the early months and years, when intellectual development is most rapid, it is not clear how great or how permanent such influence is (Hunt, 1961).

Some writers have urged that we ask how heredity and environment interact or how they contribute to behavior rather than which one is more important (Girardeau, 1971). According to Girardeau, researchers should work on answering specific questions within the following more general one: "'Given X set of biological characteristics, what procedures are necessary and sufficient to develop Y behavior, maintain Y behavior, and reduce or eliminate Y behavior?'" (p. 342). The assumption of biological deficit does not lead clearly to ideas about which factors should be changed or manipulated to improve functioning (Brown, 1980), but biological researchers can ask questions about how to change the X set of biological characteristics to make the Y behavior easier to control or develop (Girardeau, 1971).

Hormonal and Metabolic Problems

There are many hormonal and metabolic disorders and dysfunctions that may result in mental retardation in children. Carter's (1970) handbook, for example, devotes approximately forty pages to describing specific enzyme defects and their resultant disorders alone. Only the most frequent and best-known hormonal and metabolic problems are mentioned here. For more detailed discussions of these disorders and the resultant symptoms, as well as more extensive coverage of other disorders, the reader is referred to Carter (1970).

Phenylketonuria (PKU) is an inherited defect in enzyme activity which affects one in approximately 15,000 children in the United States (Carter, 1970). Infants with PKU may seem normal during the first few weeks after birth, but within six months they show marked motor retardation, which may also be accompanied by severe behavior problems and, usually, profound retardation (Mordock, 1975). Broad screening programs and diet therapy have reduced the number of individuals with this disorder from its previous level of 1 percent of the retarded population (Carter, 1970). *Tay-Sachs disease* is another inherited disorder. Jewish children are disproportionately represented among the sufferers (Carter, 1970). Children with this disorder look normal until about the middle of their first year, when nerve cell degeneration begins and associated body functions decline, until death occurs between ages two and four (Carter, 1970). *Cretinism (hypothyroidism)*, which results from a dysfunction of the thyroid gland, occurs in approximately one-half of 1 percent of the institutionally retarded (Love, 1973). Most children with this disorder suffer severe retardation, although good results can be obtained if treatment is begun early (Love, 1973).

Down's syndrome (mongolism) is a genetic disorder involving an abnormal number or pattern of chromosomes, with resultant severe retardation. Children with this disorder account for 15 percent of the institutionally retarded (Love, 1973). The risk of giving birth to a child with Down's syndrome increases with maternal age after thirty or thiry-five years (Smith and Wilson, 1973)—that is, women who become pregnant after that age are more likely to bear children with Down's syndrome. Children afflicted with this disorder have characteristic physical features, have a slower rate of mental and language development (see Figure 9.3), and have difficulty learning advanced or complex skills. According to Smith and Wilson (1973), 20 to 40 percent of such children do not live beyond the first few months or years, with heart defects causing the highest number of deaths in the first year. Their research indicated that those who received more early stimulation at home progressed more quickly on certain tasks than those in institutions. For example, of those children at home, 44 percent were walking by age two and 78 percent by age three. In contrast, none in the institutional group was walking by age two and only 6 percent by age three, although the differences were much smaller later. By age five, 95 percent of children at home and 84 percent of

FIGURE 9.3 *Early developmental performance of Down's syndrome children raised at home compared to that of normal children. The widest point in each diamond represents the average age for performance, and the spread of the diamonds represents the range. Source:* D. W. Smith and A. A. Wilson, *The Child with Down's Syndrome (Mongolism)* (Philadelphia: W. B. Saunders Co., 1973), p. 37. Reprinted by permission.

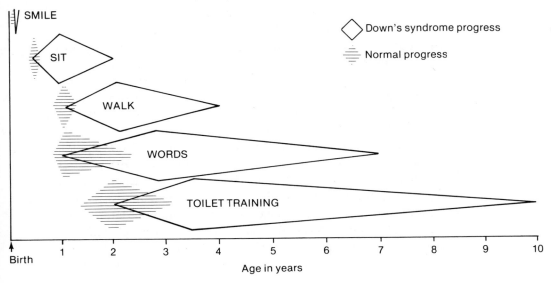

those in institutions were walking. The authors therefore concluded that the environment in which the children develop is an important influence on the timing of their developmental milestones and on early performance.

Hydrocephaly involves a fluid accumulation in the cranium which causes enlargement of the head. As the enlargement continues and skull sutures separate, infants become increasingly helpless because of difficulty supporting their head and because of brain damage (Mordock, 1975). IQs of children with this disorder are usually under 50 (Love, 1973). *Microcephaly* is the opposite of hydrocephaly anatomically; it is characterized by a small brain and head. According to Carter (1970), it can be genetically caused or can be due to various prenatal events or factors.

Prenatal Influences

Teratogenesis refers to changes that occur in the uterine environment at critical developmental periods. These changes may result from metabolic abnormalities of the mother or from viral, physical, or chemical agents or events and may result in structural defects (Carter, 1970). Examples of these agents include radiation, viruses, vitamins, hormones, and drugs (such as thalidomide). The dosage and timing of exposure are very important in determining the effect of the agents. Viruses constitute one of the most frequent causes of prenatal infection leading to retardation. Such an infection may be mild in the mother but disastrous for the fetus (Carter, 1970). Mumps and chickenpox early in pregnancy, as well as some forms of influenza and German measles (rubella), can have adverse effects, especially if they occur during the first trimester of pregnancy; the degree of retardation hinges on the extent and location of the damage (Carter, 1970).

Fetal alcohol syndrome refers to mental and physical retardation caused by heavy alcohol intake of pregnant women (APA, 1980). Poor nutrition, which might occur alone or in combination with excessive use of alcohol, can also have serious consequences for the fetus. Birth injury or insufficient oxygen during and immediately after birth (anoxia) can result in brain damage and consequent retardation. Retardation has also been associated with prematurity, perhaps because of a more difficult birth process (Telford and Sawrey, 1977). Other possible prenatal influences include lead poisoning; carbon monoxide poisoning, which can lead to anoxia; ingestion of other toxins; blood incompatibilities; and allergic reactions such as might occur with immunization during pregnancy (Carter, 1970).

Postnatal Problems

Postnatal physiological or organic problems that can result in retardation include infections such as meningitis or encephalitis, lesions, hemorrhaging, or child abuse (Carter, 1970). There can also be toxic influences, such as ingestion of lead and other poisons, or injuries. Malnutrition in infants and young children can also cause developmental problems or permanent retardation; it is often considered to be the greatest single factor in mortality and morbidity (Carter, 1970). However, correlations with nutrition decrease greatly when economic and social status are held constant (Telford and Sawrey, 1977).

CULTURAL-FAMILIAL RETARDATION

Cultural-familial retardation refers to etiological aspects in the 75 percent of retarded children for whom there is no clear organic pathology and whose retardation is presumed to be due to a combination of hereditary and environmental factors. Children in this category are usually mildly retarded (IQ of 50–70), and the incidence of retardation is higher in their families (APA, 1980). The lower socioeconomic level is disproportionately represented. The children's physiological functioning may be somewhat below normal because of less than adequate physical care; more importantly, there is often an absence of good reinforcers for intelligent behavior (Girardeau, 1971).

Characteristics found more frequently in the families of these children include a higher number of complications during pregnancy, delivery, and infancy; larger family size (five or more children); greater crowding; and unskilled or semiskilled labor as the premarital work background of the mother (Birch et al., 1970). For some children, even minimal damage in such an impoverished environment may be sufficient to lead to retardation; the same level of damage might not affect IQ nearly so much in a more enriched environment (Birch et al., 1970). Children in the impoverished environment may experience intellectual, social, or linguistic deprivation; genetic, environmental, biological, and early child-rearing influences, singly or in combination, are probably involved (APA, 1980). There is no evidence yet for genetic transmission as a major cause of cultural-familial retardation (Girardeau, 1971). A diagnosis of cultural-familial retardation is a presumptive diagnosis, not a positive one (Robinson and Robinson, 1970).

The term mental retardation, then, encompasses a very heterogeneous group of children with very diverse causal factors, adaptive and functional skills, remedial needs, and prognostic outlooks. The following case study illustrates the way in which a child may be considered retarded at one time and not at another, the kinds of problems retarded children experience, and the advantages of using many different remedial interventions.

CASE STUDY

Anne was a fifteen-year-old girl who was unable to manage many basic self-care behaviors such as shampooing her hair, shopping, making change, or helping with routine chores. Although there were suggestions of possible brain damage, no current tests revealed such damage. Overprotection and isolation of Anne by her parents contributed to her inability to function independently and to learn new skills.

Psychological assessment of Anne revealed a Full Scale IQ of 66 on the WISC-R. This score, in addition to her poor adaptive skills and her age, indicated that she met the AAMD definition criteria for retardation and was within the mildly retarded range. She also had poor motor skills, very limited language skills, and little factual knowledge of the world around her. Her drawings, one of which is reproduced in Figure 9.4, were impoverished for someone her age and were very similar to those of chronologically much younger children. Her laborious and ineffective method for attempting to arrive at the solution to a math problem (809 $\times$ 47) is illustrated in Figure 9.5. Her very concrete approach to the problem was similar to that of younger children who still count on their fingers and precluded the handling of more advanced tasks.

The main goal of her treatment was to increase her adaptive functioning, and many different techniques were used. She was involved in a behavior modification program in which she earned tokens for appropriate behavior which could then be used for special treats or outings. In addition, she was given much individual help in learning self-care skills, such as shampooing her hair, eating properly, making change, and caring for her clothes. She was also given considerable training

202

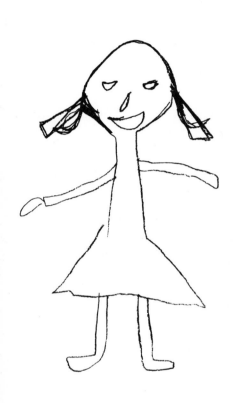

$9 \times 1 = 9$
$9 \times 2 = 18$
$9 \times 3 = 27$ $4 \times 1 = 7$
$9 \times 4 \ 36$ $4 \times 2 = 8$
$9 \times 5 \ 45$ $4 \times 3 = 12$
$9 \times 6 \ 54$ 4×4
$9 \times 7 \ 62$

$8 \times 1 - 8$
$2 \times 2 - 16$
$8 \times 3 = 27$ $3 \ 4 \ 5 \ 6 \ 7 \ 8 \ 9 \ 10 \ 11 \ 12$
$8 \times 4 = 32$

$13 \ 14 \ 15 \ 16 \ 17 \ 18 \ 19 \ 20$

FIGURE 9.4   FIGURE 9.5

and assistance in developing better basic social skills in order to improve her relationships with other children and with adults. She was given training in linguistic skills and encouraged to use language to communicate her needs and feelings. Gradually she was allowed greater independence, which she welcomed and was proud of.

As a result of her treatment program, she was able to become involved in a sheltered workshop and develop some craft skills. She gradually increased her time there until she was attending nearly full time and was deriving a good deal of satisfaction from her work and from her relationships with other people there.

Later psychometric testing yielded a Full Scale IQ of 77. The increase in IQ was largely due to her increased use of language, her greater involvement with other people, and her generally increased awareness and knowledge of the world around her. Based on the later testing, she would no longer be considered retarded according to the AAMD definition, though she was still within the borderline range of intellectual functioning.

Remediation

Although a small percentage of retarded children respond to medication, changes in diet, or psychotherapy, the main aspects of helping most of them to achieve their maximum level of functioning are education and good care (Achenbach, 1974). Various kinds of educational programs, techniques, and strategies which have been used to teach specific skills and increase overall independence and adaptive functioning are discussed in the following section. It is the responsibility of the clinician and the team of professionals involved to work out the most effective program possible, based on a thorough and careful assessment of the individual child's needs, the family, and the resources of the school and the community.

Special Education

Remedial needs vary widely at different levels of retardation. Mildly retarded children, for instance, need readiness skills and training in adaptive social behavior; the moderately retarded need training in functional skills such as self-help skills, vocational skills, and social and communication skills; and the severely and profoundly retarded need self-help and survival skills (Hallahan and Kauffman, 1978).

The most appropriate kind of educational setting and program depends in large part on the level of severity, from regular classes for the least severely retarded to institutions for the severely and profoundly retarded. The most common settings are regular classes, resource rooms where children receive specific help for part of the day, and specialized classes or schools. Some have suggested that the academic progress of retarded children is affected little by their placement (Jones et al., 1978); others consider special classes inferior to regular class placement for children with IQs below average (Carlberg and Kavale, 1980). Since the passage of Public Law 94-142 (the Education for All Handicapped Children Act) in 1975, public schools are required to provide an appropriate education for all handicapped children, designed with their unique needs in mind. Furthermore, the legislation requires that they be educated in the "least restrictive environment." That is, they must be educated in as normal an environment as their particular needs permit—with nonhandicapped children if possible. Wherever they are placed, knowledge of their particular deficits and information-processing difficulties must be used to design specific intervention programs (Schwartz and Johnson, 1981).

Behavioral Techniques

Behavior modification techniques have been used increasingly to improve social and adaptive skills of retarded children. Such skill training involves less emphasis on developing insight into reasons for behavior than on analyzing specific social deficits in terms of the particular verbal and nonverbal behaviors involved (Hersen and Eisler, 1976). It is often used with severely and profoundly retarded children because of its emphasis on task analysis and its success where other methods have failed (Hallahan and Kauffman, 1978).

Operant techniques have been used successfully to improve toilet behavior in severe institutional retardates (Giles and Wolf, 1966). Crisp and Coll (1980) taught a thirteen-year-old profoundly retarded institutionalized child to use a walking frame by applying positive tactile and verbal reinforcements and ignoring his head-banging. This skill increased kinesthetic stimulation for the child and allowed him to initiate activity and interact with others; it also decreased his motivation for stimulation through self-injurious behavior.

Operant techniques have also been used successfully in groups of children to reduce disruptive behavior (Sulzbacher and Houser, 1968; Zimmerman, Zimmerman, and Russell, 1969) and attentional problems (Zimmerman, Zimmerman, and Russell, 1969). There has also been interest not only in changing specific behaviors but in studying critical events in the environment that influence behavior in the long run (Weisberg, 1971).

Successful training in self-instruction with cognitively impulsive mentally retarded adolescents demonstrated that they, too, could use language for behavioral control (Peters and Davies, 1981). Social skills training which included instruction, feedback, reinforcement, role-playing, and modeling was also effective in raising the level of social skills in two moderately retarded boys up to or beyond that of normal controls (Matson, Kazdin, and Esveldt-Dawson, 1980).

Parent Training and Education

One of the advantages of behavioral approaches is that the techniques can be taught to parents and teachers and other nonprofessionals who can then train others—even other retardates—to apply learning principles, thus creating a "therapeutic pyramid" (Achenbach, 1974, p. 254).

When behavioral techniques are taught to nonprofessionals such as parents, it is necessary to determine whether such training has lasting results. Research data suggest a tentative yes. One follow-up study done fourteen months after a twenty-week training program (Baker and Heifetz, 1980) showed that ninety-five families had retained the knowledge they had gained of program principles, and their children had maintained their skill gains. In addition, nearly a half continued to practice "useful teaching."

Institutionalization

There is general agreement that institutionalization should be avoided if possible. When it is necessary, small residences in the community are more desirable than the large, often poorly staffed, primarily custodial institutions that have served so often in the past (Suran and Rizzo, 1979). There has been a growing tendency to view mental retardation as a problem of the family and community, and a greater emphasis is now being placed on the need to develop other forms of help within the community such as day care, educational programs, and parent training and guidance (Grossman, 1972). As more community-based help becomes available, institutional care can be reduced, especially for mildly retarded children.

Caring for retarded children at home is usually thought to put great stress on the families involved (Hallahan and Kauffman, 1978). However, Grossman (1972) has pointed out that institutionalization can have negative effects on both the retarded and the normal children in a family. He believes normal children do not necessarily benefit from institutionalization of a retarded child; in fact, unless undue demands are made on the normal children to help care for a retarded sibling, they may actually cope better if the retarded child is kept at home. This, of course, depends in large part on the characteristics, attitudes, and resources of individual families.

Vocational Training

Mildly retarded adolescents can benefit from work-study programs in which academic and vocational training are coordinated (Clark and Rosen, 1973; Hallahan and Kauffman, 1978). Many can then adjust successfully in the community. Moderately retarded individuals can also profit from vocational and occupational training which facilitates the development of greater independence. The kinds of jobs available to mildly and moderately retarded individuals depend, of course, on the level of their adaptive behavior, mental age, motivation, and training, as well as on the cooperation of the general population (Hallahan and Kauffman, 1978). Retarded individuals are frequently placed in sheltered workshops where they can learn skills and then put them to use under conditions of protection and minimal stress. They can also benefit greatly from assistance in developing skills in such job-related areas as filling out applications, proper interview behavior, management of money, and appropriate on-the-job behavior.

Infant Stimulation Programs

There has been considerable interest in early infant stimulation programs as a means by which mental retardation might be prevented or its severity lessened. In one program, special stimulation was given to infants who were critically ill and therefore had even less contact with their mothers than did other premature newborns. Intended to make them more socially responsive, the stimulation resulted in both psychological and physical benefits (Brown and Hepler, 1976). Other studies (Garber and Heber, 1973; Powell, 1974; Scarr-Salapatek and Williams, 1973) have also provided evidence for the positive effects of early infant stimulation programs in improving the developmental progress of infants.

Skeels (1966) earlier had been able to reverse the developmental direction of some retarded children through a planned program of nurturance and stimulation during infancy, followed by placement in normal and loving adoptive homes. These children attained normal intelligence levels, which they maintained as adults. As adults they were also more frequently self-supporting, independent, and married and more highly educated than a comparison group, which had higher intelligence at the start but was placed in a less stimulating environment (an orphanage) for a prolonged time. The latter group showed progressive retardation and required expensive custodial care. Skeels concluded that one cannot predict later intelligence from early observation, as many children born with sound constitutions and normal potential may become retarded without proper care.

Computer-Assisted Instruction

Lally (1981), working with mildly retarded children, used a "talking computer" to supplement conventional methods of teaching associations between written words and oral versions of those words. He found an average increase in sight vocabulary of 128 percent in the group using the computer and only 34 percent in a comparison group. The increase remained for more than twenty-three weeks following the four-week training program.

The use of computers can increase the motivation and interest of mildly retarded children who have long histories of problems in school. In addition to being a highly interesting medium, it offers immediate feedback, provides an opportunity for repetition and review, and allows individuals to work at their own rate of speed.

Psychotherapy

Psychotherapy, or verbal therapies, have usually been considered to be of little value in the remedial programs of retarded children because of communication difficulties (Clark and Rosen, 1973), difficulties with abstract thought, distractibility, and other problems, although supportive therapy with families has generally been found helpful. More recently, however, some workers have reported increasing evidence that with significant modifications, both individual and group psychotherapy can work and are desirable (Mowatt, 1970; Suran and Rizzo, 1979). Multiple family therapy, in which several families are seen together, can be useful in reducing feelings of stigma and isolation and in providing support for the families (Mowatt, 1970).

Prevention

Although mental retardation cannot be completely eradicated, much can be done to reduce the incidence and to minimize its severity. Even before pregnancy, good immunization programs and genetic counseling regarding inheritable disorders can be enormously helpful. Amniocentesis, or the study of amniotic cells, can be undertaken in cases where hormonal or metabolic disorders are suspected. Advice on and help with such problems as Rh incompatibility should be available. During pregnancy, good prenatal care is essential, including prenatal education and information regarding the physical and psychological factors involved in normal, healthy development. Good nutrition for pregnant women as well as for infants and young children is mandatory. Restraint in the use of or exposure to medication, alcohol, toxins, and other teratogenic agents during pregnancy is also essential.

Other important preventive work includes birth control for high-risk populations, biochemical screening of newborns, and parent training (Robinson and Robinson, 1970). High-risk infants should be monitored closely, and education and training in infant stimulation programs should be promoted. Widespread immunization programs and good, accessible medical care are also important.

All of these programs, if actively promoted and effectively implemented, would go a long way toward reducing the incidence and severity of retardation among children.

Discussion Questions

1. Discuss Arthur Jensen's views of the factors involved in the development of intelligence and the relative contributions of heredity and environment. What evidence exists to support or refute his views?
2. Examine the merits and disadvantages of regular and special classroom placement for mildly retarded children.
3. Which specific skills do you feel are most essential for a retarded individual to develop? Discuss how the development of those skills might best be accomplished.

CHAPTER 10 # Learning
Disabilities

Among the areas of study of children with problems, learning disabilities is one of the newest. Only within the past two decades has the term "learning disabilities" even been used, although much of the groundwork for dealing with such children had been laid much earlier. The fact that Kirk's 1962 book *Educating Exceptional Children* included only ten or twelve pages on learning disabilities out of nearly four hundred pages, compared with the many complete texts available today, is striking evidence of the newness of this field.

In the first half of this century Orton (1937) described the developmental and language disorders of children with whom he worked, including alexia (disability in reading), agraphia (disability in writing), developmental motor aphasia (delayed speech), apraxia (clumsiness), word deafness, and stuttering. At approximately the same time, Grace Fernald (1943) was using a multisensory approach with children with learning problems. The field received another boost from the work of Albert Strauss in the 1940s. Strauss and Lehtinen (1947), working with brain-injured children, noted various thinking and behavior disorders in the children they saw and suggested some general principles to be heeded in teaching them. Strauss generated a great deal of controversy by assuming brain damage in all children who demonstrated certain symptoms common to brain-injured children, such as hyperactivity or figure-ground problems (Werner and Strauss, 1941). The considerable criticism he received for this notion significantly increased the interest in and study of children with these problems. During the 1960s, partly as a result of the work of Kephart (1960) and others, study of learning disabilities mushroomed, as indicated by the proliferation of articles and books focusing on "learning disabilities."

Theoretical/Descriptive Background

There is still much controversy concerning many aspects of the field of learning disabilities, including disagreement over the *definition* of the object of study. The confusion is due in part to the fact that several kinds of handicaps or problems often overlap, such as emotional disturbance with physical handicaps (Kirk and Kirk, 1971); also, it is hard to differentiate specific learning disabilities from other learning problems. Disabilities in reading (dyslexia), writing (dysgraphia), and math (dyscalculia) must be distinguished from the more generalized learning problems that develop as a result of attentional deficits or hyperactivity, for example. Moreover, the frequent, though not inevitable, occurrence of associated problems such as behavioral problems has contributed to the terminological and diagnostic confusion in this area.

Children with the problems to be described in this chapter have been variously labeled as learning disabled, perceptually handicapped, minimally brain damaged, educationally handicapped, and neurologically impaired, depending on the orientation and biases of the diagnostician. Thus, many definitions of learning disability have been employed, some more inclusive than others.

There is reasonable agreement, however, that the term "specific learning disability" refers to the condition of those children who have average or above average intelligence and who do not have significant physical or emotional problems, but who nevertheless have great difficulty learning in the regular classroom, with conventional methods of teaching. The definition included in Public Law 94-142 (the Education for All Handicapped Children Act) has two parts. The first, adopted from the National Advisory Committee on Handicapped Children, is reproduced here:

> "Specific learning disability" means a disorder in one or more of the basic psychological processes involved in understanding or in using language spoken or written, which may manifest itself in an imperfect ability to listen, think, speak, read, write, spell, or to do mathematical calculations. The term includes such conditions as perceptual handicaps, brain injury, minimal brain dysfunction, dyslexia, developmental aphasia. The term does not include children who have learning problems which are primarily the result of visual, hearing, or motor handicaps, of mental retardation, of emotional disturbance, or of environmental, cultural, or economic disadvantage. (Lerner, 1981, p. 7)

The second part of the definition provides operational guidelines for evaluating such disorders (Lerner, 1981).

There are no clear *incidence* figures because of the terminological confusion and disagreement, but estimates range from 1 to 30 percent (Hallahan and Kauffman, 1978). The U.S. Office of Education (1975) estimated that approximately 3 percent of children under nineteen years of age are afflicted. As with most disorders, there is a highly disproportionate number of boys in the learning-disabled population.

This higher number of boys may reflect different maturation rates, different cultural expectations, or "biological vulnerability" of the male sex (Owen et al., 1971).

Areas of Difficulty

The problems faced by learning-disabled children can involve many different areas.

PERCEPTION

Although learning-disabled children have adequate visual and auditory acuity, their interpretation of the input through those modalities is often inaccurate or distorted. Within the *visual* sphere they may have difficulty with such perceptual tasks as visual discrimination (telling a "b" from a "d," for instance) and visual closure (recognizing an object with only partial clues). They may reverse letters or words; they may have poor visual memory and thus fail to remember words; or they may have visual figure-ground problems. Within the *auditory* sphere, they may have difficulty with auditory discrimination (telling one sound from another), auditory blending (putting sounds together to form words), or sequencing within words. They may have problems in the area of auditory memory and thus not recall previously learned sound combinations or words. They may also have auditory figure-ground problems which make it difficult for them to focus on one sound and inhibit attention to others.

They may also have distorted feedback from or interpretation of *tactile* and *kinesthetic* cues, which can result in a variety of problems. For example, they may have difficulty with balance, coordination, and direction. They may have problems in writing, a skill that is dependent on accurate interpretation of both the tactile cues involved in holding a pencil and the kinesthetic sensory input which accompanies hand movements during writing (Hallahan and Kauffman, 1976).

Learning-disabled children may also have significant difficulty with *spatial-temporal* perceptions. They may have problems with spatial relations (determining the position of objects in space), they may not be able to judge size or distance, and they may experience directional confusion, all of which can interfere with activities as diverse as

214

throwing a ball and writing. Children with spatial problems may have difficulty with reading or arithmetic, where they need to judge size, quantity, and position (Golick, 1969). They may also have serious problems with writing, in part because of difficulties with spatial aspects of the environment and with rhythm. The frequently observed poor planning and placement of letters and words, uneven size, and lack of organization are all apparent in Figure 10.1, a writing sample from a learning-disabled child.

Children may differ in their preferred perceptual modality—that is, the modality through which they learn best. Auditory learners, for example, learn best with auditory stimuli, such as in a phonics approach, but may have difficulty when material is presented visually. Conversely, visual learners have less trouble with written and other visual material but may have difficulty processing auditory stimuli. Figures 10.2 and 10.3 provide examples of the ways in which these preferences affect learning. The author of Figure 10.2 is more efficient at processing auditory stimuli and thus has written the words phonetically. The child who wrote Figure 10.3 relies heavily on visual stimuli and writes words on the basis of their similarity to the shape or gestalt of previously learned words.

FIGURE 10.1   *Writing sample from a learning-disabled child.*

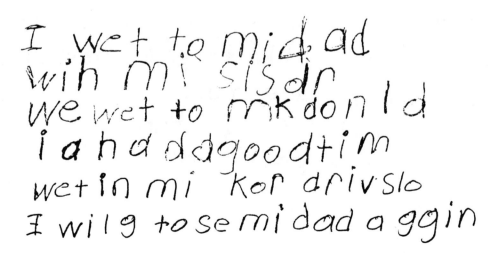

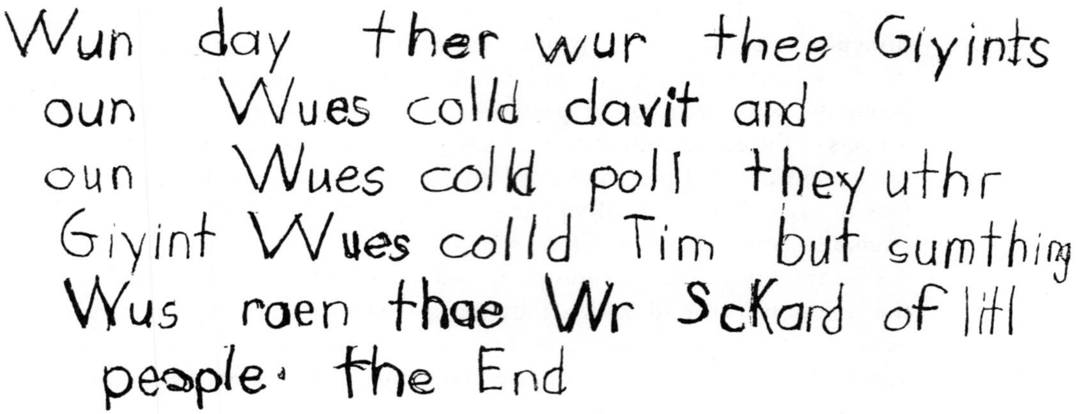

Wun day ther wur thee Giyints
oun Wues colld davit and
oun Wues colld poll they uthr
Giyint Wues colld Tim but sumthing
Wus roen thoe Wr ScKard of litl
peaple. the End

FIGURE 10.2   *Writing sample from an auditory learner.*

FIGURE 10.3   *Writing sample from a visual learner.*

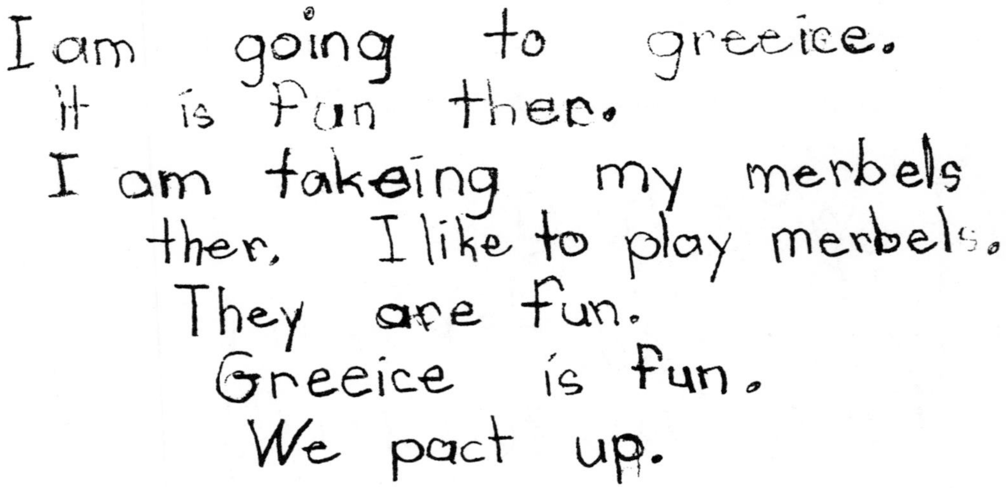

I am going to greeice.
It is fun ther.
I am takeing my merbels
ther. I like to play merbels.
They are fun.
Greeice is fun.
We pact up.

Discussion of some *controversial aspects* of perceptual difficulties and their role in learning disabilities, which some feel has been overemphasized, is included in a later section.

MOTOR FUNCTIONING

Children with learning disabilities frequently suffer from disturbances in motor functioning. Two of the most common forms of such disturbances are discussed below.

Poor Coordination

Learning-disabled children may have difficulty with gross motor or fine motor activities. A child with poor gross motor coordination may appear awkward, may stumble or fall frequently, or may exhibit underdeveloped skills in such activities as running, hopping, or playing catch. A child with poor fine motor coordination may have difficulty holding a pencil properly or writing. There may be poor coordination of the eye movements required to track across a page or poor coordination of the muscles involved in speech.

Hyperactivity

Hyperactivity is a frequent symptom of learning-disabled children, although not all learning-disabled children are hyperactive and hyperactivity can be caused by many things. It is true, however, that most hyperactive children have learning problems (Reid and Hresko, 1981). Hyperactivity does not constitute a diagnostic entity or a homogeneous group in the sense that the behavior is consistent or uniform or that response to treatment can be predicted (Loney, 1980). The correlation between hyperactivity and learning disabilities is not high enough to warrant discussing them as part of a "syndrome"; in fact, many of the behaviors often associated with hyperactivity as a syndrome are results of the kinds of reinforcements the child has received rather than symptoms of a disorder (Ross, 1976).

Hyperactive children often seem to be involved in endless activity. They move constantly about, rather impulsively, and have difficulty staying with any activity for very long. Their behavior often attracts attention because their timing is so erratic—they move when they would be expected not to (Goldberg, 1979). Hyperactivity is most noticeable in school but may appear anyplace where sitting and attention are required, such as at meals (Safer and Allen, 1976).

Hyperactivity may also be apparent in verbal behavior—incessant talking and frequent changes in topic. The hyperactive child is "always on the go"; and although there are wide variations in teacher and parent tolerance of such behaviors, there is usually little difficulty in distinguishing a clinically hyperactive child from a normally bright and curious youngster. Werry and his colleagues (1975), for instance, demonstrated that teachers could rate children very accurately using the Conners' Teacher Rating Scale (Conners, 1969).

There is no good evidence that hyperactivity is caused by identifiable brain damage or dysfunction (Loney, 1980; Ross, 1980). On the other hand, there is no strong evidence that it is psychogenically caused either; it is widely thought to be constitutional, perhaps genetic (Loney, 1980). Even if some hyperactivity is genetically based, as certain evidence seems to suggest, that factor is interwoven with family variables in its etiology and continuance (Safer and Allen, 1976).

Hyperactivity has often been attributed to low levels of central nervous system arousal and inhibition, leading to a lack of inner control of motor and sensory output and input, which in turn leads to learning and behavioral problems (Satterfield, Cantwell, and Satterfield, 1974). However, authors of one review (Hastings and Barkley, 1978) suggested that at resting levels of autonomic nervous system activity hyperactive children do not appear to be under or overaroused, whereas studies involving the *impact* of stimuli suggest that such children are consistently underaroused or underreactive to stimuli. Stimulant drugs appear to increase the arousal of such children and thus enhance the impact on the nervous system of stimuli (Hastings and Barkley, 1978).

It has also been suggested that hyperactivity might be due to additives in food (Feingold, 1975, 1976), lead absorption levels (David et al., 1977; Safer and Allen, 1976), allergies, fluorescent lighting (Ott, 1976), and other environmental factors. Feingold, for example, claims that artificial food coloring and artificial flavors which are added to most foods today can cause a wide range of adverse physiological reactions involving many body systems and lead to the learning and

218

behavioral problems, especially hyperactivity, of many children. According to Feingold, the elimination of such additives from the diet results in markedly improved behavior in as many as 30 to 50 percent of children, depending on age and neurological involvement (Feingold, 1976). He reports that younger children respond more rapidly and that the low rate of response in adolescence may be due to irreversible neurological damage.

There has not yet been widespread acceptance of Feingold's ideas in the professional community, although many parents give enthusiastic endorsement to the results they have observed after their child has had a trial period on the diet. In one study (Harley et al., 1978), for example, psychological measurements, observational data, and teacher ratings were obtained on thirty-six hyperactive school-age boys under experimental and control conditions. The researchers did not find any evidence of improvement in laboratory observations, but parent ratings indicated improvement. Nor did Conners and his colleagues (1980) find any significant difference in activity level between children ingesting active material and those ingesting a placebo, although the former group showed initially poorer performance on some measures of a learning task.

Ott (1976) studied children in windowless classrooms under two lighting conditions and concluded that hyperactivity may be due in part to "radiation stress." He further suggested that the fluorescent lighting and mercury vapors might interact with the synthetic colors added to food. Perhaps dietary practices, especially in interaction with physiological and environmental factors, may lead to hyperactive behavior for some children, but more evidence is needed.

As hyperactive children do not constitute a homogeneous group, the study of subgroups of hyperactives, differentiated along a number of dimensions, may well prove to be a more fruitful line of inquiry (Campbell, Endman, and Bernfeld, 1977a; Campbell et al., 1977b; David et al., 1977; Hastings and Barkley, 1978; Loney, 1980; McMahon, 1980). Researchers engaged in the study of hyperactive children are showing an increased interest in comparing children in different situations and at different times in an effort to identify such subgroups of hyperactive children. Loney (1980), for instance, suggested that children who are very susceptible to changes in the environment might be considered "state" hyperactives, while those relatively resistant to environmental change might be considered "trait" hyperactives; and the former group might respond better to behavioral techniques than the latter. Moreover, those who were hyperactive at home and not at school might be quite different from those who were hyperactive at school and not at home (Loney 1980).

Campbell and her colleagues (1977a, 1977b) differentiated between "situational" and "true" hyperactive preschoolers, categories which are comparable to Loney's state and trait hyperactives, respectively. They studied preschoolers at four, followed them up at six and a half, and observed them in regular classrooms at seven and a half. They found that children who were designated as situational hyperactives had more problems than normals but fewer than the true hyperactives. They were not as inattentive and did not leave their seats as often as the true hyperactives, although they were just as disruptive. The true hyperactives remained immature and active as they grew older; there was less certainty regarding the situational hyperactives because data from the mothers were not confirmed by other measures (Campbell et al., 1977b). The researchers urged more observations in the home to determine whether the situational hyperactives were actually harder to handle at home or whether there was simply less tolerance there. Thus, the isolation of more behaviorally and physiologically homogeneous subgroups would be helpful (Hastings and Barkley, 1978).

McMahon (1980) recommended the division of hyperactives into subgroups differing in symptom severity, age at onset, response to medication, and specificity or generality of symptoms.

When adolescents who had previously been diagnosed hyperactive were compared with normal controls on cognitive and social-emotional dimensions, the hyperactives did significantly less well on attentional, visual-motor, and reading tasks and rated themselves lower on some of the sociability and self-esteem items (Hoy et al., 1978). Thus, although activity and distractibility levels may decrease during adolescence, inattention and processing problems often continue, resulting in the persistence of academic and social problems (Hoy et al., 1978; Safer and Allen, 1976).

COGNITION

Learning-disabled children may have problems with some of the most basic psychological processes. For example, they often have a very

220

short *attention span*. This problem is so common that the newer term "attentional deficit" is preferred by many clinicians. The DSM-III (APA, 1980) uses "Attention Deficit Disorder" to replace such labels as minimal brain damage, minimal brain dysfunction, hyperkinetic syndrome, and hyperactive child syndrome, because virtually all of the children with those diagnoses demonstrate attentional problems as a prominent symptom. Attention is an active process which depends on other cognitive processes, is influenced by the meaningfulness of stimuli, and is associated with physiological correlates (Reid and Hresko, 1981). Reid and Hresko note that attention generally improves with age, and impairments in children's ability to attend may be due to limitations or problems in the amount of information that can be dealt with and in ability to organize material and relate it to past experience.

Attentional deficits may or may not be associated with hyperactivity. In cases where they coexist, the attentional problems tend to persist during adolescence long after hyperactivity of children with this disorder has decreased (APA, 1980; Hoy et al., 1978; Safer and Allen, 1976).

Attentional problems affect the functioning of children in many ways. They may not find it possible to stay with a task nearly as long as their peers. They are very distractible; attention may shift within a short period of time among events as diverse as a teacher's instruction, someone walking past the door, and another child's behavior. Because of poor initial learning of material, there is also poorer retention. If basic concepts and skills are poorly learned and therefore not easily recalled, higher-order concepts can be only partially learned or learned in a distorted manner, and the children's learning problems begin to multiply.

Although attentional deficits have been demonstrated frequently in learning-disabled children, explanations as to why they develop and their import are still lacking. Reid and Hresko (1981) suggest, however, that deficits which are observed may be better viewed as problems in "...efficiency of processing after information has reached short-term memory" (p. 100).

Children with learning disabilities frequently cannot bring one aspect of the environment into focus while minimizing other aspects. This difficulty with *figure-ground discrimination*, noted long ago by Werner and Strauss (1941) in brain-injured children, can be in the auditory or visual sphere. Learning-disabled children may not be able to inhibit attention to paper rattling, foot shuffling, and other background noise in order to focus on the teacher's voice as distinct from the background noise. Hence, they may respond to all noises more or less equally. Similarly, when visual perception is required, they may have difficulty focusing on relevant stimuli and inhibiting response to others.

A child's *cognitive style* is also related to learning ability. Kagan (1966) first described the reflection-impulsivity dimension differences in problem-solving strategies, and considerable research has been done in this area since. For example, Blackman and Goldstein (1982) reported that reflective children showed better attentional behavior and did better in school, and many have demonstrated that children can be helped to become more reflective (Blackman and Goldstein, 1982; Meichenbaum and Goodman, 1971). Similarly, children who are field independent (that is, can use relevant cues and ignore irrelevant ones) perform better in school, whereas children who are underachieving tend to be more field dependent (Blackman and Goldstein, 1981). Blackman and Goldstein maintain that this field independence can be taught and that learning can be facilitated by modifying instructional methods to better fit a child's cognitive style.

Learning-disabled children often show more impulsivity than their peers and siblings, both motorically and cognitively. Their impulsivity can be seen in frequent stops and starts of various activities, in darting about (perhaps into streets or other potentially dangerous situations), in sudden and unpredictable behavioral or verbal outbursts, and in fast and disorganized approaches to problems or tasks. Such impulsivity can result in negative reinforcement from the environment, in disturbed interpersonal relationships with peers, and, perhaps, in a greater number of accidents, as well as in poorer learning and school performance. Ross (1976), however, contends that the whole notion of impulsivity could be reformulated in terms of selective attention, and that if such children could be taught to attend selectively the impulsive behavior would disappear.

Difficulties with long- or short-term *memory* in learning-disabled children are frequently reported. These include difficulty in handling sequences within words, remembering sequences of stimuli, remembering words and proper spelling, and remembering a sequence of directions given by the teacher. Such memory problems can also result

222

in more perseverative errors and poorer recall of complex or unusual sentences (Wiig and Roach, 1975). That some researchers (Lyle and Goyen, 1968) did not find evidence of short-term memory problems in retarded readers may be due to the differences in the ages of the subjects studied and the complexity of the tasks assigned, making direct comparisons inappropriate.

Reid and Hresko (1981) point out that retention may be related to depth of processing. They believe that adults do not remember separate words or sentences, but rather abstract relations between sentences. Encoding involving semantic and cognitive operations thus is retained longer than that involving sensory and perceptual stimuli; however, the potential for problems appears to be greater also. In one study Cermak et al. (1981) showed that the interference of similar material hindered retention of verbal material to a greater extent among learning-disabled children than among normals.

There is considerable evidence that when children with reading problems are confronted with memory tasks, they may use less efficient strategies (Torgeson and Goldman, 1977; Wong, 1982). That is, there appears to be a problem in how they *perform* rather than a structural deficit (Reid and Hresko, 1981). For example, Wong (1982) found that learning-disabled children had lower self-checking ability than others and used less thorough and efficient organizing strategies when searching for and selecting retrieval cues. Poor readers have shown improvement in both total recall and verbalization or rehearsal when the task was changed to facilitate rehearsal (Torgeson and Goldman, 1977).

Children with learning disabilities are frequently reported to be less able to deal with tasks requiring *abstract thought,* often performing better on more concrete tasks. Concept development may thus be affected, as concepts require abstract thinking and a capacity to generalize from one situation to others, as well as to make necessary discriminations. As a result, such children may overgeneralize or undergeneralize when categorizing objects, numbers, or experiences. They may not see similarities that are obvious to others and thus fail to carry over learning from one situation to another, causing the parents to claim in exasperation that the child "just never seems to learn." Or a child may feel unable to do one set of math problems even after successfully completing a similar one because the similarities in the two are not apparent.

LANGUAGE

Language is undoubtedly the most troublesome area for learning-disabled children—and the most highly researched. Problems and delays may occur during the early stages of language development or with later, higher-order communicative skills such as reading and writing. Difficulties can vary from minor deviations to severe disorders.

Delays in Language Development

The normal course involves first the development of inner language, in which the child makes sense of his or her experience even before it can be communicated to others. Receptive language develops next, by which the child learns how to decode messages sent by others and, as a consequence, to understand their meaning and the symbolic use of words. Finally, expressive language develops, whereby the child learns to take thoughts and put them into a symbolic code (that is, a word), or encode them, so that they can be communicated to someone else. As increasing competence in language acquisition is based on previous acquisitions (Menyuk, 1969), the earlier a child develops a problem or the earlier the delay, the more serious and pervasive the difficulty will be. A child who is competent in understanding language may still have problems in production of language or, for some reason, may not use language frequently. However, a child who has disturbances in inner language or in making sense of the environment will have a more profound language disorder than a child who has adequate inner and receptive language but has difficulty with expression.

Reading Problems

Children with language problems are at high risk to develop *reading problems* as well. These reading problems may or may not include dyslexia, a disorder in which incoming visual or auditory stimuli are scrambled, reversed, or distorted and very difficult for the child to decode. Children may also experience general delays in reading or a lack of fluency. The complexity of the problem facing researchers and educators is underscored by the findings of Lyon and Watson (1981). Using a cluster analysis, they identified six homogeneous subgroups

224

of children with specific reading disabilities on the basis of eight language and perceptual tests. The battery showed that the subgroups performed significantly differently from one another and from normal readers in a comparison group; the subgroups also differed on oral reading and reading comprehension measures. That is, the groups had different patterns of deficits, a finding which has implications for better matching of teaching methods and materials to a child's abilities. As reading is very basic to all other learning, reading problems are often pervasive and proper treatment is crucial.

SOCIAL-EMOTIONAL FUNCTIONING

Learning-disabled children may also experience a number of *social-emotional* difficulties. They are frequently described as emotionally labile or unstable, being "up" one day and "down" the next. Poor self-concepts may prevent them from exerting full effort on some learning tasks, which in turn adds to their unhappiness. They may withdraw to avoid further failure or may act out some of their frustration in various kinds of problem behaviors. They often experience isolation and alienation from their peers because of their hyperactivity, reading peculiarities, and general school problems; often they are set apart as "strange" or different. Finally, they may be subject to a wide range of emotions within their families, including frustration, rage, shame, guilt, and anxiety, depending on individual family members' reactions to their particular problems.

Sometimes such children can "get by" and remain undiscovered as long as tasks are simple and demand only skills that they have acquired. However, as more complex functions such as memory, sequencing, and intricate grammar are required, their performance may get considerably worse or appear quite uneven, depending on which skills are involved.

Causal Explanations

Medical (organic, neurological, biochemical), psychological (environmental, cultural, emotional), and educational causal explanations have been offered in an attempt to unravel the mystery of learning disabilities.

225

NEUROLOGICAL–BIOCHEMICAL–GENETIC EXPLANATIONS

Although some children are retarded in reading and learning because of actual brain damage and clear neurological deficits (Rabinovitch, 1959), a more frequently used explanatory concept has been that of *minimal brain dysfunction* (MBD). This term refers to a dysfunction that is inferred from such behavioral signs as poor coordination, language difficulties, perceptual deficits, and reversals. These signs are referred to as "soft neurological signs" because dysfunction is only inferred from them: it does not show up on such neurological tests as electroencephalograms (EEGs). EEG findings were not helpful as they were not consistently associated with language or learning problems or familial incidence (Owen et al., 1971). Studies with EEGs have yielded contradictory findings, and the behavioral significance of any abnormal EEGs that are found is questionable (Feuerstein, Ward, and LeBaron, 1979). Feuerstein and his colleagues noted that some physiological measures have indicated deficits in attention/arousal as manifested in both central and autonomic nervous system activity, but more research is needed.

The notion of minimal brain dysfunction has come under increasing criticism as inaccurate, misleading, and of dubious educational value. Ross (1977), for instance, criticized the term as unnecessary and confusing because it emphasizes the brain without evidence for its involvement and uses a medical analogy for an educational problem. Such a label can mislead and result in unfortunate consequences for the child, and research has not supported the idea of an actual behavioral syndrome (Ross, 1976; Routh and Roberts, 1972).

Learning disabilities have also been attributed to *biochemical disturbances.* Levy (1973), for instance, maintains that an altered structure or a changed chemical balance leads to distorted feedback in the child, with resultant developmental immaturity. This causes poor self-control, distorted body awareness, and confused time/space orientation, which in turn lead to the activity and behavior disorders characteristic of learning-disabled children.

There appears to be little evidence to support the role of *genetic* factors in learning disabilities, although genetic factors may predispose a child to maturational lag, which could then lead to delayed reading skills (Satz and Sparrow, 1970). Although there may be familial aspects in some cases (Owen et al., 1971) and although a genetic hypothesis may provide at least a partial explanation of the problems of hyper-active children (McMahon, 1980) and dyslexia (Finucci, 1978), the research is generally weak methodologically (Coles, 1980; McMahon, 1980). Studies investigating such physiological factors as chromosomal abnormalities have been largely negative (Reid and Hresko, 1981). There is a need for more research into the ways in which environmental factors interact with genetic predispositions (McMahon, 1980), and delineation of more homogeneous subtypes within families might be helpful (Finucci, 1978).

PERCEPTUAL OR VERBAL DEFICITS

Although children with learning problems often perform poorly on various visual perceptual tasks, the *nature* of the relationship between academic and perceptual success is not clear (Reid and Hresko, 1981). Many researchers (Kinsbourne, 1973; Lyle and Goyen, 1968; Myklebust, 1968; Rosner, 1973) have stressed the central role that visual and auditory perceptual problems play in learning disorders. Others have concluded that although perceptual difficulties may characterize young children, such processes as language, attention, and auditory functioning are also of central importance (Bryan and Bryan, 1978). In support of this, Satz and Sparrow (1970) have argued that younger reading-disabled children (seven to eight years of age) show more visual-motor problems than older ones (nine to twelve) because of delays in maturation of the earlier skills. Older children show more impairment on conceptual problems, which involve later-maturing, language-related skills (Satz and Sparrow, 1970; Satz, Rardin, and Ross, 1971). Thus, Satz and his associates urge more longitudinal studies regarding delays in developmental patterns which might predict later reading acquisition problems. Bryan and Bryan (1978) suggest that there is much more evidence, both direct and indirect, for verbal deficits than for perceptual explanations. For example, they found differences between retarded readers and normal readers in the processing of auditory linguistic material but not strictly visual perceptual material.

The role of auditory perceptual factors is still controversial, however. Reid and Hresko (1981) concluded that auditory *perceptual* abilities appear to be quite unrelated to academic achievement, though some other auditory factors may be significantly related to reading.

227

They determined further that problems with cross-modal integration actually reflect a more general processing problem. On the other hand, after reviewing and statistically integrating the findings of 106 studies, Kavale (1981) concluded that auditory perceptual skills are importantly related to reading ability.

As there is a high incidence of delays and difficulties in language acquisition, during preschool years the emphasis should be on study and analysis of children's language ability rather than their perceptual-motor skills (Bryan and Bryan, 1978). Golick (1973) even maintains that the idea of a perceptual handicap has done a disservice to children by serving as a catchall for professionals, by confusing parents, and by hindering teachers. In any case, many of the studies yield only correlative data regarding reading problems and perceptual deficits, so a causal relationship cannot be assumed (Hallahan and Cruickshank, 1973).

DEVELOPMENTAL DELAY

Many researchers have attributed the problems of learning-disabled children to delays in their development. There have been descriptions of neurological immaturity (Owen et al., 1971), a disturbed neurological organizational pattern (Rabinovitch, 1959), a "pervasive organismic immaturity" (De Hirsch, 1975), and a developmental lag in maturation (Ross, 1976). This immaturity interferes with integration in many areas of functioning and can result in lags in the ability to selectively attend to complex stimuli and to sustain that attention (Ross, 1976) and in poorly patterned perceptual experiences (De Hirsch, 1975). The impact of these, however, depends on how well the child can adapt, on the environment, on prenatal and postnatal stress, and on other factors (De Hirsch, 1975).

It has been suggested that developmental dyslexia is not a unitary disorder; rather, it reflects a central nervous system maturational lag or immaturity which results in delayed acquisition of the skills that normally develop at different ages (Satz et al., 1971). In other words, the deficits of dyslexic children resemble patterns of behavior seen in younger children, and the early maturational lag presages immaturity in the skill development that occurs at later stages as well (Satz et al., 1971).

228

PERCEPTUAL-MOTOR WEAKNESSES

Other explanations of learning problems come from the perceptual-motor theorists. Although there are important differences among them, the basic idea they share is that good motor functioning and development underlie good academic functioning. Therefore, any academic difficulties that a child experiences must be due to problems with perceptual-motor coordination, development, and functioning. One of the motor theorists, Kephart (1967), maintains that accidents during the developmental period may interfere with the child's development of certain basic assumptions about the world and thus result in a disturbed orientation to the physical environment.

Other perceptual-motor theories include Barsch's (1967) movement approach or theory of movigenics; Getman's (1965) visuomotor complex, which he enthusiastically claims can lead to progress with children on whom others have given up; and Cratty's (1971) emphasis on active motor learning and the use of games to remediate coordination difficulties. Undoubtedly the most controversial of the perceptual-motor theories is that of Doman (Doman et al., 1967) and Delacato (1959; 1963; 1966) and the Institute for the Achievement of Human Potential in Philadelphia, which they founded. Their theory is based on the idea that children with reading problems have experienced inadequate neurological development because of a lack of clear cerebral dominance. Their remedy for such neurological inadequacy is to use various patterning exercises which are intended to re-create missed neurological stages and lead to improved neurological organization and cerebral dominance and, therefore, enhanced neurological functioning.

This notion has come under heavy criticism as a technique that purports to change the actual functioning of the brain when in fact there is no proof that it does. In addition, recent studies suggest that reading and lateral dominance are not related (Kirk, Kliebhan, and Lerner, 1978). The controversy over their method is not over the assumption of a relationship between neurological events and behavior but over the claim that external exercises can predictably change those events (McCarthy and McCarthy, 1969). The theory has also been criticized for offering false hope to parents who are desperately searching for help for their child and who then delay seeking other kinds of help.

ENVIRONMENTAL AND PSYCHOLOGICAL FACTORS

Environmental variables have been implicated in the etiology or exacerbation of learning problems. Included among the list of such variables are family environments that are rated as disorganized and less than stable emotionally, factors which may particularly affect learning-disabled children (Owen et al., 1971); neurotic disturbances (Pearson, 1952); limited schooling; and other external influences (Rabinovitch, 1959). Where such psychological and external factors are involved, treatment may include psychotherapy as well as remedial work, and there may be rapid progress (Rabinovitch, 1959).

It has been suggested that some learning problems may be due to inadequacies of the educational system or inappropriate teaching (Golick, 1973). That these actually *cause* learning disabilities is not clear—and not likely—but they are very important factors in determining how a child's problem is dealt with, how the child's feelings are handled, what kind of remedial approaches are used and how effective they are, and to what degree further problems are prevented or minimized.

SUMMARY

Because of the frequency with which learning-disabled children suffer multiple problems or handicaps (Kirk and Kirk, 1971) and the likelihood of multivariate causes (Hallahan and Cruickshank, 1973), some writers (Lerner, 1976; Wallace and McLoughlin, 1975) have emphasized the need for a multidisciplinary approach to learning problems. Among the professional specialists who might be involved in such an approach are regular and special education teachers, psychologists, pediatricians, neurologists, ophthalmologists, and speech and language specialists, depending on the child and the specific problems involved.

The following case study illustrates many of the characteristics of children with learning problems and the interactions of various behavioral and learning patterns. It illustrates how such children may act out their frustration and how the family dynamics and attitudes interact with, and contribute to, the child's problems. It also illustrates the need for multidisciplinary approaches to such a child and the need for cooperation among various professionals.

CASE STUDY

Kevin was an eleven-year-old boy who was referred because of academic and behavioral problems at school, very uneven functioning, and low motivation.

Although Kevin's developmental milestones were average, he had shown some difficulties in the form of easy distractibility, reversals, hastiness, and difficulty associating numerals with number words as early as grade one. He was strong in other areas, particularly social and verbal areas, but increasing problems were noted in grades three, four, and five, particularly in math and in his work habits and behavior.

Kevin's school performance was inconsistent. At times he did the work, but at other times he became disruptive and aggressive and was becoming increasingly isolated from the class.

Psychological testing revealed superior language skills but difficulties in the perceptual-motor area and problems with math, spatial relations, abstract designs, and sequencing. It was not clear whether some of his low scores were due to hastiness, insufficient checking, perceptual difficulties, or lapses in concentration. However, as his reading had not been hampered, it seemed less likely due to perceptual problems than to difficulties in the *reproduction* of forms and in coordination. There were also suggestions in the test results of problems with social behavior, perception, controls, and aggressive behavior. It seemed possible that perhaps his good language skills were not as well rewarded by his home environment as physical prowess, and that the aggressive models he saw (TV violence, parent use of physical punishment) may have contributed to his aggressive responses.

The program designed to help Kevin and his family included a recommendation for a neurological examination to assess his neurological status because of his history of explosive and violent outbursts, lapses in attention, and perceptual-motor difficulties. It also included counseling for the parents regarding their handling of Kevin. At school Kevin became involved with a resource room teacher for a part of each day for specific help in areas in which he was weak or showed significant deficits. His increased interest and involvement in baseball was encouraged and reinforced and resulted in considerable positive feedback from peers, with fewer aggressive episodes. As his level of frustration decreased, his social and classroom behavior improved, and his academic performance became more consistently satisfactory.

Remediation

Since the passage of PL 94-142, a comprehensive and individualized plan of intervention, including an Individualized Educational Program (IEP), must be worked out for all handicapped children before educational services are begun (Lerner, 1981). There are also several general principles of remediation to consider, as well as specific remedial techniques from which to choose in planning the most effective program. Many of the techniques are controversial, and they have met with varying degrees of success. Both the basic general principles and the most frequently used specific intervention strategies are discussed in the following paragraphs.

General Principles of Remediation

Among the general principles that need to be considered in planning for a child, regardless of the specific strategies selected, are the following.

Begin early. Waiting for the child to "grow out of it" or hoping that somehow the problems will simply go away can waste valuable remedial time and may also result in the development of additional problems. Early intervention tends to be less extensive and, therefore, less expensive. Intervention after years of difficulty, considerable frustration, and damaged self-esteem is likely to be more intensive and costlier in terms of therapeutic efforts and is also less likely to be totally successful.

Begin at the child's level. Obviously, treatment that is begun beyond the functional level of the child will be ineffective and will result in more wasted time. If a child is having difficulty with receptive language, for example, efforts directed at expressive language will not be helpful. If basic reading skills have not been acquired, assigning more and more reading tasks or increasing repetition of material will not be of help either.

Work on the child's problem areas while maintaining and encouraging success in areas of relative strength. When a child is receiving remedial help in problem areas, it is very important to seek out areas of relative strength so that success experiences can occur concurrently with remedial efforts. This is essential to sustain the child's self-esteem and motivation to continue.

232

Use varied and interesting methods of presentation which are tailored to meet the child's particular needs. If a child learns best through the auditory modality (that is, if the child is an auditory learner), phonics, oral work, and taping might be emphasized. If a child is a visual learner, less emphasis might be placed on phonics and more use made of visual tasks and learning aids. In order to restore the lost interest of a child who has had a long history of problems with schoolwork, teachers need to select material carefully and make it as interesting and as relevant to the child's interests as possible. An adolescent with a serious learning problem will be more likely to work at reading if the task involves reading a drivers' training manual rather than a difficult geography text. Games such as those described in Golick's *Deal Me In* (1973) and other inventive techniques should be tried as well to increase interest and motivation. Working with computers can often provide enough novelty to rekindle interest and motivation in children with a long history of negative school experiences.

Use multisensory techniques. Many writers have advocated the use of several sensory modalities simultaneously to help a child acquire basic reading skills. This approach may be quite effective with many children; some, however, may be distracted when they are in a situation where several kinds of stimuli are impinging on them. For them, stimulation in a preferred modality may be more desirable. Again, thorough knowledge of an individual child's strengths and weaknesses is essential if one is to plan the most effective, individualized remedial intervention program.

Specific Intervention Techniques

The general considerations just discussed are relevant to planning for virtually any learning-disabled child; the issues below involve individual decisions as to which of many specific remedial techniques available would be most useful with a particular child.

BEHAVIORAL AND COGNITIVE TECHNIQUES

Behavioral and cognitive techniques that have been used successfully include operant conditioning (Leviton and Kiraly, 1976), self-instruction (Meichenbaum and Goodman, 1971), and modeling (Denny, 1972; Hallahan and Kauffman, 1978; Ridberg, Parke, and Hetherington,

1971; Ross, 1977). In one study (Meichenbaum and Goodman, 1971), training in overt and then covert verbal self-instruction was effective in improving both cognitive and motor performance of impulsive children. In another study, practice and attentional training allowed high-anxious children to function as well as a low-anxious group, whereas those with a placebo and those in a control group continued to make more errors (Ribordy, Tracy, and Bernotas, 1981).

Modeling techniques in which children observe problem-solving strategies in others, sometimes combined with self-instructional training (Hallahan and Kauffman, 1978), can significantly affect response latency. In one study (Denny, 1972), subjects who observed a reflective model took longer to respond than those who observed an impulsive model. In another study (Ridberg, Parke, and Hetherington, 1971), exposure of grade-four boys to a film model using a cognitive style opposite to their own was found to alter their response latency and reduce the number of errors they made. Training in more reflective behavior appears to intensify concentration and thus increase efficiency (Reid and Hresko, 1981).

There is disagreement, however, as to the overall value of behavioral techniques. Gittelman-Klein et al. (1979) claim that there is little empirical evidence of their effectiveness alone or in combination with stimulant medication. Others enthusiastically endorse their use as productive across a wide spectrum of behaviors. Still others observe that they help with some behaviors more than with others.

Although behavioral techniques have been reported to be effective in changing some behaviors (Denny, 1972; Meichenbaum and Goodman, 1971; O'Leary and Pelham, 1979; Wulbert and Dries, 1979) and were judged superior to stimulant drugs in several studies, at least in research classrooms (Backman and Firestone, 1979), the evidence for their value in bringing about *academic* improvement is weak. A lack of improvement may be due to a lack of generalization from experimental situations to other situations (Wulbert and Dries, 1979), particularly regular classrooms. For example, there may be a lack of generalization from training activities to such classroom behaviors as sitting still, cooperating, and remaining task-oriented (Ross, 1976), or from the nature of the academic tasks studied in the laboratory to those assigned in the classroom. In addition, only the most basic academic behaviors have been studied so far, whereas classroom study of such subjects as creative writing, music, art, and geography, is very complex (Kauffman, 1975).

234

Backman and Firestone (1979) concluded that it is likely that behavioral techniques influence one set of behaviors and medication another; they suggested that it may be too much to expect everything from a single intervention. Rather, it would be more realistic and effective to use such treatments as medicine, family therapy, behavior therapy, and educational strategies in combination.

MEDICATION

The use of drugs with learning-disabled children is controversial and has generated a voluminous body of research. Stimulant drugs, of which Ritalin (methylphenidate) is probably the most common, have frequently been administered to hyperactive children in varying dosages and for varying lengths of time. In one study, for example, medication was found to be the most frequently prescribed intervention for children who had been identified as hyperactive, although it was usually used with other treatments (Lambert, Sandoval, and Sassone, 1979). Decreased hyperactivity in children has even been reported as a result of the ingestion of the stimulant caffeine in the form of two cups of coffee daily (Paluszny, 1977). The use of stimulant medication with children who are hyperactive may seem odd. Such medication, however, stimulates the central nervous system, and as a result the child experiences greater alertness, is less distractible, and is better able to focus attention. The medication may also enhance short-term memory and persistence (Werry, 1977), thus facilitating task performance.

Although medication can be helpful in the overall program of a child, many factors influence a child's response to drugs (Conners, 1971). There is evidence that different dosages may be required for maximum improvement in learning and for maximum improvement in social behavior, for example. If a lower dosage is optimal for enhanced learning and one increases the dosage to a level recommended for maximum improvement in social behavior, learning performance may go down (Sprague, 1977). The selection of target behaviors is therefore very important in determining the dosage for a given child (Sprague, 1977).

Drugs should be used only with careful management and follow-up and only after or in conjunction with other forms of intervention (Conners, 1971; Paluszny, 1977). Whether a child is started on medication at all may depend largely on the severity of the symptoms and the tolerance level of the environment (Goldberg, 1979); a team approach involving the child, family, school, and physician should be used (Paluszny, 1977).

Although short-term effects on impulse control, attention span, and other behaviors are well documented, there is little evidence that drugs improve a child's academic functioning (Backman and Firestone, 1979; Loney, 1980). Long-term follow-up studies have failed to show significant differences between those children treated and those untreated (Backman and Firestone, 1979).

Stimulant medication may have negative effects. Some children may get worse (Ross, 1976); and other, desirable, exploratory and social behavior may be reduced along with activity level and inattention (Barkley and Cunningham, 1979). Other negative side effects which may occur include insomnia, stomachaches, growth suppression, and personality changes (Goldberg, 1979; Werry, 1977).

Thus, although stimulant medication has proven useful in the treatment of many children, it does not appear to be universally or consistently effective. Further research is required into its varied effects on children, taking into account differences in dosage levels, age of the child, target behaviors, and interaction with other factors.

Minor tranquilizers may help children whose hyperactivity is caused by emotional factors, but they are less effective with learning-disabled hyperactive children (Paluszny, 1977).

In any case, the successful use of medication should not take away from the importance of environmental and psychological characteristics; and psychotherapy may still be in order for secondary problems such as low self-esteem, disturbed relationships with peers, and depression (Satterfield, Cantwell, and Satterfield, 1974).

PERCEPTUAL-MOTOR TRAINING

The motor theorists as a group recommend physical activity as a means to improve not only physical coordination and functioning but also academic performance. Some of their ideas and methods have been discussed previously so they will not be repeated here. There is no proof to date that such motor or movement training can in fact improve the academic functioning or behavior of learning-disabled children. Most of the reports of research in this area, both in support of and in opposition to perceptual-motor training, have been very

236

weak methodologically (Hallahan and Kauffman, 1976), yielding only correlative data. However, the increased self-esteem that accompanies improved coordination and the resulting increase in motivation encourage advocates of this approach (Mordock, 1975), as a child's performance may be indirectly affected.

SPECIFIC READING REMEDIATION PROGRAMS

Much has been written about specific reading remediation programs as well as assumptions underlying their use. Generally, there are three approaches to remedial procedures, as described by Kirk and his colleagues (1978): (1) skill or task training in which specific skills and subskills are developed; (2) process training in which the underlying processes involved, such as visual discrimination and sound blending, are developed rather than task skills; and (3) a process/task approach where there is an integration of the first two. According to Kirk and his colleagues, no one method has been clearly shown to be superior; very important variables are the teacher's enthusiasm and effective presentation. An example of the marked effects one's presentation can have is the strategy of hyperlearning (Prichard and Taylor, 1981). This involves the use by the teacher of peripheral cues, relaxation, and a number of other techniques to make the children feel good about themselves, to increase motivation, and to help convince them that they can learn faster than they thought.

Although learning-disabled children *can* learn, they do not if appropriate procedures are not used (Bryant, 1967); and most language remediation programs can be adapted to a particular child's problem regardless of the etiology of that problem (Hammill and Bartel, 1975).

Specific programs which place varying emphasis on skill and process training include the VAKT (visual-auditory-kinesthetic-tactile) or multisensory approach (Fernald, 1943; Gillingham and Stillman, 1960), the DISTAR method, the Cloze technique (in which missing words are filled in), the Rebus approach (in which pictures are substituted for some words), and the neurological impress method (Kirk, Kliebhan, and Lerner, 1978).

An example of a skill training program is the DISTAR method, which grew out of the work of Bereiter and Engelmann (1966). It is a very detailed remedial reading program in which children learn specific subskills through various exercises before actually beginning to

237

read books. Process training includes teaching approaches in which training is done in the modality in which the child is deficient. However, Reid and Hresko (1981) concluded that there was little support for the notion of matching instructional techniques to a preferred modality.

There have been suggestions that perhaps children should be separated into subgroups, as different skills are being acquired rapidly at different age levels (Guthrie and Siefert, 1978). In the early stages of reading (grades one and two), there is a heavy demand for perceptual, decoding, and memory skills. By grades four to six, there is more emphasis on comprehension and application of prior knowledge to written material (Guthrie and Siefert, 1978). As reading disabled children learn the necessary skills and processes more slowly, a significant amount of time should be spent on formal instruction in reading (Guthrie and Siefert, 1978).

Techniques such as overlearning, the arrangement of frequent success experiences, and frequent review should be used in the remediation of reading problems including dyslexia (Bryant, 1967). Fay and her colleagues (1981) suggested that there is a hierarchy of cognitive strategies associated with reading. They found that good readers can attend to more cues simultaneously and select the most productive ones. They argue that their findings support the idea of a cognitive-developmental model of disability, and that a focus on reading subskills only may not meet the needs of some children who have a developmental delay in other skills.

Current Issues

PREVENTION AND EARLY DETECTION

To avoid or minimize current problems and to prevent greater problems in the future, it is essential that teachers, parents, and professionals working with children have a good grasp of normal developmental and learning principles. Such knowledge permits realistic expectations and increases the likelihood that they will detect potential problems. Training in early detection and progress evaluation as well as in sound educational planning is necessary. Although all problems cannot be avoided, preventive efforts and early detection can ensure that problems are dealt with early and that children are taught as effectively as possible.

MAINSTREAMING

Several controversies over remedial issues have already been discussed. Another is the swirl of controversy over the concept of mainstreaming in the wake of the introduction of PL 94-142.

At first glance, the idea of programming for and remediating children's learning problems while maintaining them in the regular classroom, in the "least restrictive environment," sounds like an unequivocally good idea, and there are strong proponents of mainstreaming. Some of the advantages claimed by its supporters are that it reduces the stigma (Jones et al., 1978) and isolation of special classes, that it provides positive behavioral and academic models for learning-disabled children, and that it is more economical.

However, there has also been considerable criticism. Critics maintain that teachers are frequently ill prepared and hence ineffective, that the children compare themselves unfavorably with others in the class who do not have learning problems, and that it is not equally effective for disorders of all degrees of severity. In one analysis of fifty studies, special classes were found to be superior to regular classes for children with learning disabilities and emotional or behavioral disturbances, and inferior for children with subaverage IQs (Carlberg and Kavale, 1980).

Successful mainstreaming requires that instruction for the child with special needs be compatible with that being given others in the classroom, that the teacher be willing to accommodate children with varying abilities and learning styles, and that cooperative relationships exist between regular and special education teachers (Vander Zanden, 1980). The effectiveness of mainstreaming also depends on the teacher's ability and attitudes (Jones et al., 1978). Finally, Myklebust (1980) warns against oversimplification and overgeneralization in this matter because the child's cognitive problem still exists regardless of classroom placement; a study of the learning process is still required.

Discussion Questions

1. How did the perceptual, integrative, personality, and environmental characteristics interact in the case study of Kevin to produce the academic and behavioral picture that resulted in his referral?
2. Look over an elementary school reader and discuss the perceptual

modalities it emphasizes. What problems might it cause for a child with a learning disability? What aspects of its content and presentation might be confusing or distracting?

3. Discuss the pros and cons of mainstreaming. Which kind of program would you prefer for your own child if a learning disability were present? Why?

CHAPTER 11   # Mild to Moderate Cognitive-Affective Disorders

The disorders included in this chapter are frequently referred to as neurotic disorders. As the term neurotic has a psychoanalytic flavor, however, they are here designated as cognitive-affective disorders to emphasize that individuals with these disorders show maladaptive behavior or disturbances in the way in which they perceive, feel about, think about, and interact with the world and the people around them. The four most common mild to moderately severe disorders are discussed in this chapter. In the next, severe disorders involving marked impairment in these areas will be dealt with.

The overall incidence of mild to moderate cognitive-affective disorders is not known; estimates vary from 5 to 20 percent of the child population (Chess and Hassibi, 1978). The range of behavior is wide, extending from essentially normal with a few "neuroticisms" to incapacitating and immobilizing dysfunction.

A symptom can best be seen as a compromise behavior or solution, regardless of one's theoretical perspective. From a psychoanalytic viewpoint, a neurotic symptom develops as a result of conflict between the ego and the id, between reality and libidinous impulses. For that reason, some writers suggest that neurotic disorders are not seen in prelatency children who have insufficient structuring of personality and ego development (Shapiro, 1973). In any case, symptoms are neither healthy nor growth-producing. They are temporary solutions that ease somewhat the individual's discomfort and anxiety for brief periods of time. However, much energy is required to maintain defenses, and therefore the child has less energy for other, more growth-producing activities. The fact that symptoms provide only temporary and partial relief, however, in no way diminishes their importance or minimizes the ease with which they become part of a person's habitual way of responding to situations.

A behavioral point of view suggests that a person's disordered behavior is simply learned behavior. It may be dysfunctional, interfering with learning and other tasks, but its occurrence has ameliorated an unpleasant state (that is, anxiety). Such moderation of an aversive condition is reinforcing, thereby increasing the likelihood of its recurrence in the future when the anxiety returns. It can, therefore, fairly quickly become a habitual way of responding, and its habit strength is increased until its reinforcing properties change. The key to decreasing dysfunctional behavior, according to the behaviorists, does not lie in clarifying the nature of internal conflicts, or seeking their origin, as in a psychoanalytic approach; rather, it lies in the iden-

tification of maladaptive behaviors, followed by a change in the reinforcement contingencies surrounding those behaviors. Rhodes and
Paul (1978) put it succinctly as follows:

> Since the practitioner's concern and empathy focus more directly on the
> individual child and his particular needs, the practitioner operates differently
> within the predominant behavioral model than within other major explana-
> tory models of emotional disturbances. He would not, for instance, concern
> himself with inner processes or conditions of the child who is being labeled
> maladaptive. Rather, his empathic concern would be with the fact that the
> child's current activities are not gaining maximum benefit from the environ-
> ment. He is not sharing fully in the stimulation and reinforcements available
> in the environment. In a sense, the child is being grossly deprived of the envi-
> ronmental benefits in relationship to other children within the same settings.
> His deprivation stems from the fact that he has learned certain kinds of behav-
> iors and these are being maintained by the conditions which exist at the pres-
> ent time in his own personal interactive exchange with that environment. The
> deprivation is being maintained by a maladaptive coupling system, or con-
> necting arc, between the individual and the environment. (Rhodes and Paul,
> 1978, p. 45)

Discussions of some of the most common types of disorders follow.
They include both analytic and behavioral components.

Obsessive-Compulsive Disorders

Theoretical/Descriptive Background

Incidence estimates range from as low as 1 percent of clinic populations (Erickson, 1978) to as high as 17 percent (Despert, 1955), though
wide variations may be due in large part to differences in definition
and labeling. What some refer to as a specific fear or habit disturbance
may be labeled an obsession or compulsion by someone else (Kessler,
1966). Furthermore, although classical obsessive-compulsive disorders
in childhood are usually thought to be relatively rare (Achenbach,
1974; Hollingsworth et al., 1980; Yates, 1970a), they usually appear at
between nine and twelve years of age and can be disabling unless
properly treated (Hollingsworth et al., 1980). Many adults with the
disorder date their symptomatic onset to preadolescence (Chess and
Hassibi, 1978), and obsessive-compulsive symptoms have been
reported in the parents in approximately 10 percent of the families of
children with these problems (Fine, 1973).

In obsessive-compulsive disorders there are irresistible, irrational thoughts (obsessions) or actions (compulsions) which intrude into a person's consciousness and interrupt thought and behavior. Obsessions include irrational ideas, doubts, or fears. For example, one who has an intense fear of dying of cancer despite the absence of any evidence whatever of its developing might be said to have an obsession. The hallmarks of obsessions and compulsions are their irrationality, repetition, and ritualistic quality. The person experiencing them knows, intellectually, that they are irrational and unrelated to his or her usual behavior, and may have a strong desire to be rid of them, but is unable to shrug them off. In the case of compulsions there is an inability to stop the irrational action or behavior. If forcibly stopped from completing an action, the individual becomes very anxious. For example, excessive handwashing is a compulsive symptom; although the person may know that there is no objective need to wash hands forty times a day, and that such behavior may even be injurious, acute anxiety results if the person is forced to stop before that magic number is reached. Some so-called compulsive behaviors are totally within the normal range of behavior and are, in fact, desirable, but become neurotic and dysfunctional when they become too intense, too frequent, or incapacitating. A good student must be somewhat compulsive—for example, checking work to make sure it's correct and exercising care. On the other hand, if the student feels compelled to check it ten or twelve times or redoes the whole assignment quite unnecessarily "just to be sure," the behavior is less functional. The subjective distress felt by obsessive-compulsive children further distinguishes them from children who may show obsessional interests in leisure activities and experience resultant isolation from peers, but who are content with their situation (Chess and Hassibi, 1978).

As with other disorders, there are important differences between children and adults in the nature of their obsessive-compulsive disorders. First, it is probably more accurate to speak of obsessive-compulsive *tendencies* in children, rather than obsessive-compulsive personalities or characters, as a child's entire personality is fluid at this point. Second, all children manifest certain compulsive behaviors from time to time which are completely within the normal range and represent common behaviors of specific developmental stages. The ritualistic bedtime behavior of most two- and three-year-olds, in which the number of bedtime drinks, stories, and trips to the bathroom far exceeds any objective necessity, is an example of such normal but compulsive behavior. If, however, a child's ritualistic behavior persists far beyond the usual age and becomes more frequent, intense, or incapacitating, it is not normal. Third, unlike that of adults, a child's obsessive-compulsive behavior frequently involves the participation of other people (Kanner, 1972), as, for instance, when a mother has to spend considerable time arranging things in just a specific way to prevent excessive anxiety in the child.

According to a psychoanalytic view, the basic mechanism involved in these disorders is represssion. The individual represses an unpleasant memory or impulse and keeps it unconscious by continual rumination on an unrelated topic or by repetition of a meaningless act. If these repetitive thoughts or acts are prevented, the memory or impulse threatens to become conscious and the person becomes anxious. Obsessions and compulsions are not good solutions. They interfere with the person's normal functioning and often lead to increasing seclusion or isolation as a consequence of efforts to avoid being conspicuous and to avoid criticism by parents and ridicule from peers (Kanner, 1972). They are, however, a lesser evil than expression of a forbidden impulse and are fraught with less guilt. Hence, they are reinforced and repeated. They are frequently seen in children whose parents are very strict and perfectionistic, with a strong sense of right and wrong (Kanner, 1972). Obsessive-compulsive children are likely to put a high emphasis on cleanliness, orderliness, and conventional behavior and manners and often appear to be quite constricted (Achenbach, 1974). Fine (1973) surveyed the literature and concluded that obsessive-compulsive children are very ambivalent toward their parents but are not allowed to express anger toward them. In one study (Hollingsworth et al., 1980), most of the subjects had parent models with severe problems and one-third of the parents had serious medical illnesses. The symptoms of the children were seen as defenses against the anxiety of serious life stress as well as modeled behavior.

CASE STUDY
Daniel was referred to the clinic at the age of 13 by a teacher who noted that he withdrew from many activities, daydreamed, needed a good deal of prodding, was indecisive, and appeared nervous and tired. She felt, however, that this represented considerable improvement over his earlier episodes of acute anxiety. He did remain, however, extremely inhibited in the expression of hostility and aggression.

Daniel was reserved and guarded and did not initiate any comments. Some of his responses suggested, however, that his father's expectations of him were unrealistic for his age and ability, and that the resultant pressure on him threatened, frightened, and angered him. His father appeared to be hostile and authoritarian in his handling of Daniel, and was insensitive to Daniel's needs. He conveyed the strong impression that he was too busy to be bothered with Daniel or with Daniel's brothers and sisters, and he continually shifted the responsibility for Daniel's care to outside agencies.

Daniel's initial demeanor was constricted, reticent, and inhibited. Occasional relaxation was consistently followed by a return to more inhibited behavior during the next session. Daniel often compulsively chose solitary "projects" in the playroom which served both to keep him busy and to alleviate any need to talk. He was distant, seemingly indifferent, and rather flat in his affective expression. At one point he became obsessed with the notion that somebody was watching the sessions through the one-way mirror, despite repeated statements and reassurances to the contrary, and could only function after he was allowed to actually inspect the room each time.

During treatment the therapist tried to create as permissive an atmosphere as possible to encourage Daniel to relax and verbalize his feelings. He had numerous sessions with the father in order to help him adjust his expectations of Daniel to a more reasonable level and to show him other ways of handling situations. Activities which Daniel and his father could enjoy together were encouraged and reinforced. As their relationship gradually improved, much of Daniel's compulsive behavior disappeared.

Spontaneous change seemed improbable. Without intervention, Daniel's obsessive-compulsive tendencies and behaviors would likely have become more marked, more frequent, increasingly maladaptive, and perhaps more solidified and disabling, given his background and the nature of his behavior. His symptoms would probably require increasing time and energy; as a result, there would be decreased involvement in other, more constructive activities.

Treatment

In spite of the clear need for intervention, there has been relatively little research on the specific treatment of obsessive-compulsive dis-

246

orders in children until recently, and what has been done is contradictory. Some studies espoused traditional individual psychotherapy as the most effective treatment for classical neurotic conditions such as obsessive-compulsive disorders (Belmont, 1973); others espoused behavioral techniques; and still others concluded that no traditional therapy has been shown to result in significant improvement in these disorders (Yates, 1970a).

Chess and Hassibi (1978) reported complete recovery in 50 percent of treated cases, worsening in 30 percent (some of whom were later diagnosed schizophrenic), and marginal adjustment in 20 percent. A less optimistic report came from Hollingsworth and his colleagues (1980), who reported that of ten cases treated with "intensive" psychotherapy and followed up from one to fourteen years later, seven still showed symptoms and reported serious problems with peers and with social relationships. Prognosis, then, depends at least in part on the nature of the underlying disorder (Adams, 1978).

A psychodynamic therapist, taking either an analytic or a nondirective stance, would work with the parents toward better understanding and more realistic expectations of the child (Kanner, 1972). Behavioral therapists would attempt to decrease the reinforcement value of obsessions and compulsions, interfering with or punishing the intruding thoughts and behaviors and rewarding incompatible responses. Preventing the compulsive behavior—that is, response prevention—has been found to be effective in reducing ritualistic behavior (Foa, Steketee, and Milby, 1980; Rachman, DeSilva, and Roper, 1976; Stanley, 1980), with gains maintained at one-year follow-up and with no symptom substitution. Others have found exposure to be effective in decreasing anxiety in compulsives (Foa, Steketee, and Milby, 1980), with gains usually maintained over follow-up of several years (Marks, 1981). However, relaxation was not helpful, and obsessive ruminations were less responsive to behavioral therapy (Marks, 1981).

Fine (1973) has combined psychotherapy and behavioral methods in his family therapy/behavioral approach, which is briefer and more goal-directed than traditional treatment. He recommended that families interrupt the rituals and then allow the child to express the ensuing anxiety and anger. More follow-up evaluative research will be necessary to assess the long-term effectiveness of the various intervention strategies.

Phobias

Theoretical/Descriptive Background

Unlike fears, which are usually defined as normal responses to genuine danger or threat and are reasonable, phobias refer to an unreasonable, excessive, and persistent maladaptive response to more vague or benign stimuli (Graziano, DeGiovanni, and Garcia, 1979; Miller, Barrett, and Hampe, 1974). Most studies of children's fears are laboratory studies focusing on mildly or moderately fearful subjects; little research has been done on severe fears within a naturalistic setting (Graziano, DeGiovanni, and Garcia, 1979). With the exception of school phobia, phobias are not particularly prevalent among children (Graziano, DeGiovanni, and Garcia, 1979). Phobias must be distinguished from childhood fears, which are seen fairly frequently at various developmental levels. Separation anxiety, for example, is very common around one year of age, but it disappears spontaneously. The intensity, disruptiveness, and generally intractable and irrational quality of phobias suggest a more severe disturbance. Moreover, phobias are beyond voluntary control, cannot be reasoned away, lead to avoidance responses, and are not age or stage specific (Miller, Barrett, and Hampe, 1974).

The analytically oriented psychologist perceives phobias to be instances of anxiety displaced from an original object onto another one, which can then be avoided. For example, someone who has a fear of sexual impulses might project and displace this fear onto birds or heights or some other object and then avoid that object. Sometimes the feared object is clearly related to the child's conflict, but more frequently it is not.

The behaviorally oriented psychologist perceives the development of phobic conditions as a conditioning process. Phobic fears are believed to develop through a process of classical conditioning in which previously neutral stimuli become paired with a fear response and then elicit the fear response in the future.

There is general agreement among both analysts and behaviorists that phobic fear can generalize, causing increasing withdrawal. A child who initially fears crowds or closed spaces may become anxious during a shopping trip but later develop fears about driving into the shopping plaza, leaving the yard, or even going outdoors. Such gen-

248

eralization is well illustrated in the description of John, the school phobic, later in this chapter.

The specific phobia most frequently seen by clinicians is *school phobia*, a term coined by Johnson et al. (1941). Incidence estimates range from 1 to 8 percent of clinic population (Erickson, 1978), a considerably higher figure than Eisenberg's (1958) 17 per 1000, which was based on 4000 clinic admissions. It is more common in early elementary grades (Kessler, 1966), with a peak incidence at age eleven or twelve (Chess and Hassibi, 1978). Again, differences in definitions affect the incidence figures. The DSM-III (APA, 1980), for example, distinguishes between school refusal, which may be due to separation anxiety, and school phobia, where the child fears the school situation whether or not a parent is present. Some note a reversal of the usual tendency of boys to outnumber girls (Kessler, 1966); but Gordon and Young (1977), after reviewing seventeen studies reporting sex differences, concluded that despite reported differences in both directions, the total figures were actually very close. Intelligence levels are usually average or above, with the majority in the superior range (Johnson et al., 1941).

It is often suggested that the feared situation in school phobia is not the school itself, but separation from the mother (Johnson, 1941) and a general inability to be comfortable away from home. The anxiety the child feels is then projected or displaced onto the school. However, not all school refusals are due to separation anxiety (APA, 1980); multiple factors including marital problems of the parents, fear of failure and rejection, and conflicts over increasing independence can all contribute (Chess and Hassibi, 1978). In most school phobic cases, the mother subtly encourages the child to stay home; the mother and the child may have an intense need to be near each other and so communicate separation anxiety to each other (Eisenberg, 1958). As Kessler (1966) and Gordon and Young (1977) point out, however, most of the research lacks adequate controls to explain or take into account mothers with similar conflicts whose children are not phobic, or children with separation anxiety who do not become phobic. The father may also play a role in the development of overdependency by not helping to weaken the mother-child attachment, as the child matures, in order to reestablish the primacy of the marital relationship (Skynner, 1974).

Somatic complaints among school phobic children are common and include headaches, stomachaches, sore throats, and a host of other symptoms. The mother may supply excuses freely and with minimal justification to keep the child at home, such as insisting that the weather is too hot or too cold or that the child has a slight cold.

Some writers (Coolidge, Hahn, and Peck, 1957; Kennedy, 1965) have suggested that it may be useful to make a distinction between two types of school phobias, neurotic and characterological. Kennedy (1965), for example, distinguished between Type I (neurotic crisis) and Type II (way-of-life) school phobics on the basis of such differentiating symptoms as health of the mother, communication between parents, number of incidents, and type of onset. The neurotic type would typically include younger children (kindergarten through grade four) who showed an acute onset, generally good functioning in nonschool areas, and a better prognosis; the characterological type, made up largely of early adolescents, would show a generally deeper level of disturbance, a more gradual onset, and a poorer prognosis (Gordon and Young, 1977).

According to Kennedy, the Type I school phobic may spontaneously return to school in any case, but the rapid treatment program that Kennedy developed can hasten or facilitate that return. His program for Type I phobics includes good public relations so that cases are referred early; matter-of-fact handling of somatic complaints; mandatory school attendance; structured interviews with parents to encourage them to persist in the program; intervention with the child, which involves stressing the transitory nature of the problem and the advantage of facing the fear; and follow-up. All of his Type I subjects responded with complete remission of symptoms and with no symptom substitution.

The following case study is illustrative of the second or more severely disturbed school phobic.

CASE STUDY
John was referred to a community clinic at age fourteen because of continuing nonattendance and threatened court action. His original refusal to attend school began when he was thirteen and had been absent for two months because of surgery. After his surgery, he became extremely anxious at the thought of returning to school and facing peers' questions about where he had been, despite the legitimacy of his absence.

250

Although his original fears were focused on a return to his classroom, they soon generalized to the school in general, then to the walk between home and school, and finally to his own yard, where he feared someone would see him, stop, and ask where he had been. Even his brother could not entice him outside to play football as they had frequently done before. He was clearly immobilized.

School refusal was only one of John's symptoms. He also suffered from extremely low self-esteem, poor body image, an emaciated look, extreme anxiety attacks, a slight speech impediment, frequent somatic complaints, a lack of peer relationships, underachievement in school, and depression. Getting him to attend school or to see his therapist was a major task, made more difficult by the parents' excuses for John that permitted him to stay at home.

In spite of these problems, John did make very slow but real progress at the clinic. He gradually became more involved in activities, and occasionally initiated activities with peers. Schoolwork was no problem for him, and he was never a disruptive influence in the classroom. It was difficult, however, for the parents to assimilate such progress. They often minimized it and pointed out other problems or some negative aspect of the therapy. Despite his healthier behavior at the clinic, John rarely showed it in the company of his parents, or in family meetings, where he more often showed his previous, less functional self. Communication among family members was covert and confused, and any attempts to make it more straightforward were met with overt agreement but covert subterfuge.

As the parents' initial complaints about the clinic's work gradually changed to condescending tolerance, and later to more explicit hostility and dissatisfaction, John's absences once again became more frequent. A decision was reached that nothing more could be accomplished at least for the time being because of his erratic attendance, and the therapist terminated the treatment.

The prognosis for significant change was poor.

Treatment

Treatment of school phobic children is clearly a family affair; much work must be done on the intrafamilial relationships as well as on the child's school attendance. Frequently, however, the parents resist or even undermine the treatment. The mother, especially, may have a strong need of her own to keep her child near and dependent. The primary goal of treatment is to get the child back into school—to get him or her involved with the outside world before nonattendance has become a firmly entrenched habit. On the practical side, extended absence from school may become a legal problem as well as a psychological one.

Treatment of school phobia may include group, individual, or family therapy and other kinds of activity simultaneously. Behavioral techniques have been shown to be especially helpful in the treatment of phobias. A gradual desensitization program (Wolpe, 1969; Wolpe and Lazarus, 1966), relaxation training, and other behavioral therapeutic interventions may be necessary to enable a school phobic to reenter school or to help children with other phobias to decrease their fear. Rose (1972) concluded that a group desensitization procedure was at least as effective as individual desensitization and more effective than no therapy, insight therapy, or placebos in treating various kinds of phobias. On the other hand, Miller and his colleagues (1972) found that treatment effectiveness was a function of age. Their factor analytic comparison of reciprocal inhibition, psychotherapy, and waiting list control showed that treatment was most effective for children from six to ten regardless of the therapists' experience or technique, whereas neither of the treatments worked with eleven- to fifteen-year-olds.

Others claim that little progress has been made over the past sixty years. Graziano, DeGiovanni, and Garcia (1979) concluded that there is scant evidence to support the effectiveness of systematic desensitization and that cognitive and developmental factors should be studied more, with cognitive and verbally mediated approaches appearing the most promising.

Windheuser (1978) demonstrated that simultaneous treatment of the child and the mother, including modeling therapy, was more effective than treating the child alone. Modeling appears to be the most frequently used and reliable strategy for decreasing fear (Graziano, DeGiovanni, and Garcia, 1979).

Research on treatment effectiveness suggests that promptly instituted treatment is most effective (Chess and Hassibi, 1978; Waldfogel, Tessman, and Hahn, 1959) and that the prognosis for older children is poorer than that for young children (Chess and Hassibi, 1978). In support of this, Coolidge and his colleagues (1960) posited a direct relationship between severity of disturbance and age. In one study (Rodriguez, Rodriguez, and Eisenberg, 1959), 89 percent of clients under eleven returned to school, whereas only 36 percent of those over age eleven did so. Others (Hersov, 1960; Skynner, 1974), however, found no relationship between age and outcome of treatment.

Differences in outcome criteria may account for some of the apparently discrepant findings. Caution is suggested in the interpretation of outcome studies that do not differentiate between simple return to school and overall emotional and social adjustment as criteria for success, as the former criterion typically yields much higher, more optimistic rates (Gordon and Young, 1977). Erickson (1978), for example, cited a 72 percent rate of return to school for school phobic children who had received psychotherapy, and a 90 percent rate if psychotherapy was combined with pressure to return. It appears that a combination of psychotherapy and behavior therapy is most effective; some conflicting results regarding long-term change may be due in part to reliance on only one mode of intervention.

Gordon and Young (1977) concluded that although dynamic theory leads in etiological explanation and questions, learning theory has made a considerable contribution toward treatment; they stressed the need for empirical validation to supplement the largely clinical experience base on which both viewpoints now depend. For a more extensive description of studies of school phobics along several dimensions, the reader is referred to Gordon and Young's excellent review.

Anxiety Attacks

Theoretical/Descriptive Background

Probably one of the most distressing of human conditions is acute anxiety. When a child faces an attack, his or her attempts to defend are overcome by the anxiety, which then breaks through in a kind of panic. If the panic occurs at night, it may take the form of night terrors or other sleep disturbances (Chess and Hassibi, 1978; Kanner, 1972). The child may experience dizziness, trembling, and nausea, as well as such physical symptoms as cardiac, respiratory, or digestive distress (Langford, 1937). At times there may be severe cardiac distress; Kanner (1972) noted the frequency with which an anxiety attack is mistaken for cardiac illness. A child may or may not know what has triggered the attack. An original attack is often precipitated by an experience such as a death or serious illness in the family for which the child was ill prepared (Kanner, 1972). Later attacks may be completely subjective responses to internal signals, so that a helpless onlooker has no clue as to the child's sudden distress. There is no obvious, objective danger. The attacks vary in length from a few moments to as long as half an hour, perhaps two to three times in a week. They occur more frequently in girls than in boys (Kanner, 1972). The subjective experience of an anxiety attack is vividly described in the following quote from Chess and Hassibi (1978):

> Anxiety is an unpleasant sensation that, in milder forms, is experienced by children as a feeling of apprehension and general irritability accompanied by restlessness, fatigue, and such visceral components as headaches, a "funny feeling" in the stomach, or in the chest. In an acute anxiety attack, the apprehension is intensified, the child is in terror, cries, looks frightened, is not easily reassured, and may believe that his death is imminent. He may complain that he cannot breathe, that his heart is stopping or going too fast, that people look different to him, and that he has changed into another person. He may be pale or perspire profusely, cling to whoever is around, ask for his mother, and altogether present a pitiful picture of a helpless child. An older child, in search of an explanation for his fear, may accuse people around him of wanting to harm him, strike out at peers, overthrow whatever is in his way, and behave as if he is having a temper tantrum. However, he may be crying while violent and may cling to the trusted person who tries to stop him. He may accept whatever excuse or explanation is offered him, or he may halfheartedly try to find a cause in what somebody else had done to him. (pp. 241–242)

CASE STUDY

Bob was a fourteen-year-old boy referred because of occasional bizarre and odd behavior in school, difficulties in learning, fearfulness, and very low self-esteem. He was very guarded and tense and extremely concerned with how well he was doing. He attempted to use an extensive vocabulary in highly intellectualized discussions of various news events, seemingly to impress the examiner with his intellect and knowledge. The overall impression was of someone attempting to appear self-assured and competent to cover thinly veiled insecurity.

As soon as it became clear that he would be unable to answer many of the items or do some of the tasks, he became increasingly anxious. His speech became more rapid, he became visibly agitated, and he soon began to pace up and down. He was no longer able to concentrate, and quickly left the room, perspiring and trembling. His anxiety level had very quickly gone from barely controlled to completely out of control and disrupted entirely his capacity to function. The threat of being made to look "stupid" or inadequate was so great for him that the only way he could handle the situation was to leave entirely.

After being in treatment for a year, however, Bob had had more frequent success experiences, and his self-esteem had improved significantly. He could tolerate making some mistakes, and he was able to function for much longer periods of time.

He appeared to use obsessive-compulsive behaviors initially to maintain very precarious control of his anxiety. When stress and the level of perceived threat became too high, the behaviors were ineffectual and the anxiety surfaced. Treatment focused on efforts to reduce stress where possible and to reinforce behaviors which were adaptive for him in the face of stress.

Treatment

Calm, authoritative reassurance often provides quick and relatively permanent symptomatic relief (Kanner, 1972). In some cases, medication may be required for immediate relief, and continued therapy may be necessary to discover what associations exist between the individual's life experiences and internal conflict or reaction tendencies to bring about such extreme anxiety. Behavioral techniques might include such procedures as relaxation techniques, as well as systematic desensitization if the precipitating events, thoughts, or fears can be discovered.

Depression

Theoretical/Descriptive Background

The incidence and nature of depression in children are rather controversial; clearer diagnostic criteria are needed (Pearce, 1977). Many writers agree that classic depressive disorders are relatively uncommon in children, but major depressive disorders can begin at any time, including infancy (APA, 1980; Spitz and Wolf, 1946), and they may be underdiagnosed in childhood (Lefkowitz and Burton, 1978). There is considerable lack of agreement regarding symptoms and any cause-effect sequence (Levitt and Lubin, 1975), as well as whether some depression is masked. Although a depressive mood is seen in virtually all acute states of depression, many do not show obvious sadness—hence the term "masked" or "smiling" depression (Klerman, 1974).

The range of symptomatology in depressed children is wide and there are marked differences with age (Lefkowitz and Burton, 1978), though Pearce (1977) claims that the changes in symptom patterns with age are due primarily to changes in frequency rather than symptoms.

The varied symptoms include those commonly recognized—disinterest, unhappiness, low self-esteem, and uninvolvement—as well as those which some feel mask depression—acting out or delinquent behavior, somatic complaints, school phobia, and underachievement (Glaser, 1967; Hollon, 1970; Weeks and Mack, 1978). Still other symptoms of depression are pessimism (which is not natural to children), self-punitive or self-injurious behavior, and preoccupation with death or suicidal threats or attempts. Some researchers feel that since the evidence does not suggest a syndrome of depression, diagnosing a condition as such is unwise, because it may mask other problems (Lefkowitz and Burton, 1978), or it may be masked by a variety of other symptoms (Lewis and Lewis, 1979). Levitt and Lubin (1975) suggest that if depression were not diagnosed unless there was an expressed depressive mood, individuals so classified would constitute a more homogeneous group, and that masked depression is inferred and speculative.

A developmental perspective is necessary to understand childhood depression, as it may be manifested differently at successive maturational stages (Boverman and French, 1979; Pearce, 1977). Moreover, as the future development of children may be affected, it is necessary to identify areas of development that are blocked or distorted (Boverman and French, 1979). There may also be a lowered threshold for depression with increased maturity, which in turn may be lowered further by psychological and biological changes during puberty (Pearce, 1977).

Depression is considered an affective rather than a cognitive disorder (APA, 1980; Levitt and Lubin, 1975), though it can clearly interfere significantly with cognitive funtioning, as is illustrated in the case study of Janet in this section.

Depressive feelings are present in many children and adolescents as a symptom secondary to such other problems as learning disabilities and child abuse. It is difficult to differentiate between primary depression and depression that develops secondary to chronic illness, and developmental aspects further confound the issue (Lewis and Lewis, 1979). While depressive symptoms are significantly more frequent in children with the DSM-III "affective disorder," they often occur with other disorders, so the term "childhood depression" should be used with caution (Carlson and Cantwell, 1980). At best the disorder is hard to classify, given the difficulties in operationally defining it and establishing criteria for it (Lewis and Lewis, 1979). Some feel that depression is so common even in normals that it should not be considered deviant (Lefkowitz and Burton, 1978).

In normal persons a depressed mood is relatively temporary and is frequently a response to an objectively burdensome life situation such as a death in the family or a divorce. Clinical depression refers to a longer-lasting, usually more intense depression, which often seems unrelated to life events and which is more disruptive of a person's ongoing life experience. According to Brumback and Weinberg (1977), one should not diagnose depression unless it has persisted for at least a month and is different from the child's usual personality.

Depression may, of course, end in suicide. According to Garfinkel and Golombek (1977), suicide before age fourteen occurs rarely, but the rate increases quickly thereafter, peaking between fifteen and nineteen. Some suicidal threats or attempts in young children may reflect efforts to alter or escape difficult situations (Chess and Hassibi, 1978), express anger, punish certain persons, or force change, rather than an actual wish to die; children may have an immature comprehension of death and its finality, perceiving it as reversible (Glaser, 1971; Garfinkel and Golombek, 1977).

Etiological explanations have included psychological, genetic, and biochemical views. Family influences and interactions, early separation, events that predispose individuals to low self-esteem, and other adverse environmental factors have been implicated (Pearce, 1977). Lewis and Lewis (1979) find promise in a psychobiological approach—looking at the effects of psychological factors on biological functioning, and biological factors on mood changes. In other words, multicausal views are recommended (Boverman and French, 1979).

A frequent analytic explanation of depression is that it is aggression that has been turned inward. A person who is very angry toward someone but cannot express it may turn that anger inward and become actively self-destructive or may suffer feelings of worthlessness. Others view depression as a reaction to loss (of a person, of a relationship, of a goal)—a kind of mourning process in which the person can see no reason to go on or feels completely alone. The depressed behavior of very young children and even infants whose parenting has been interrupted or seriously disturbed has also been interpreted as a reaction to the loss (Spitz and Wolf, 1946). Some behaviorally oriented workers, however, have suggested that the real import of a loss or deprivation may lie in the fact that it constitutes removal of a significant reinforcer (Eastman, 1976).

A behavioral explanation is that depression results from inadequate or decreased social reinforcement (Eastman, 1976). Nay (1976) suggests that "depression" may be a result of people's inability to meet the inappropriate and overly stringent standards they have set for themselves, with the result that they experience very little self-reinforcement. Depressed individuals are too hard on themselves; they never pat themselves on the back.

Seligman (1974) suggested that when children feel helpless to effect change in their environment or feel that they have no control over what happens, depressive feelings may result. Finally, organic components such as genetic or biochemical factors may predispose specific children to depression (Poznanski, 1979).

Manic-depressive disorders, which are very serious affective disorders found most frequently in adults, involve extreme mood swings, in which an individual vacillates between serious, even immobilizing depression and periods of high activity and euphoria. Although some writers (Anthony and Scott, 1960; Feinstein and Wolpert, 1973; Varsamis and MacDonald, 1972) maintain that such manic-depressive disorders can appear before puberty, there is fairly widespread agreement on the rarity of this disorder in preadolescent children (Achenbach, 1974; Alderton, 1977; Despert, 1968; Group for the Advancement of Psychiatry, 1974; Hall, 1952; Poznanski, 1979), and so it will not be discussed in any detail here. When manic-depressive illness does appear, it seems to be of the same type as that seen in adults (Anthony and Scott, 1960).

The following case study illustrates many manifestations of depression, including somatic complaints, low self-esteem, confusion, anxiety, and unhappiness.

258

CASE STUDY

Janet was referred at age fourteen for an investigation of severe headaches for which no physical cause could be found, shortness of breath, chest pains, and anxiety. She was hospitalized and, while there, behaved quite submissively and became very tense about discharge plans.

Her family background included an alcoholic, borderline-abusive mother and an absent father. She sometimes threatened suicide or left the home for varying lengths of time. The father had left after trying unsuccessfully to persuade the mother to seek treatment for her drinking. He expressed a willingness to have Janet live with him if she wanted to after her hospitalization.

Prior to her referral she had had difficulty at school, especially in math, despite average or above-average ability, and she began to express considerable hostility toward school and her teachers. She also became more difficult to handle at home.

During psychological testing she was anxious, depressed, and confused. She was worried about her physical health and where she would live, and she was unable to concentrate, articulate, or use normal cognitive functioning. She described it best: "I just can't think clearly—my mind is all clouded. I can't think at all."

She expressed a strong need for help and felt that no one had been effective in efforts to help her. She felt alone and worthless and unlovable and said her physical symptoms frightened her. Treatment involved antidepressant medication and sessions with an accepting therapist with whom she could explore her feelings of worthlessness and anxiety. Gradually she began to feel better about herself and, with the help of the therapist, began to set some specific short-term goals for herself. Her father was seen in therapy and was encouraged to allow Janet to live with him. He was also given some specific behavioral guidelines for more effective response to and handling of Janet's behavior.

Treatment

The choice of treatment for depression depends on one's theoretical point of view. There is controversy over the effectiveness of antidepressant medication. Some say that there is a lack of evidence to show that it is beneficial for children (Garfinkel and Golombek, 1977), while others have found such antidepressant drugs as Tofranil (imipramine) to be effective (Frommer, 1967). The data suggest that perhaps such medication is more useful with adolescents and older children (Halpern and Kissel, 1976; Rutter, 1975); some of the contradictory findings may be due to age differences among subjects in various studies.

Depressed children may also be involved in psychotherapy or play therapy, where they can learn to express their feelings and concerns and develop new ways of coping with their problems. Learning to express anger in an acceptable way and becoming involved in activities that provide success experiences can improve self-esteem and lessen despression. Behavioral techniques can be used to help children to become more involved with various activities and to reduce such behaviors as self-deprecatory statements. If one adopts the behavioral explanation of decreased social reinforcement, therapy should include social skills training and involve the whole family, as it is a major source of reinforcement (Eastman, 1976).

Discussion Questions

1. Discuss each of the case studies in this chapter from a psychodynamic and/or behavioral point of view. Questions which you might ask include:
   a. What are the child's behaviors telling you?
   b. What conflicts or maladaptive learning is involved?
   c. What does the child need?
   d. What is maintaining the behavior in the environment?
   e. What further information would you like or need to have to make a good assessment of the problem?
   f. What program or therapeutic interventions would you recommend?
2. Discuss what kinds of life experiences, parent behaviors, or other factors might lead to the development of the various disorders.
3. Explain why specific therapeutic techniques discussed previously may or may not be effective with children suffering from each of the disorders discussed in this chapter.

CHAPTER 12   # Severe
Cognitive-Affective Disorders

Children who suffer from severe cognitive-affective disorders, frequently referred to as childhood psychoses, are less functional generally, less independent, and more disturbed than children with most other disorders. Their behavior is frequently bizarre, and their thought processes and judgment are often seriously impaired. Motor peculiarities or physical concomitants may also be involved. Their contact with reality seems more precarious, and their treatment is usually of greater intensity and longer duration. They are a greater problem for their families and frequently require institutionalization. They are very needy and unhappy children.

The actual numbers of children with disorders as severe as those discussed in this chapter are relatively low. Despite their rarity, however, they have generated an extraordinary amount of research because of the challenge their problems pose in terms of diagnosis, etiology, and treatment. A testimonial to this widespread interest was the emergence in the 1970s, of a journal devoted entirely to these disorders, *Journal of Autism and Childhood Schizophrenia.* (Its title was changed in 1979 to *Journal of Autism and Developmental Disorders.*)

Discussions of severe disorders of childhood usually distinguish among three major types: early infantile autism, childhood schizophrenia, and symbiotic infantile psychosis. There is some semantic and clinical confusion in regard to this classification, however, as not everyone agrees on the three main types or views them as three separate diagnostic entities. There are those who view autism as a subgroup of schizophrenia (Eisenberg, 1956; Eisenberg and Kanner, 1956); who see it as a separate and highly specific category, distinguishable clinically from childhood schizophrenia (Despert, 1968; Rimland, 1964; Ross, 1980; Rutter, 1965, 1968; Treffert, 1970); who use the terms synonymously (Goldfarb, Mintz, and Stroock, 1969); who suggest that the three are variants of the same disorder (Ornitz and Ritvo, 1968); and who distinguish only between autism and symbiotic infantile psychosis (Mahler, 1969).

Many behavioral writers (Blackman, 1974; Craighead, Kazdin, and Mahoney, 1976; Ross, 1974) assert that one can observe and discuss autistic behavioral characteristics without assuming that they indicate any underlying syndrome or unitary disorder that can be clearly distinguished from other serious behavioral disturbances. They question the usefulness of such labels as schizophrenic and prefer to describe such children in terms of their serious behavioral deficits. In this chapter, the three types of disorders will be discussed separately, although it is recognized that there may be considerable overlap and many similarities among them.

Generally, children with severe disturbances can be distinguished from less severely disturbed children in a number of ways. Their contact with reality is more precarious, and they frequently appear to be responding to internal cues or responding exaggeratedly to external events. Their affect and behavior often bear little relationship to what is actually going on around them. Rather, their behavior appears to be in response to their own esoteric thoughts, fantasies, or distorted perceptions. They are usually highly anxious and may experience panic in response to seemingly minimal provocation. Their behavior is noticeably strange, bizarre, or inappropriate, and prognosis is guarded.

Early Infantile Autism

Theoretical/Descriptive Background

Early infantile autism, a term coined by Leo Kanner in 1943, is used to describe children who display a particular pattern of behavior in responding to their environment. They typically show little or no eye contact with others. Although they are usually quite healthy physically, they often engage in odd motor behavior such as whirling around, rocking, flapping their hands in front of their faces, or banging their heads. If they talk at all, their speech often has an odd, mechanical quality and often involves pronoun reversal. They do not use language to communicate but often have superior rote memories. They frequently insist on absolute sameness in their environment and may panic at even very minor changes. They are typically profoundly out of contact with their environment and unable to communicate with other people, but often show a relatedness to objects. At times they may perform at unusually high levels or show above-average ability or interest in specific areas, quite inconsistent with deficits in most other areas of functioning (Rimland, 1964). Nadia, for instance, was an autistic but extraordinarily talented artist; at the age of three she could make drawings and sketches of advanced complexity and skill but could not speak (Gardner, 1979). Her rooster sketch is reproduced in Figure 12.1.

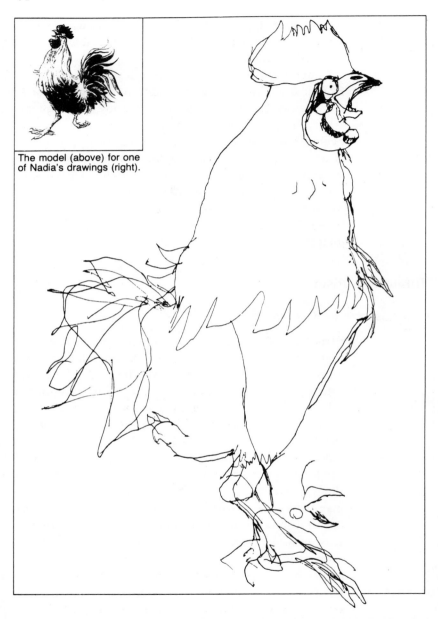

The model (above) for one of Nadia's drawings (right).

FIGURE 12.1   *Source:* Reprinted with permission from *Nadia: A Case of Extraordinary Drawing Ability in an Autistic Child* by Lorna Selfe. Copyright by Academic Press Inc. (London) Ltd. 1977.

The key characteristics of this disorder are autistic aloneness, disturbed language, and insistence on sameness in children without demonstrable physical deficits (Ross, 1974). Children who manifest such symptoms because of clear organic damage are usually not diagnosed autistic (Eisenberg, 1972).

Although varying definitions make the actual incidence hard to determine, autism is rare (Rimland, 1964; Ross, 1974). Estimates range from four or five out of 10,000 (Lotter, 1966; Wing, 1972) to seven out of 10,000 (Treffert, 1970), with a preponderance of boys (Kanner, 1971b; Lotter, 1966; Treffert, 1970), as is true of most childhood disorders. Unlike the case of schizophrenia, incidence of psychopathology in the families of autistic children is low (Eisenberg, 1956; Rimland, 1964).

There is considerable disagreement regarding the etiology of autism. Some maintain that it is caused by psychological or environmental factors or characteristics; others attribute the disorder to biochemical, neurological, or other physiological causes. When Kanner (1943) first identified the syndrome, he reported autistic disorders to be " . . . *inborn affective disturbances of affective contact"* (p. 250). He also pointed to the number of parents of autistic children who were highly intelligent, highly educated, intellectual, rather cold, and showed some obsessiveness in their background. This was frequently interpreted to indicate that Kanner espoused a large psychogenic component in the etiology of autism. Others (Bettelheim, 1967) have maintained that autism is precipitated by negative or ambivalent responses of the caretaker and "the parent's wish that his child should not exist" (Bettelheim, 1967, p. 125)—or as a result of some attachment deficit or disturbance in mother-child bonding (Zaslow and Breger, 1969). Years later, however, Kanner (1971b) maintained that his early assumption of an inborn deficit in the child's ability to form normal contact with others had been confirmed by later studies and that autism *is not* a psychogenic disorder.

While some writers (Bettelheim, 1967; Szurek, 1956) have taken a highly psychodynamic stance, a number of behavioral theorists have postulated a strictly environmentalist view. Ferster (1961), for example, argued that the main difference between autistic and normal children lay in the relative frequency of specific behaviors, with "normal" behaviors having occurred only infrequently in the child's reinforcement history. He maintained that a child exhibits autistic behavior because in earlier years acceptable behavior was not reinforced and disturbed behaviors were (Ferster, 1961). The very reinforcement adults use to terminate such aversive behavior as self-destructive acts or tantrums actually maintains and strengthens it, so the child suffers cumulative deficits in his or her behavioral repertoire (Ferster, 1961). According to Yates (1970a), such a reinforcement framework translates the concept of the "refrigerator parent" into operational terms.

One result of such psychogenic and environmentalist theorizing is that guilt is frequently added to the already heavy emotional burden of parents, and more recent studies have indicated that a purely psychogenic hypothesis is inadequate to explain the disorder. Although parents of autistic children do often have higher educational levels (Kanner, 1943; Lowe, 1966), they are not systematically different from others emotionally, except perhaps in experiencing greater stress in living with an exceptionally difficult child. Schopler and Loftin (1969) found impaired thinking in parents as a result of situational test anxiety in association with their psychotic child; such anxiety was not present when they were tested regarding their other, normal children. Pitfield and Oppenheim (1964) found no evidence of excessive hostility, detachment, rigidity, or rejection in the mothers. They did find the mothers to be more indulgent and uncertain, but these characteristics easily could have resulted from the problem, rather than having caused it. In any case, the existence of a correlation between certain parental characteristics and the presence of autism in children in no way proves a causal relationship (Rimland, 1964).

Among those writers who have attributed autistic disorders to various neurological, biochemical, genetic, or attentional problems are Folstein and Rutter (1978). They concluded from their twin study that a genetic factor and perinatal biological events might be important, possibly in combination. In one study Etemad et al. (1973) found severe EEG abnormalities to be a negative prognostic sign, although mild EEG abnormalities in children without clear organic disorders were not critical prognostically. Hutt et al. (1965) found the EEGs of autistic children to be very similar and of a type rarely found in nonautistic children.

Others (DesLauriers and Carlson, 1969; Ornitz and Ritvo, 1968) have implicated a dysfunction of the arousal system. Autistic infants can be hypoactive or hyperactive (DesLauriers and Carlson, 1969). While some children may appear to be overly sensitive and try to reduce the

266

intensity of incoming stimuli or engage in stereotyped behavior to prevent further stimulation (Hutt et al., 1965), others may try to increase stimulation or may require a higher intensity of stimulation to learn than normals. In one study Hutt et al. (1965) found less stereotyped behavior in an empty room with low sensory input, whereas in another study Metz (1967) determined that autistic children preferred higher volume settings for recordings than normals, which suggests that they would act to sustain higher levels of stimulation than normals.

One explanation comes from Lovaas and his colleagues (1971), who suggested that autistic children suffer from stimulus overselectivity. When presented first with complex stimuli involving tactile, visual, and auditory cues, and then presented with each stimulus separately, they attended to only one, whereas normals responded to all three. This disparity may have been due to differences in intensity of stimulation, however, and there was no support for the notion of impairment in any one sense modality. Such partial and overselective attention may lead to impoverished learning, resulting in greatly reduced language ability and a very limited behavioral repertoire (Lovaas et al., 1971). A related but not yet adequately tested hypothesis is that of a "receptor-shift failure" (Yates, 1970a, p. 258). This attributes an autistic child's problems to a failure to shift from "near-receptors" such as touch or contact to more visual and auditory ones, a shift that occurs in normal children at about six months of age and is critical for cognitive development. It would be interesting to know whether the subjects in Lovaas's study responded significantly more frequently to tactile cues. If so, perhaps the stimulus overselectivity he noted was due to their attention to near-receptor stimuli and a failure to shift to the other, developmentally more mature ones described by Yates. This hypothesis might also be used to explain the high inverse relationship between self-stimulating behavior and discrimination learning described by Koegel and Covert (1972), which they attributed to the child's selective attention to the self-stimulating behavior and failure to learn the desired discrimination as long as the self-stimulating behavior continued.

Another explanatory view, arising from a cognitive perspective, focuses on the child's impaired capacity to process incoming stimuli. There may be difficulty organizing sensory impressions (Eisenberg, 1956), processing symbolic material (Kanner, 1971a; Rutter, 1968;

Yates, 1970), or relating new stimuli to past experience (Rimland, 1964). Such difficulties would result in fragmented memory and an inability to perceive and understand relationships and abstractions, which would interfere with language and cognitive development (Rimland, 1964). Ungerer and Sigman (1981), for example, found that in the play of autistic children, unlike that of normal children, equal time was spent in immature and mature forms of play. However, those autistic children with better language comprehension showed more symbolic and functional play and more integrated play for longer periods. This relationship of play impairment to language comprehension supports the idea of a " . . . generalized symbolic impairment in autistic children" (Ungerer and Sigman, 1981, p. 336). According to Ungerer and Sigman, autistic children did not separate objects from actions on the objects enough to symbolically represent them in thought. Perceptual disturbances are also fundamental to other problems with relationships, motility, language, and rate of development and are manifested in an early inability to distinguish self from the environment, to imitate, and to regulate sensory input (Ornitz and Ritvo, 1968). Rutter's (1968) review led him to rule out retardation and psychogenic factors as central and to suggest that explanations involving perceptual and cognitive deficits are most promising. Social and behavioral problems are then secondary to these primary deficits (Kanner, 1971).

Many writers of varying theoretical persuasion (Ross, 1974; Eisenberg and Kanner, 1956; Kanner, 1971) agree that an interaction of environmental, neurophysiological, innate, and experiential aspects is most likely involved in the etiology of autism. The type of parental handling and the child's emotional relationships may well affect how well the child is able to cope and whether the problems are eventually overcome (Rutter, 1965).

Ornitz and Ritvo (1976), after an exhaustive review of the literature, summarized the diverse findings on autism as follows:

1. Autism is a specific syndrome.
2. It shows up at birth or very soon after (before thirty-six months) and lasts a lifetime.
3. Symptoms reflect " . . . underlying neuropathophysiological process that affects developmental rate, the modulation of perception (sensorimotor integration), language, cognitive and intellectual development, and the ability to relate" (p. 618).

268

4. It is not psychologically caused.

5. It may occur alone or with other central nervous system disturbances.

6. It is normally distributed across all population groups.

Some of the contradictions in the findings that have been reported may be due to the fact that controls for age and developmental level were not included (Freeman et al., 1981). Perhaps subgroups of autistic children should be compared, as autistic children with IQs under 70 show different behaviors from those with IQs over 70 (Freeman et al., 1981).

The following case study, which clearly illustrates many of the specific characteristics noted in the previous discussion, comes from an article comparing childhood aphasia and autism.

CASE STUDY

Boy G was the second of four children. . . . The pregnancy was marked by vomiting and nausea. Labor was $3\frac{1}{2}$ hours and uneventful. G was healthy at birth. The parents note that their chief concerns during the first weeks of life were his loud screaming for no known reason, intense fear of lights, and abnormal sleeping patterns. He struggled against being held by arching his back and bending back his head. The acquisition of developmental milestones other than speech was normal. . . . Until age 3 years, he learned certain words and then stopped using them. At age 3;1, he was prescribed phenobarbital to regulate his sleep. Language production rapidly increased between ages 3 and 4; his first meaningful vocalization was a sentence, "It looks like a flower." Following this, his language development was marked by delayed echolalia (of sentences and whole conversations) and repeated questions. His memory for dates and names was truly remarkable.

His preschool years were marked by several unusual behaviors: odd posturing and mannerisms, flicking, severe hyperactivity and distractibility, rituals, gaze aversion, perseverative behaviors, and little thought to personal safety. He attended special nursery school from age $3\frac{1}{2}$ to 5 years, where slight progress in social interaction was made. At age 5, a thorough neurological examination suggested he suffered from autism, and the neurologist added that this was complicated by a severe learning disability associated with visual-motor retardation. An EEG performed at age 5 years was normal. He was begun on phenothiazine (thioridazine) and stimulant (methylphenidate), with subsequent decrease in activity and improvement in sleep. From ages 5 to 6, he attended a school for learning-disabled children; at age 7 years he was placed in a school for emotionally disturbed children. During this period his social behavior improved; severe withdrawal and aloofness were absent by age 7 years. His speech, although rich and well articulated, remained marked by delayed echolalia and fixation on certain topics. Hyperactivity, distractibility, and short attention span had become serious problems both at school and at home. He attended a special school for brain-injured children from ages 8 to 10 years. At age 9;11 years, physical examination revealed an attractive, slim boy who was noticeably active and distractible. His speech was generally good, but had an odd mechanical quality and was marked by frequent repetition of questions and poor use of pronouns. He moved a great deal in an exploratory and curious way, acknowledging others and relating socially in an immature fashion. Neurological examination revealed no abnormalities. He could easily carry out commands and answer complicated questions. Routine laboratory studies, human genetics and ophthalmology consultations, and urinalysis and urine for genetic screening were all normal. An EEG was abnormal due to mild generalized slowing. . . . At age 11 years, he remained socially quite deviant, but had an amazing capacity to remember names and dates, and to do rapid calendar calculations. (Cohen, Caparulo, and Shaywitz, 1976, pp. 627–628)

Treatment

Various kinds of treatment have been tried with autistic children, including medication, perceptual training, educational approaches, individual psychotherapy, and learning approaches both to lessen self-destructive behavior and to teach positive behavior (Shapiro, 1978). The choice of technique follows and depends on one's etiological view. For example, those who feel that language and cognitive deficits are central, such as Rutter (1965; 1968; 1972), stress the importance of offering special education therapeutically, with the main goal of aiding social skill and language development where these skills have been impaired because of such cognitive deficits.

Those who attribute the problem to arousal dysfunction may emphasize high levels of involvement in the child's world and high levels of stimulation, especially of a kinesthetic and tactile nature, in which parents and teachers can participate (DesLauriers and Carlson,

1969). Zaslow and Breger (1969) described a "rage reduction method" of treatment, based on their hypothesized attachment deficit, which depends heavily on sensorimotor exchanges between therapist and child to allow the child to move into more appropriate language and social learning that has been blocked. This method also involves high levels of stimulation of "near-receptors" (tactile and kinesthetic receptors) and may succeed for that reason rather than because of a "rage reduction."

Medical treatment has not been very helpful with autistic children, but it may be used for target symptoms such as extreme hyperactivity or anxiety. All of the medications, however, can cause short-term and long-term effects, some of which are probably unknown (Campbell, 1978), so the risk-benefit ratio needs to be carefully considered.

Psychotherapy usually plays a limited role because of the severity of the cognitive, language, attentional, and relationship difficulties present, though some have (Phillips, 1957) claimed that it can help the child develop better control of the environment. However, psychotherapy for parents may be very helpful, and changes in the parents may then alter the child's disturbed behavior (Berlin, 1978). Families also require a good deal of support because of the extreme stress and pressures, and they need help with specific problem behaviors of the child such as tantrums, dependency, and self-destructive behavior (Wing, 1972).

Behavior modification has been advocated as an effective way to decrease negative behaviors and to develop new and more desirable ones in order to correct specific deficits in cognitive, language, and social skills (Hersen and Eisler, 1976; Lovaas et al., 1973; Lovaas, Schreibman, and Koegel, 1976; Risley, 1968; Yates, 1970a). Many (Hewett, 1965; Lovaas, 1966; Lovaas, Schreibman, and Koegel, 1976) have found that the basic principles of operant conditioning can be used to help autistic children learn complex language and self-help skills and to increase their imitation of adult behaviors (Metz, 1965). These methods can be taught to parents (Yates, 1970), who can then maintain treatment gains with the child in the home (Lovaas, 1978; Lovaas et al., 1973). Establishing imitative ability in the child, followed by modeling of new behaviors, is also a very efficient way to develop new behavior (Sherman and Baer, 1969). In one study (Egel, Richman, and Koegel, 1981), observation of normal peers modeling correct responses led to a dramatic increase in the discrimination learning of autistic children which persisted when the model was removed, a finding that has clear indications for treatment in a more normal setting.

There is some controversy over the effectiveness of treatment; progress appears to be very slow regardless of the intervention technique that is used. Eaton and Menolascino (1967) found no significant relationship between type and length of treatment and improvement. Ornitz and Ritvo (1976), after a review of the literature, concluded that no rational treatment based on etiological factors alters the course of an autistic disorder, though special education, residential treatment, and behavior therapy can help ease symptoms in most cases.

Although the outlook does appear to be slightly better when intervention is early and intensive, most writers agree that prognosis for improvement appears to be highly related to language functioning (Bettelheim, 1967; Eisenberg, 1956; Despert, 1968), as language is one indicator of the extent of disturbance and isolation (Eisenberg, 1956). In Eisenberg's study, half of the children who had speech at age five showed a fair to good social adjustment, whereas only one of thirty-one nonspeaking children showed such improvement. Kanner and his colleagues (1972) considered speech before five and noninstitutionalization to be positive prognostic indicators, in sharp contrast to Bettelheim's (1967) contention that treatment should usually be done within an institutional setting except perhaps with very young children who have a relatively mild disturbance.

Follow-up data are inconsistent but generally indicate a very guarded prognosis. The approximately three-quarters of Eisenberg's (1956) sixty-three children who were followed up at adolescence showed little improvement; most were functioning at a severely retarded level. Although the eleven children whom Kanner had originally described as autistic were functioning as adults with varying levels of psychotic behavior, they seemed somewhat duty bound regarding jobs and friends and were enjoying more success with the former than with the latter (Kanner, Rodriguez, and Ashenden, 1972). Follow-up of children treated with behavior therapy techniques suggests that there may be large differences among the children one to four years after treatment, depending on their environment after treatment. Institutionalized children regressed; those children whose parents were trained to continue the therapy continued to improve (Lovaas et al., 1973).

Bettelheim (1967) claimed much higher rates of success for his

272

intensive psychoanalytic treatment regime at his Orthogenic School, with only 20 percent of the forty children included in his follow-up study showing a poor adjustment. Those who showed a fair or good adjustment and functioned rather well retained characteristics that set them apart and made them appear odd, and they had lower than normal empathic capacity. Bettelheim's data, however, are very much at odds with the much more prevalent view that children with disorders as severe as autism retain residual problems throughout their lives. According to Ornitz and Ritvo (1976), as many as two-thirds of them retain sufficient cognitive and intellectual deficits to be considered retarded throughout life.

Childhood Schizophrenia

Theoretical/Descriptive Background

As with autism, incidence estimates vary widely because of varying definitions, with a higher proportion of boys than girls typically reported. Historically, schizophrenia has been considered rare before puberty (Bender, 1953; Rutter, 1965), but 12 percent of Bender's 626 children diagnosed as schizophrenic were under five. Hall's (1952) youngest was nine.

Many of the general symptoms of childhood schizophrenia resemble those of autism, among them withdrawal, bizarre and inappropriate behavior, language disturbances, stereotypy, and poor social relationship. However, some writers have made distinctions between autism and schizophrenia in terms of onset, history, and course of the disorder (Eisenberg and Kanner, 1956). Schizophrenic children usually have a later onset and may have had some normal development previously; they do not manifest extreme aloneness and isolation or insistence on sameness in the environment, nor do they show the marked islands of unusual abilities in music, memory, and other areas that are seen in autistic children (Rimland, 1964). Schizophrenia, unlike autism, does not occur in a disproportionate number of twins (Rimland, 1964); and the hallucinations of childhood schizophrenia are very rarely seen in autistic children (Eisenberg, 1956).

One of the most important differences and the most positive prognostically is the age of onset (Kanner, 1943). Unlike autistic children, with their fundamental and extreme inability to communicate normally from the beginning, schizophrenic children usually have had relationships and normal functioning previously from which they have withdrawn and to which it is hoped they can be restored. However, even where early normal functioning was alleged, in retrospect signs of peculiarities of functioning even before the onset of the disorder can often be recalled (Despert, 1968; Kessler, 1966). Although the schizophrenic child uses language more frequently than the autistic child, it may be incomprehensible or highly egocentric and hence not a communication tool. The schizophrenic child's speech is often flat, with many oddities and idiosyncrasies which lead to further social rejection and isolation (Goldfarb, Braunstein, and Lorge, 1956). An excerpt from the conversation of one of Lauretta Bender's (1947) child schizophrenic patients illustrates well the unusual quality of the language and its peculiar, highly personalized content:

> I say, hello, doctor, have you any new toys? Let me open your radiator with this screwdriver. I say let me open it. I say, so what! Can I copy your animals? I am in a doctor's office. You and I are twins, aren't we? I am coloring this camel brown. I said I am coloring it brown. I said I am coloring it brown. Have you a little scissors? Have you a big scissors? I say, have you a big scissors? Well, here's what I will use. What do you think? It is called a knife. How does my voice sound? What? Judy, what? Is that your name? I'm cutting out this camel. Is it pretty enough to hang on the wall? Can you cut as pretty as this? My sister says, camel talk. Isn't that funny? Camel talk. My voice sounds like up in the library. Doesn't it? In the hospital my voice sounds like up in the library. Can you say li-bra-ri-an? The library is where you get books. (pp. 49–50)

And it continues in that fashion. At the other extreme the schizophrenic child may exhibit mutism (Despert, 1968).

Thought processes may be disorganized and difficult to follow or may contain highly symbolic content. The logic is not readily apparent to others; however, there may be a kind of peculiar logic for the child, which can sometimes be discerned through careful attention to situational variables (Goldfarb, Mintz, and Stroock, 1969). Social awareness and judgment are usually poor, and there may be inappropriate affect as well as behavior. For instance, a schizophrenic child may laugh when describing something very sad, such as a death, or may appear very flat and show very little affect even when describing an event that would evoke horror or fear in normal children, such as a murder. The child may be overactive or aggressive, usually inappropriately and impulsively so, or very withdrawn. There may be difficulty separating real from imaginary events, or differentiating oneself from others and from the environment. That is, the child may have trouble making "the I–not I distinction" (Despert, 1968, p. 116). This blurring of boundaries is sometimes seen in the drawings of schizophrenic children; they may be unable to contain the person within the outline of a figure, or there may be unclear personal boundaries, as illustrated in Figure 12.2.

The child may seem to show more interest in fantasies than in the real world, thus appearing very withdrawn, although what appears to be fantasizing may actually be preoccupation with various physical sensations which involve little cognitive content (Kessler, 1966).

As with autism, there is disagreement between those who stress psychogenic causes of childhood schizophrenia and those who argue that there are biochemical, neurological, or genetic difficulties involved. On one side are the environmentalists, who see parental influence as primary. Blame has been directed at a so-called schizophrenogenic mother who is said to behave in such a way as to lead her child to psychosis. Also implicated have been confused or distorted communication (Bateson et al., 1956; Goldfarb, 1964) and negative family interactions (Wolman, 1970), which are alleged to have interfered with normal parent-child relationships. However, other researchers have argued that the important pathological antecedents found in the histories of schizophrenic children are too varied to have had a specific relationship to the schizophrenic syndrome (Despert, 1968). Creak and Ini (1960) concluded that their study of families failed to support the notion of a psychogenic cause.

On the other side is Bender (1953), for example, who suggested that childhood schizophrenia is based on a maturational deficit. The biological developmental lag then leads to other symptoms, though there must be a hereditary predisposition and a physiological crisis that precipitates the disorder. Similarly, Taft and Goldfarb (1964) interpreted their finding of more reproductive problems and complications in schizophrenics than in normals as a demonstration of the contribution of brain damage to a child's adaptive difficulties. However, even theorists who stress such factors recognize the importance of environmental factors, which interact with the physiological ones either to precipitate a disorder or to influence its course and the *pattern* of symptoms (Bender, 1953; Taft and Goldfarb, 1964).

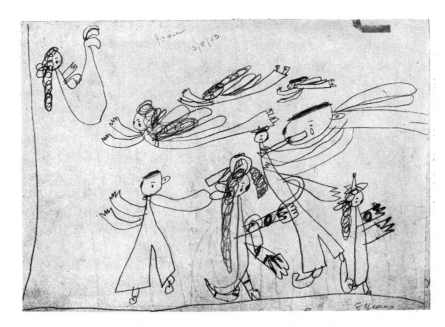

FIGURE 12.2   *Drawing by an eight-year-old girl. Source:* J. Allison Montague, "Spontaneous Drawings of the Human Form in Childhood Schizophrenia" in *An Introduction to Projective Techniques,* Harold H. Anderson and Gladys L. Anderson, eds., © 1951, p. 383. Reprinted by permission of Prentice-Hall, Inc., Englewood Cliffs, N.J.

One's stance on this controversial etiological issue is central to one's perception of the nature of the disturbance and consequently to one's choice of treatment.

CASE STUDY
When Janice was first seen at the clinic, she was 13 and unable to relate to other people at all. She was very angry and highly anxious and either used language in a very ineffectual manner or became severely withdrawn. Her behavior was highly inappropriate and unpredictable. She sometimes became almost assaultive, sometimes behaved very seductively but was totally unaware of the inappropriateness of her behavior. She seemed to have no social sense whatever. She sometimes appeared retarded. At other times she seemed capable of understanding situations and appeared to be somewhat manipulative. She had frequent crying spells and often giggled and laughed for no apparent reason. She screamed frequently, and sometimes let

out loud whoops and whirled away from others. Her language, which was very limited, had an odd echolalic quality to it. She was clearly set apart from even her disturbed peers and showed virtually no functional behavior for the first three months of therapy. She needed help with such basic routines as dressing and washing her hair; she could not do laundry, shop, or do other age-appropriate things; and she did not know her birthdate or other factual information about her environment.

Her background was one of almost total isolation from other people and a very confined life with an extremely hostile mother, a younger sister, and an ineffective father. The mother, a professional woman, was frequently verbally abusive. At the same time she discouraged her children from developing any outside interests and, therefore, learning and practicing social skills. The mother resented the demands that the children made on her time. Her father, though concerned about her, was intimidated by his wife and unable or unwilling to intercede effectively on Janice's behalf or on behalf of her sister.

After a lengthy period of treatment during which she gradually came to trust other adults in the environment and, later, peers, she was able to begin to develop more appropriate social skills and relationships with others. She began to use language more frequently, and her episodes of uncharacteristically high functioning suggested that she may have had above-average intellectual potential at one time which had been inadequately developed because of her serious disturbance. She remained grossly immature, at times still inappropriate in affect, and retained very odd language mannerisms. It appeared likely that residual effects of her severe early disturbance would persist throughout adulthood.

Treatment

Like that of autism, the treatment of childhood schizophrenia varies widely. Some feel that treatment is best approached in a therapeutically managed and arranged residential setting (Goldfarb, Mintz, and Stroock, 1969), while others advocate as normal an environment as can be achieved and the avoidance of institutionalization if at all possible (Wolman, 1970). There is widespread agreement that the very first priority is to bring the child to better reality testing and that other symptoms must take a back seat to this goal (Wolman, 1970). For example, Despert's (1968) first therapeutic goal was to break into the child's symbolic and unintelligible world and establish "affective contact" (p. 193). Goldfarb and his colleagues (1969) emphasized "corrective socialization" in which schizophrenic children would be helped to

193). Goldfarb and his colleagues (1969) emphasized "corrective socialization" in which schizophrenic children would be helped to attend to and respond to stimuli in the environment in a more effective and organized way and to distinguish themselves from and communicate with others in the environment. Others stressed the need to try to restore equilibrium in an individual whose development had been well established previously (Rutter, 1972a), or to stimulate maturation, relieve anxiety, and strengthen the child's defenses (Bender, 1953).

Medical intervention may be helpful, especially during an acute phase, in making the child more amenable to other therapy, but it is best used as an adjunct form of treatment (Kanner, 1972).

The value of psychotherapy with schizophrenic children is unclear: it is difficult to evaluate treatment because of diagnostic problems, poor controls for such factors as spontaneous remission, and different objectives depending on the theoretical approach (Werry, 1979a). Although psychotherapeutic intervention is likely to be a slow, gradual process, sessions with a therapist, regardless of the method or theoretical perspective, may bring improvement because of the therapeutic effect of such attention (Wolman, 1970). In addition, eliciting *expression* of affect may itself lead to a more genuine response in the therapist, which in turn may lead to genuine affect in the child and a feeling of attachment (Ney, 1967).

Behavioral techniques used with schizophrenic children appear to have been successful in changing specific behaviors. Operant conditioning has been used, for example, to develop specific social and language skills and other complex behavior (Ney, 1967; Hersen and Eisler, 1976). In general, the behavioral techniques do not aim to "cure" a disorder; they are designed rather to help the child decrease undesirable behavior and increase basic skills in order to achieve a more normal adjustment. They also help the child order the environment enough to begin to manipulate it successfully, which leads to growth (Leff, 1968).

Although operant techniques can bring improvement in specific behaviors, some feel that the building of normal human relationships and attachment requires a prolonged interpersonal experience as with a therapist (Goldfarb, Mintz, and Stroock, 1969). Some also question the generalization of effect, wondering whether the child will be able to use the newly acquired skills outside the training environment in other situations. It is important not only to transfer behaviors from the training medium to the life situation but also to transmit control from the experimenter to the child (Yates, 1970a). Before genuine success can be claimed for behavioral procedures, it is necessary to determine whether generalization occurs (Leff, 1968), to demonstrate that the specific procedures were in fact responsible for the behavior changes noted (Sherman and Baer, 1969), and to find which factors determine the generalization (Leff, 1968).

Therapy can be directed at changing factors in the environment that exacerbate the problem or add to the child's stress. Some researchers (Bender, 1953; Goldfarb, Mintz, and Stroock, 1969; Peck, Rabinovitch, and Cramer, 1949; Wolman, 1970) have emphasized the need to treat the parents in order to change the family's interaction patterns, helping them deal with feelings of guilt, isolation, hostility, and anxiety, and to help the child adapt to life in the family and community (Peck, Rabinovitch, and Cramer, 1949). Although such work with parents is important, it may be quite difficult to carry out because of the parents' frustration, the high levels of hostility in both the parents and the child, and frequent parental pathology (Wolman, 1970).

Spontaneous remission can sometimes occur with puberty (Bender, 1956). Prognosis, however, remains rather poor, and treatment consists primarily in producing symptomatic change through behavior modification, education, and medication (Werry, 1979a). In one follow-up study of seventy-one children diagnosed psychotic as preschoolers, Havelkova (1968) found that the intellectual deficit of the children was only partially alleviated by treatment. The data also suggested that there is a critical period for treatment and that earlier intervention is most helpful for those whose disorder is mild and whose recovery may thus be aided by maturation.

Symbiotic Infantile Psychosis

Theoretical / Descriptive Background

Margaret Mahler (1952) first described symbiotic infantile psychosis as one of two "developmental psychoses" of childhood which occur in the first five years of life, the other being early infantile autism. The two have in common a primary disturbance in object relations and ego boundaries—that is, in the child's relationship to the environment. According to Mahler (1969), children normally go through autistic, symbiotic, and separation-individuation developmental phases. In the first phase distinctions are not made between self and mother, and in the second phase there is a close, dependent relationship with the mother. Only in the latter phase, when the infant becomes increasingly aware of physical separateness from the mother, does a sense of a separate psychological self and its boundaries develop. The whole process of separation (leaving mother) and individuation (assuming one's own characteristics) is referred to as the infant's "psychological birth" (Mahler, Pine, and Bergman, 1975). The main aspects of this psychological separation occur between five and thirty-six months, when a normal child is able to function separately and enjoy independence; but progress is markedly disrupted in the seriously disturbed and symbiotic child.

Symptoms of this disorder often do not become apparent in the first year because the relationship between mother and child is normally close then and the infant is expected to be dependent on the mother. However, as Mahler and Gosliner (1955) pointed out, symptoms begin to appear in the second year, when maturation characteristically brings greater mobility and exploration, and hence greater possibilities for separation of mother and child. This threatened separation causes intense anxiety, which overwhelms the symbiotic child and may result in panic and very disturbed behavior. The child identifies too closely with the mother, an identification that distorts perception of the world, precludes growth and independence, and leaves the child with no interests or ambitions of his or her own (Wolman, 1970). There is low frustration tolerance and an inability to grow out of a totally dependent stage to attain the independence of a normal preschooler; "his ego is borrowed from his mother" (Kessler, 1966, p. 274).

Mahler and Gosliner (1955) have suggested that pathogenic factors involved might be a constitutional predisposition or sensitivity on the part of the child, as well as a mother who is overprotective or who infantilizes the infant and hence interferes with the infant's individuation. Mahler perceives autistic children as having gone no further than the first stage of development, whereas children with symbiotic psychosis have begun to progress to the next stage, but have panicked during the separation-individuation phase and regressed to the symbiotic stage. Much of their behavior may then be very disturbed, and they may in fact look like the autistic child in many ways (Erickson, 1978).

Symbiotic infantile psychosis is a very rare disorder, and there is not unanimous agreement as to whether it warrants separate classification. Eisenberg (1966), for instance, reported that he had seen only one symbiotic patient and that few clinicians use that category. The Group for the Advancement of Psychiatry (1974) has included in their classification scheme an "interactional" disorder which includes children with symbiotic psychosis but also embraces those children who show symbiotic relationships and unusual dependence on their mothers as a function of other disorders. The disorder is included here as a separate category simply to provide a symptomatic picture of one other severe childhood disturbance in both cognitive and affective functioning.

The following excerpt from B. B. Wolman (1970) illustrates well the disturbed separation process and overdependence described above.

CASE STUDY
When Johnny came with his mother, he held on to her and refused to leave her hand. He followed her everywhere; when she sat down, he stood next to her chair. She sat down with a sigh and a moan. She was a heavy, talkative, verbose woman, and described in great detail her troubles with her husband and son. She was the self-sacrificing martyr who had married a "selfish, inconsiderate man" and had had with him this "poor, mentally retarded child."

Johnny was six years old, pale and obese. He pulled her hand and interrupted her speech with questions not related to mother's story. His speech was blurred; he swallowed syllables, and his voice did not carry well. He was definitely overdressed. He wore three sweaters. According to mother, Johnny was susceptible to common colds.

Whenever a question was directed to Johnny, his mother answered for him. She was vehemently hostile to her husband but not overtly hostile to her child. To the contrary, during the session, she hugged and kissed Johnny, and whenever she burst out in tears, her affection for Johnny seemed to grow.

Johnny cried together with his mother, although one could not be sure whether he was really moved by the content of her story. Most probably he automatically responded to her tears irrespective of their cause and with little attention to the content of her story.

Johnny had no friends or playmates. On weekends his mother took him to the park, but she never allowed him to play with other children because "they were dirty," and

Johnny was a "sensitive child" and easily caught diseases. No child was allowed to visit Johnny's home; nor was Johnny allowed to visit other children. The reason given by the mother was the danger of infectious diseases and her conviction that Johnny was unable to defend himself against other children who (all of them) are aggressive.

Johnny liked dogs but his mother seemed to be jealous even of animal friends. Her excuse was that dogs bite and have fleas and poor Johnny might get bitten by dogs and fleas.

In reply to my question, the mother maintained that she wished Johnny to become more outgoing and independent. At this moment Johnny asked her to tie his shoelaces. She refused. Johnny repeated his demand; he raised his voice and screamed. His mother called him "monster," but yielded to his whim and tied the laces. I imagine that such battles have occurred daily. Johnny was taught to rely on his mother in everything; he was repeatedly told how incompetent and inadequate he was. He was discouraged from doing anything on his own; whenever he dared to try, he was criticized for his clumsiness. Gradually he gave up trying. *The only way to please mother was to depend on her* and make her believe that she was an indispensable, generous, and most kind person. Johnny was afraid to alienate his mother and ceased to live his own life. He somehow knew that he was expected to ask mother's help in everything. Though occasionally his mother protested, her anger was at a minimum as compared with her malicious, venomous criticism whenever Johnny dared to do anything on his own without referring to his mother. (pp. 97–98)

Treatment

Mahler (1969) has as her first aim of treatment involvement of the child in "a 'corrective symbiotic experience'" (p. 167) in which the child relives earlier developmental stages to reach a higher one that allows independent functioning. The two aspects of treatment which must go together, according to Mahler, are, first, that the child must be helped to test reality very slowly, gradually, and at his or her own rate; and second, that there must be ongoing, continuous support from a therapist who takes the role of a surrogate mother. If the separation goes too fast or occurs without continuing support from a therapist, there may be panic and further regression. The mother also needs supportive therapy simultaneously (Mahler, 1952). Even with long, careful treatment, however, the prognosis is only moderately good for arresting the process and even poorer for a "cure" (Mahler, 1952, 1969). Furer (1971) was somewhat more optimistic; he reported that when treatment began at ages two to four, the child could enter school at six or seven, which would help introduce reality to the child and facilitate gradual weaning from the treatment center.

Most behavioral theorists do not deal with symbiotic infantile psychosis separately, as they view it as well as the other severe disorders in terms of behavior clusters rather than syndromes with distinctive intrapsychic dynamics. Hence, their approach would be directed toward specific behavior changes in the mother and child, aimed at increasing the child's skills and level of independent functioning.

Discussion Questions

1. Discuss the case study of autism from the various theoretical perspectives included in the chapter. Try to explain the symptoms from both psychodynamic and behaviorist points of view.
2. Which therapeutic interventions would you choose if you were responsible for the autistic child's treatment? Support your choices with research findings wherever possible.
3. Try to generate some hypotheses which would help to clarify some of the confusion regarding the etiology of childhood schizophrenia.

CHAPTER 13   Psychosomatic
Disorders

Interest in the interaction of biological and psychological events has a long history. As far back as ancient Greece, philosophers such as Aristotle and Plato contemplated the relation of mind to body—their unity or separateness. Even Hippocrates observed the interaction of psychological factors with disease in his statement, "It is more important to know what sort of person has a disease than to know what sort of disease a person has" (Wittkower and Warnes, 1977). Over the centuries various ideas developed about the effects of psychological events on physical functioning and about the reverse interaction in which one's physical ailments led to "madness."

In more recent times many explanations have been espoused for the apparent connections and associations between psychological and physical events. This entire area of study has usually been subsumed under the heading of psychosomatic disorders, but it includes highly disparate views about the processes involved. Even the label "psychosomatic" is not universally agreed upon. Achenbach (1974), for example, prefers "psychophysiologic" because of the negative connotations attached to "psychosomatic." The DSM-III manual (APA, 1980) lists the usual "psychosomatic disorders" under "Psychological Factors Affecting Physical Condition" (p. 303) and describes such factors as those that " . . . contribute to the initiation or exacerbation of a physical condition" (p. 303), which may be a disorder or a single symptom.

Researchers disagree on the relative importance of physical and psychological factors in the etiology of these disorders. Some maintain that various factors such as illness, constitutional weakness, and other physical characteristics may cause weakness in a particular body system and thus increase its susceptibility to damage (Knopf, 1979); some have taken the view that certain physical disorders can be caused almost exclusively by specific psychological events and experiences. Others give only contributory and precipitatory status to psychological events, while still others consider such psychological events or factors to be the *result* of physical disorders—that is, consequent events. The interaction of physiological and psychological factors can be circular, with physical problems leading to greater stress, which can then exacerbate the physical problems. Interestingly, one recent review indicated that referring patients simultaneously to a psychologist and a physician reduced the amount of medical service necessary (Rosen and Wiens, 1979).

286

Physical problems that are related to psychological events but are not considered to be genuine psychosomatic disorders include self-injury, hypochondriasis (overconcern with one's health), malingering (conscious faking), and conversion symptoms (symbolic expressions of unconscious conflicts).

In this chapter the various views of psychosomatic disorders will be detailed and tentative conclusions drawn. Some general methodological considerations relevant to psychosomatic disorders will be dealt with first, followed by more detailed discussion of frequently studied specific disorders which are often thought to have important psychological or psychosocial features in their etiology and clinical course.

Methodological Considerations

Available studies of psychosomatic disorders have frequently been criticized for their methodological weaknesses and errors (Achenbach, 1974; Karasu and Plutchik, 1978; Mendelson, Hirsch, and Webber, 1956; Rees, 1964; Werry, 1972). One problem is that many of the studies have been done retrospectively: individuals who already suffer from such disorders as asthma and ulcers are selected for more extensive study to see what kinds of psychological variables exist in their backgrounds. However, it is impossible to determine whether prevailing psychological variables or factors contributed to the development of the disorder (antecedent conditions) or developed in reaction to and as a consequence of the disorder (consequent conditions). Thus, to assume that psychopathology precedes the physical problem, as is frequently done, is to wrongly infer causation from correlation. More rigorous experimental studies of the functional relationship between psychological states and physiological responses are needed (Achenbach, 1974), as well as more predictive studies.

Studies have also been criticized for such methodological weaknesses as overgeneralizing from too few cases or on the basis of insufficient or questionable evidence, biased selection of data, oversimplification of highly complex data (Lidz and Rubenstein, 1959), exclusive emphasis on either physiological or psychological factors without regard for the other (Rees, 1964), and poor controls. Without adequate controls, contradictory findings often cannot be explained, because differences could be due to age, sex, personality, methodology, or problems of definition (Karasu and Plutchik, 1978).

Theoretical Explanations

Explanatory models developed for the interaction of physiological and psychological events tend to concentrate on either the organic/physiological factors or the psychological factors.

Physiological and Genetic Factors

In the first category of explanations, the emphasis is on somatic weakness, inherited autonomic nervous system patterns or differences, genetic vulnerability, and other kinds of physical predisposition, as well as such physical agents as chemicals and allergens. Such physiological factors may, however, require a precipitating psychological event to become manifest as a disorder.

Psychological Factors

In the second category of explanations, primary etiological significance is attributed to psychological factors or events. Within the range of such primarily psychological theories or explanatory models, however, there are specific and nonspecific theoretical explanations of the course of psychosomatic disease development.

SPECIFICITY THEORIES

The specificity theories hold that specific psychological factors or events lead to specific physical disorders or are highly associated with them; for example, a person with dependency conflicts is likely to develop an ulcer (Weiner et al., 1957). That is, particular conflicts are specific to a disorder and are always found in individuals who have that disorder (Werry, 1972). Alexander (1950), for instance, maintained that specific psychological conflicts or events have consistent effects on specific body organs, usually via innervation of the autonomic nervous system, resulting in dysfunction and organic changes in susceptible individuals whose conflicts remain unresolved.

288

NONSPECIFICITY THEORIES

The nonspecific theories maintain that psychosomatic disorders may arise in association with psychological events, but not in a specific one-to-one association which holds for everyone. According to these explanations, disorders develop as a result of general stress reactions which can arise from various psychological stimuli (Kaplan and Kaplan, 1959). No direct correlation is assumed between the nature of the psychological stress and the nature of the organ involved in a disorder, though characteristic patterns of responding to stress may be genetically or biologicaly determined (Wolff, 1950). With stress, a reaction at the psychological level causes one to feel upset, and a reaction at the physiological level activates the autonomic nervous system (Simmons, 1977). Although such psychophysiological responses to stress are normally adaptive, they can lead to damage if they are elicited inappropriately, too frequently, or in an exaggerated way (Werry, 1972).

EVALUATION

The weight of empirical support falls on the side of the nonspecific point of view. Specificity theories have become less popular because empirical tests have simply failed to support them (Werry, 1972). Widely varying personality characteristics can be found in people suffering from the same disorder, and some with a "classic" pattern do not even develop the disorder (Lachman, 1972). Rather, whether a disorder develops depends on the intensity, frequency, and duration of the emotional arousal in relation to the person's biological or physiological resistance or "assets" (Lachman, 1972). Stressful events may also be the trigger which precipitates psychosomatic disease (Heisel, 1972) or acute episodes in chronically ill children (Bedell et al., 1977). Study of covert muscular activity accompanying mental activity, which can give important information about how an individual processes information, must be interpreted in the context of other physiological activity as well as environmental demands on the person (Caccioppo and Petty, 1981). Finally, continued efforts to link specific affect, conflicts, or parent characteristics to specific symptoms diverts attention from the complexities of individual children (Dowling, 1973).

Immunological Considerations

Related to the models emphasizing stress are explanations that focus on the importance of the immunological system. For example, children with arthritis, hernias, appendicitis, and psychiatric problems have been found to have experienced more stressful events in the year prior to onset than had controls (Heisel et al., 1975), and stress has been associated with increases in susceptibility to certain viruses and infections (Black, Humphrey, and Niven, 1963) and even cancer (Greene and Miller, 1958; Jacobs and Charles, 1980).

Newer reports (Jacobs and Charles, 1980; Rogers, Dubey, and Reich, 1979) suggest a relationship between the effectiveness of the immunological system and psychological factors such as one's capacity to cope with stress. Psychological factors may have an effect through endocrinological changes, through autonomic nervous system changes, or through separate mechanisms such as are suggested in immunosuppression conditioning (Rogers, Dubey, and Reich, 1979).

There is some evidence that immunosuppresion can be conditioned, at least in rats (Ader and Cohen, 1975; Rogers et al., 1976). Researchers have succeeded in inhibiting even a tuberculin skin test (Mantoux reaction) in positive reactors with the use of hypnosis (Black, Humphrey, and Niven, 1963), controlling various physiological processes through biofeedback techniques (Shapiro and Surwit, 1976), and directly altering the immunological response through stimulation of the brain (Rogers, Dubey, and Reich, 1979). Rogers and his colleagues, however, concluding that stress is a risk factor which is significantly but not always associated with disease, caution against oversimplified notions of stress and psychological factors as the "cause" of disease. Rather, they advocate viewing stress " . . . as having a complex interaction with the personality and biology of the host and hence with the expression of disease" (p. 154).

This interaction is a very complex one, because while stress may suppress the immune system, it may also enhance it and hence may sometimes have a protective effect; and a variety of related behaviors that change with stress, such as diet and sleep, may also affect the immune system (Rogers, Dubey, and Reich, 1979). Rogers and his associates noted further that the effects of stress depend in part on the nature of the stress, its timing and duration, the life cycle of the person, and other factors; its special importance in children may be that it can affect the *development* of the immune system.

Family Interaction Patterns

The role of the family is often given central importance in discussion of psychosomatic disorders. Minuchin and his colleagues (1975) developed their "open systems model" to extend the focus from the child to the child within the family. They argued that certain family organizations are associated with the development of psychosomatic symptoms, that somatization is encouraged by the family process in some families, that these symptoms maintain the family equilibrium, and that the illness is used as a vehicle for communication in such families. According to their model, symptom choice is related to the family's history and organization and to the complaints of other family members. Therapy, then, is directed toward the family's pattern of interaction and feedback in an attempt to change these processes. They reported that when treatment changed the family organization, the child improved greatly.

Burbeck's (1979) empirical study of the open systems model, however, led him to question its validity. He criticized the research of Minuchin and his colleagues as limited and inconclusive, with too few cases, single-case designs, and a select population (most severe).

The most common conclusion (Long et al., 1958; Purcell, Weiss, and Hahn, 1972; Rees, 1964; Simmons, 1977; Weiner et al., 1957; Werry, 1972; Yorkston, 1975) is that many disorders develop as a result of the combination and interaction of genetic, physical, environmental, and psychological events and characteristics, although the mechanisms by which this happens are still unclear. Assuming that physiological and emotional factors are involved, disease may develop when the sum of all of these factors hits a critical level, regardless of their relative contributions, which vary among children (Finch, 1977).

Many of the psychological variables singled out as significant in specific disorders may in fact be nonspecific and important in any child who suffers a chronic illness (Lipton, Steinschneider, and Richmond, 1966; Neuhaus, 1958; O'Malley et al., 1979; Purcell, Weiss, and Hahn, 1972).

In the next section, aspects of these various explanations and viewpoints, as well as relevant literature, will be explored in the context of specific disorders which have frequently been considered to have large psychological or psychosocial components. The section on asthma is lengthier than the others, both because of the amount of research it has generated and because it exemplifies many of the problems and controversies involved in research into the intriguing area of psychosomatic disease. Therefore, descriptive, case study, and treatment material on asthma will be discussed in detail, followed by a briefer discussion of other disorders.

Specific Disorders

Asthma

THEORETICAL / DESCRIPTIVE BACKGROUND

Chronic bronchial asthma has probably generated more research and more controversy than any other disorder in terms of the relative involvement of physiological and psychological factors. Sixty percent of asthmatics are under seventeen, and boys are afflicted roughly twice as often as girls (Purcell, Weiss, and Hahn, 1972). There is fairly widespread agreement that most children with asthma have a genetic allergic predisposition, but that other important mechanisms and variables may be involved as well and that psychological factors may trigger asthmatic attacks or may even be the underlying cause in some cases (Lipton, Steinschneider, and Richmond, 1966). The agents involved differ for different people or at different times for one person and include microorganisms, physical or chemical irritants (heat, humidity, smoke), allergens, and psychological factors (Yorkston, 1975). Additional etiologically relevant factors are age and sex, family incidence of asthma and related problems, infections, personality characteristics, psychological disturbances or symptoms, pent-up tension, allergies, events preceding or coinciding with onset, and environmental factors such as climate and physical stimuli (Rees, 1964). Regardless of what determines the onset of asthma (usually a combination of factors), any agents, including stress and anxiety, may precipitate later attacks (Purcell and Weiss, 1970; Rees, 1964; Simmons, 1977).

Stress often seems to be one of the most important precipitants. The psychological factors may be obvious, as when attacks follow an incident or experience in which the person becomes very upset or anxious; or they may operate less obviously, as when thoughts provoke or worsen the attack—for instance, when individuals *think* they are in the presence of an allergen or are inhaling one, even though the sub-

292

stance in question is neutral (Yorkston, 1975). In one case (Mackenzie, 1886), for example, an asthmatic attack and hay fever were induced in a woman by showing her an artificial but very realistic rose. Tieramaa (1979) reported that when childhood onset of asthma occurred in the context of an unfavorable psychological environment, improvement after separation from close friends or relatives was frequent. In addition, psychological factors have an important influence on the *course* of the disorder, in that the illness may meet needs that are not met directly and hence may be maintained in a variety of ways, such as through noncompliance with medical recommendations (Matus, 1981).

Many differences in personality and psychological characteristics between asthmatic and normal children have been reported in the literature. Asthmatics have been described as more neurotic (Neuhaus, 1958; Tieramaa, 1979); more inhibited in their crying (Lipton, Steinschneider, and Richmond, 1966); more anxious, insecure, and dependent, and less adaptable (Neuhaus, 1958; Rees, 1964); less healthy and less aggressive but more tense (Rawls, Rawls, and Harrison, 1971); and more sensitive, perfectionistic, and compulsive, all tension-producing traits (Rees, 1964). Their mothers have been described as overprotective or rejecting (Lipton, Steinschneider, and Richmond, 1966; Rees, 1964), as well as anxious (Long et al., 1958); and disturbed family characteristics have been implicated. However, there is no evidence to suggest that families without asthmatic children do *not* have similar characteristics (Burbeck, 1979). Overprotection in the mother and dependency in the child have been used to explain such a diversity of disorders that they may no longer be useful explanations (Hetherington and Martin, 1972). In any case, such characteristics as overprotection and anxiety in parents could well be *responses* to a child's chronic and unpredictable illness rather than causally related (Parker and Lipscombe, 1979).

In one study of 1190 six- to eleven-year-old children with and without allergic histories (Rawls, Rawls, and Harrison, 1971), comparisons were made on a number of variables, including intellectual ability, psychological test responses, academic work, medical history, and social interaction patterns. Although the researchers found children without allergies to be healthier and rated them as superior on some measures, other measures did not differentiate between them. Where higher anxiety or dependence or other "neurotic" symptoms are present in these children, they may be as a result of or in reaction to the physical disorder (Franks and Leigh, 1959) and are probably characteristic of all children with chronic illness, not specific to asthma (Lipton, Steinschneider, and Richmond, 1966). Much earlier findings of similar personality characteristics and higher levels of disturbance in children with cardiac problems (Neuhaus, 1958) lend support to this notion.

Most studies involving personality factors are methodologically weak and rely too heavily on subjective psychological measures (Franks and Leigh, 1959; Werry, 1972). Werry concluded that there is no evidence of significant psychopathology, specific conflicts, or deviant parenting in the lives of asthmatic children as a group, and that there is only circumstantial evidence for the effects of anxiety and other psychological states. More rigorous studies are needed.

In an effort to explain some of the confusing and contradictory findings, many workers have urged the delineation of subgroups of asthmatic children who show different etiological factors, rates of remission, and levels of dependence on medication. In one study (Alexander, 1972), when ten- to fifteen-year-old asthmatic children were divided into two subgroups according to whether or not emotional factors were prominent in precipitating an attack, the effect of relaxation was shown to be greater in the group for which emotional factors were most important. In another study Purcell and his colleagues (1969) experimentally separated twenty-five asthmatic children, ages five to thirteen, from their families. Based on various kinds of information gleaned from careful diagnostic interviews, including the number of emotional precipitants of asthmatic attacks, they predicted quite accurately which children would show improvement with the separation. Although there were some confounding variables, they concluded that such interviews may help to determine or assess the relevance of psychological variables. In another study, sixty-two children with asthma were divided into two subgroups based on their scores on an Allergic Potential Scale (APS). Those with lower allergic potential scores showed more psychopathological factors, as did their mothers in relation to both child and spouse (Block et al., 1964). Since the children studied were similar in severity level, the authors stressed the importance of looking at subgroups to reconcile contradictory findings in the literature. In addition, perhaps the separation and investigation of various behavioral expressions and levels

294

of severity—rather than lumping together such factors as amount of school missed, type of medication, and severity of attacks—would help in detection and clarification of significant associations (Burbeck, 1979). In any case, cases in which psychological factors appear to play an important role should not be dismissed as less significant, as they can still be fatal; nor should other serious cases be dismissed as "nonpsychological" (Pinkerton, 1967).

Behavioral explanations and approaches to asthma abound in the literature. Early writers (Dekker, Pelser, and Groen, 1957; Franks and Leigh, 1959; Moore, 1965; Purcell et al., 1969) noted the role of conditioning in some bronchial asthma attacks. Others (Purcell, et al., 1969; Purcell and Weiss, 1970; Purcell, Weiss, and Hahn, 1972) have stressed the need to focus on events just before onset and reinforcement contingencies, as well as allergic potential, in order to better understand what stimuli trigger attacks. However, Purcell and Weiss (1970) concluded that conditioning of asthma had not been adequately demonstrated.

Thus, there are no unequivocal findings. The literature indicates that the etiology and course of asthma are very complex and involve the interaction of many variables, both physiological and psychological. The most promising line of inquiry appears to be the study of subgroups of asthmatics, as the term "asthmatic" encompasses too wide a range of problems and levels of severity. Age, sex, and personality differences in the clinical picture and in the course of the disorder and variations in allergic potential and reactions to stress, as well as the role of conditioning, need to be investigated further.

During an asthma attack the airways contract and the victim has difficulty breathing normally. Anxiety usually follows, and the person may go to great lengths to seek relief (Yorkston, 1975). Situations that are perceived—rightly or wrongly—as capable of provoking an attack may be avoided. Such behavior may disrupt normal functioning by interfering with school or work, family life, social relationships, and other aspects of the individual's life (Yorkston, 1975). An example of the interaction of many variables in an asthmatic condition is demonstrated in the following case study by Simmons (1977).

CASE STUDY
Six-year-old John, an only child, had a history of bronchitis, beginning at age one year and progressing to clinical asthma by age four. Allergy testing showed him to be mildly sensitive

to house dust and tobacco smoke. Many of his attacks were precipitated by infection, usually of viral origin. The parents were in their early forties. With each attack, his mother would panic and John's wheezing would become worse in spite of medication. He would be rushed to the hospital, where he would be admitted because he was so ill, only to clear with minimal treatment within twenty-four hours. The situation was becoming worse, with multiple hospital admissions, a great deal of time absent from school and the parents becoming more upset and feeling increasingly inadequate.

Discussion with the parents revealed how anxious they were about this child who meant so much to them. The physician also learned that the father resented having to give up smoking because of the child. He did not criticize them by telling them that they were overprotective, as this would have increased their feelings of inadequacy. The father was helped to recognize some of his feelings and was shown how he could continue smoking in a way that would not affect John, who was only mildly sensitive to tobacco smoke.

In discussion with the physician, much of the family stress in response to the illness was relieved. John continued to have asthmatic attacks with every severe cold, but these became less distressing to all members of the family, to the point where they usually could be handled at home without hospitalization and with less time off school. (pp. 196–197)

TREATMENT

Treatments discussed in this section are used to *supplement* medical treatment. The assumption is made that the child has had or is receiving appropriate medical treatment. Even in cases in which psychological factors have demonstrated significance, good medical care of the physical problems is essential.

To supplement medical treatment, many interventions have been tried, singly or in combination. Varying claims have been made for their success; however, many reports of treatment procedures and their effects have methodological weaknesses (Purcell and Weiss, 1970). In an assessment of the effectiveness of various treatments, it is necessary to include both objective and subjective estimates of improvement and to address the adjustment problems which have resulted from the asthma (Purcell and Weiss, 1970). Physiological improvement is not enough; the child's feelings about the asthma as well as the feelings of those around the child need to be dealt with.

Psychotherapy may be helpful in bringing some relief and minimizing emotional factors (Purcell and Weiss, 1970; Simmons, 1977). Counseling in combination with treatment of allergic factors can decrease the severity and frequency of attacks (Simmons, 1977). *Family therapy* may also be helpful (Liebman, Minuchin, and Baker, 1974; Purcell and Weiss, 1970). Liebman and his coworkers (1974), for example, claim to have successfully used weekly family therapy sessions to alleviate symptoms, or to prevent worsening of symptoms, by changing family patterns of overinvolvement and overprotection. They maintain that the symptoms serve as a focus which diverts attention from other family problems. The breathing techniques which they taught to abort attacks were insufficient to prevent relapses, and they concluded that family therapy was an effective and necessary part of the treatment of severe asthma.

Because anxiety can affect the asthma in several ways, its reduction can have important therapeutic effects. *Hypnosis* has been used successfully with some asthmatics to help the person relax. It can be used as an adjunct to psychotherapy or to change a physiological response (Purcell and Weiss, 1970). *Behavioral techniques,* particularly desensitization and relaxation training, have reportedly been used successfully to bring about both objective and subjective improvement (Alexander, 1972; Alexander, Miklich, and Hershkoff, 1972; Moore, 1965; Yorkston (1975). However, in a more recent study, Alexander and his colleagues (1979) reported that although training in relaxation did have some effect on heart rate and muscle tension, and did help reduce fear responses to the asthma itself and thus alter maladaptive anxiety, which can significantly interfere with an asthmatic child's life, it did not significantly affect pulmonary function in children with severe asthma. They suggested that such relaxation may even be counterindicated because it decreases certain physiological activities in a way that is detrimental to asthmatics.

Feldman (1976) reported success in using *biofeedback* techniques to train four severely asthmatic children to lower their airway resistance; he obtained results comparable to those found after bronchodilator inhalation.

Institutionalization is often associated with a favorable result, but there is disagreement on the reasons for the rapid improvement that is noted in many cases. Some children may need psychotherapy combined with temporary removal from the home environment (Pinkerton, 1967), or a "parentectomy" (Peshkin and Abramson, 1959). When removal from the home results in improvement, it is difficult to assess the role of psychological and allergic factors, as the removal changes both.

Conclusions regarding the relative effectiveness of the many treatment combinations with different subgroups of asthmatic children await more rigorous and methodologically sound research.

Gastrointestinal Disorders

Ulcers in adults have frequently been considered to have a large psychological component. Pictures of a hard-driving executive or a harried worrier developing ulcers are common in the mass media and in cartoons. Peptic ulcers in children are thought to be much less common (Tarboroff and Brown, 1954) and may be quite different clinically from those of adults (Lipton, Steinschneider, and Richmond, 1966). Lipton and his colleagues estimated the number of cases in children to range from .5 percent to 10 percent, in part depending on the diagnostic approach used (X-ray, retrospective studies, and others). They noted that the disorder is least common between the ages of five and ten, occurring more frequently before and after those ages, more frequently in the families of children with ulcers, and more frequently in boys. However, others have reported that duodenal ulcers are more common and are only slightly more frequent in boys (Purcell, Weiss, and Hahn, 1972).

Although there is fairly general agreement that psychological and emotional factors can influence gastric secretions (Lipton, Steinschneider, and Richmond, 1966; Purcell, Weiss, and Hahn, 1972) and can, over time, lead to damage, the level of gastric function *before* the emotional factors or events should also be considered as a potential determinant of later response (Lipton, Steinschneider, and Richmond, 1966). In addition, experimental and observational procedures in themselves may alter gastric function (Lidz and Rubenstein, 1959). Finally, some of the psychological aspects of ulcers may be a consequence of having a chronic illness (Purcell, Weiss, and Hahn, 1972).

Ulcerative colitis in children is a very serious disorder which can begin in early infancy (Engel, 1954). It has been variously regarded as an infectious, allergic, and psychological disorder and has been associated with many personality characteristics as well as with a dis-

298

turbed mother-child relationship. However, as with asthma, when psychological features are associated with the disorder, they may have nonspecific effects or appear as a result rather than a cause, though they may still affect the course of the disorder (Purcell, Weiss, and Hahn, 1972). Psychological factors may even be necessary for the disorder to become manifest, but its development likely depends on constitutional and genetic factors, prenatal influence, and critical events, as well as psychological factors (Finch and Hess, 1962). Although there is wide variation in the severity and course of the disease, it consistently requires long-term treatment (Finch and Hess, 1962) and may require surgery (Finch, 1977).

The complexities of gastrointestinal disorders and the interplay of physiological and psychological factors are illustrated in the following case study from Kanner (1972).

CASE STUDY
James L., an only child, was brought by his mother at seven and one-half years of age. He was described by her as "a very tense boy, a good kid." She added: "It's just the environmental set-up." James weighed less than five pounds at birth. "He vomited continuously for the first fourteen months; it was like pyloric stenosis in some ways but it was not typical. He was sick as a dog with every tooth he cut." He had "chronic bronchitis" until he was five years old; he was found to be allergic to green beans, fish, cod liver oil, and dried prunes. Any dietary indiscretion brought on an attack of asthma and high temperature. He did not talk until three years of age. He presented a feeding problem, had temper tantrums, cried a great deal, and had a specific reading disability. Mucous colitis began when he was four years old. There was a history of measles, mumps, scarlet fever, cervical adenitis, otitis media, and tonsillectomy.

The mother, a graduate nurse, continued working after the child's birth. She ran a hospital for two years. "Then I had a nervous collapse, nervous fatigue. I flopped again last year. I was on a slide before that. I was taking strychnine and kept going. I still get jittery. It was a complete fatigue. My legs went out from under me." She was disappointed matrimonially: "I have had the misfortune of marrying a man who has an endocrine disturbance. He makes an ass of himself and everybody else in the group. He has an awful temper. He is really crazy about James, but he thinks he should jump the minute he is spoken to, and gets mad as three hornets if he doesn't."

James, IQ 121, was demanding and boastful during the first interview. In the following play sessions, he released a flood of hostility against both parents. He presented the dolls who stood for them as extremely coercive, then turned the tables and with great delight had the boy doll order them around constantly and "punished" them if they did not "obey."

While James was being treated at our clinic, the father had himself examined and responded well to a combination of endocrine and psychiatric therapy. The mother was seen frequently by the social worker. James, after some remedial reading instructions, was sent to a boarding school for which the mother paid out of her earnings. The asthma and the colitis faded away without medication. (pp. 395–396)

Cancer

Although cancer is not usually considered a psychosomatic disorder, there has been interest in the psychological factors which are involved and which might affect a person's response to treatment and possible remission. Increasing numbers of studies have begun to suggest that psychological factors may also be important in the etiology of cancer or in a person's resistance or immunity to cancer. That is, psychological factors may significantly affect the immunological system in children and may affect whether neoplastic changes begin at all, or, if they do, how well they are tolerated (Rogers, Dubey, and Reich, 1979).

Greene and Miller (1958) studied the role of emotional and psychological aspects in the development of leukemia. After observing thirty-three children and adolescents with leukemia, they suggested that stressful psychological experiences such as separation from a significant person or object may be accompanied by various physiological ones, such as immunological or biochemical changes, which trigger the leukemia. They also pointed to the possible significance of prenatal experiences and suggested that prenatal stress in the mother may modify the fetus's physiological development, though genetic factors may also interact with prenatal and postnatal experience.

In a more recent study (Jacobs and Charles, 1980), twenty-five children with leukemia or other cancer were compared with a control group of children as to family characteristics and life events (for example, separations, changes in health of family members, family moves, marital discord, etc.) over a two-year period. In addition to finding a higher incidence of cancers in the families of children with cancer,

300

they found that 72 percent of the children with cancer had moved within the two years preceding the cancer, which was three times the rate in the control group. They assumed that moving constituted an emotional upheaval and affected the immunological and other biological systems. Such psychological events, then, may *precede* the cancer. Jacobs and Charles urge the further study of the role of conflict and negative emotion in creating a situation where malignancy might develop, especially in children who are predisposed biologically because of immunological defects or variables that make them more vulnerable to stress or who have difficulty coping with negative emotions. They also suggested that shifts of hormonal levels, which are influenced by normal growth and stressful experiences, may affect the immunological system. The role of viruses in various forms of cancer deserves more study, and emotional factors may play a significant role in increasing one's vulnerability or susceptibility to such viruses.

Emotional factors also play an important role in one's adjustment to a serious disorder such as cancer. One study of 114 individuals who survived childhood cancer (O'Malley et al., 1979) indicated that there was a high rate of adjustment difficulties in survivors, but the initial period was important in predicting long-term adjustment.

One problem that Jacobs and Charles point out is that of determining when the cancer began or was manifest clinically. They conclude that cancer may develop in the *context* of certain events, but causal explanations cannot be made. Another problem is that similar events have very different meanings and significance for different people. They do assert, however, that cancer might also be considered a psychophysiological disorder in a very broad sense.

Other Disorders

Psychological factors have been associated with many other childhood physiological problems. In some cases researchers have found frequent changes and stressful events in the backgrounds of children with various problems. This relationship has been found, for example, in children with juvenile rheumatoid arthritis (Heisel, 1972; Monaghan, Robinson, and Dodge, 1979), in children who are accident-prone (Padilla, Rohsenow, and Bergman, 1976), and in children with the disordered breathing of hyperventilation (Wahl, 1966).

In a disorder such as acne, emotional or psychological factors are not necessarily causal but are undoubtedly involved in exacerbations and hence contribute to the condition, as it also contributes to emotional factors in circular fashion (Cohen, 1965). Emotional factors and their physiological counterparts may also be important in *triggering* disorders such as infantile eczema which are associated with allergies (Lipton, Steinschneider, and Richmond, 1966). In illnesses such as diabetes, the psychological *effect* of having a disorder is most important (Pyke, 1965). The need for a restricted diet and for insulin injections intrudes on the diabetic child's life. The increased dependency that is required to some extent at least may result in a mother's overprotective behavior or infantilization, which in turn may lead to psychological upsets in adolescent diabetics (Pyke, 1965).

In order to more accurately assess the contribution of such psychological factors as stress to the development of physical disorders, more predictive studies must be done. One needs to study children who experience varying types and degrees of stress and then attempt to predict which ones are likely to develop physical disease. Such instruments as the Children's Life Events Inventory can be helpful in studying the effects of stress, especially in predictive work, where knowledge of a disorder does not bias results (Monaghan, Robinson, and Dodge, 1979).

Regardless of the causal or contributory relationships between physical and psychological factors, social and environmental influence are clearly important in the psychological adjustment of children with chronic illness; and ultimately psychological adjustment depends on the interaction of environmental and medical factors (Bedell et al., 1977). Among these factors, Cobb (1976) considers social support to be of critical importance. Moreover, cognitive and behavioral changes serve an important intermediary role in producing physiological changes such as a decrease in blood pressure (Schwartz, 1978).

Conclusions

The literature on psychosomatic disorders in both adults and children is vast. Studies cited in this chapter span nearly a century, and there is still much controversy over the relative contributions of physiological and psychological factors or events in the etiology and course of many disorders.

Among those who agree on the significance of psychological factors, there is disagreement regarding the role of specific conflicts, family dynamics, personality characteristics and response patterns, and conditioning. Most writers agree that disorders develop as a result of a combination and interaction of factors, including genetic, allergic, physiological, and psychological factors in varying degrees. In addition, there is evidence that many personality and psychological factors surface as a *result* of having a chronic illness rather than as causal factors or as factors peculiar to specific disorders. There is, however, a need to study the occurrence and role of such psychological factors or characteristics in children who do *not* develop physical disorders. To this end, more predictive studies would be helpful.

As supplements to good medical management of the various disorders, many treatment procedures have been used with varying success, including psychotherapy, family therapy, behavioral therapy, hypnosis, biofeedback, and institutionalization. Studies into etiology and into the relative effectiveness of the many treatment methods have been plagued with numerous methodological problems and weaknesses. Methodologically sound and experimentally rigorous studies are needed before definitive conclusions can be reached in this area.

Discussion Questions

1. How might psychological factors interact with physiological factors to play a significant role, as either antecedent or consequent events, in physical problems not mentioned in this chapter, such as low back pain or headaches?
2. Discuss some of the changes in experimental design which might be necessary for more definitive studies. For instance, what variables need to be controlled? What kinds of control groups are necessary? What are some of the essential elements of good research that are lacking in many available studies?
3. Do you feel that psychological factors or events have been given too much prominence or significance in the study of physical disorders in children? Too little? Why? What other psychological variables might be involved?

CHAPTER 14   Juvenile Delinquency

Juvenile delinquency is not a psychological term; it is a legal term which defines a child's or an adolescent's relationship to the state (Copel, 1973). Although justice and mental health systems are parallel, they exist separately and youths in one system get quite different treatment from those in the other (Sobel, 1979). Psychology has primarily been involved with the mental health system. Historically the role of psychologists in the justice system has been largely to assess offenders and to present the results of such assessment in court (Sobel, 1979). Now, however, increasing attention is being directed toward both treatment and preventive aspects of the problem of juvenile delinquency.

Theoretical/Descriptive Background

Definition and Incidence

Definitions of delinquency differ according to state and include a variety of behaviors (Phelps, 1976). In some areas the term is used to refer to antisocial behavior, whether or not the offender is actually apprehended (Achenbach, 1974). Even when the term is used narrowly to encompass only those children who actually appear before the courts, it covers many behaviors, from relatively minor to very serious offenses. The list of offenses may, for example, include acts such as running away, which is a problem but which would not violate the law if committed by an adult (Bakwin and Bakwin, 1972).

Ambiguity and confusion regarding the meaning of juvenile delinquency are reflected in varying incidence figures, which depend on the definition one uses. The 1967 Task Force on Juvenile Delinquency estimated that one in nine children would end up in juvenile court before age eighteen, and two out of three of those would appear in court again (Stuart, 1969). Boys exhibit more conduct problems (Peterson, 1961) and are more often delinquent than girls (Haney and Gold, 1973), though the *rate* of delinquency among females is increasing faster than among males (Erickson, 1978). As only a small percentage of offenders are actually apprehended and therefore referred to the court and legally labeled delinquent, official statistics and incidence figures are misleading at best and seriously underestimate the problem at worst (Empey and Erickson, 1966). Socioeconomic differences often further distort the incidence figures, as middle-class offenders may be perceived differently or may be "bought off" by parents (Haney and Gold, 1973).

According to Bakwin and Bakwin (1972), juvenile delinquency has always been with us, but some current aspects are disturbing:

> The disturbing elements in the present picture are the rapid increase in the number of juvenile transgressors, the spread to middle and upper income groups, the extension to rural communities and small cities, and the frequency with which crime is committed without any apparent advantage to the offending youth. The crimes are more vicious than formerly, and many of the young people appearing before the juvenile courts go on to commit one or more serious crimes as adults. (p. 573)

In order to circumvent the problems inherent in official statistics, Haney and Gold (1973) used self-report data as a measure of actual incidence. They used measures of both frequency and seriousness of offenses as indications of *degree* of delinquent behavior. They recognized no arbitrary cutoff between delinquent and nondelinquent adolescents but, rather, conceptualized a continuum along which all adolescents fell, from no illegal behavior to frequent and serious crimes. Although there are quantitative differences among children and adolescents, most do not engage in illegal or antisocial acts (Achenbach, 1974; Haney and Gold, 1973). Haney and Gold's (1973) chart of the incidence of illegal or delinquent behavior as it is distributed across the general adolescent population is reproduced in Figure 14.1.

Classification

Considerable heterogeneity within the group labeled "juvenile delinquent" has led to many attempts to identify subgroups. There is fairly widespread agreement on the existence of three basic types, which have been discussed theoretically and demonstrated empirically. These types, as well as some additional classificatory schemes, are discussed in the following paragraphs.

NEUROTIC DELINQUENT

The neurotic delinquent is considered to have a personality problem, often characterized by withdrawal and low self-esteem (Peterson, 1961), that is reflected in deviant behavior. This type is also referred to as impulsive delinquent (Ross, 1980), disturbed-neurotic delinquent

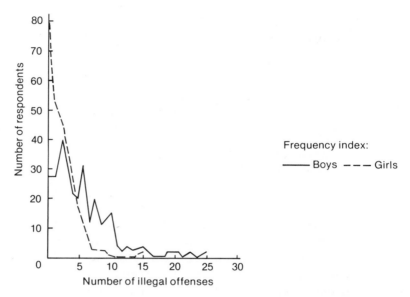

FIGURE 14.1 *Delinquency is a matter of degree, and most teenagers are not very delinquent. Source:* B. Haney and M. Gold, "The Juvenile Delinquent Nobody Knows," *Psychology Today,* September 1973, pp. 49–55. Copyright © 1973 Ziff-Davis Publishing Company. Reprinted by permission.

(Achenbach, 1974), personality disorder (Quay, 1972), neurotic socio-pathic personality (Lykken, 1957), or a Type I overinhibited person-ality (Glueck and Glueck, 1970). These youths are not the "hard-core" delinquents; they are seen as in need of psychiatric more than puni-tive response, and they frequently end up in mental health facilities rather than correctional ones. They score higher on measures of anx-iety (Lykken, 1957; Van Evra and Rosenberg, 1963) and are likely to experience genuine remorse following deviant behavior.

SOCIALIZED DELINQUENT

The socialized delinquent engages in antisocial behavior because of strong involvement with delinquent peers. This type is also referred to as a socialized-subcultural delinquent (Achenbach, 1974), as socially delinquent (Ross, 1980), or as a Type III "pseudosocial" delinquent (Glueck and Glueck, 1970). These young people have usually

308

advanced through the normal personality developmental patterns, but have modeled their behavior after delinquent peers. They have essentially normal personalities, but their loyalty to their subculture associates precludes a sense of loyalty to outgroup members; any guilt they feel is in relation to their subgroup rather than to society in general (Glueck and Glueck, 1970).

Although delinquent subcultures do exist, they are more heterogeneous than previously portrayed and manifest themselves in complex and varied ways which need to be studied (Cloward and Ohlin, 1960; Short and Strodtbeck, 1965).

UNSOCIALIZED DELINQUENT

The unsocialized delinquent is probably the most disordered and the most difficult to treat. Such a youth is also referred to as psychopathic delinquent, primary sociopath (Lykken, 1957), conduct disorder (Quay, 1972), or Type II underinhibited personality (Glueck and Glueck, 1979). These children and adolescents are typically antisocial in the sense that they have not internalized society's norms and mores about deviant behavior. They manifest less anxiety, less avoidance of punished responses, and less physiological responsiveness to a conditioned stimulus (Lykken, 1957). They are often described as lacking remorse, as being unable to empathize with others, and as having only superficial relationships with others.

OTHER GROUPINGS

Sometimes subjects in the last two categories are grouped together. MMPI profiles of legally delinquent adolescents revealed fewer differences between the unsocialized or psychopathic and socialized or subcultural delinquents than either of these groups and the neurotic group (Genshaft, 1980). The neurotic type showed a weak ego, much inner conflict, and many neurotic behaviors, whereas the others were more psychopathic, with little anxiety and few neurotic symptoms. These findings are consistent with those of much earlier studies (Peterson, Quay, and Tiffany, 1961; Quay and Quay, 1965; Van Evra and Rosenberg, 1963; Whitehill, DeMyer-Gapin, and Scott, 1976).

Haney and Gold (1973) concluded that most delinquent behavior is shared with others but not within a gang context, as few of the subjects they interviewed fit the image of either a gang member or a "troubled loner." Interestingly, they also found that delinquents consistently characterized their friends as being less delinquent than teenagers generally, regardless of how serious or frequent their own offenses were.

Clearly juvenile delinquency is not a unitary category but includes a very heterogeneous group (Hetherington, Stouwie, and Ridberg, 1971).

Causation

The list of variables that have been implicated in the etiology of delinquency includes genetic, physical, biological, hormonal, psychological, and environmental. Antisocial behavior has been attributed to chromosomes, genetic inferiority, inadequate ego and superego development, single-parent families, divorce, poverty, TV, movies, poor academic performance, disciplinary techniques, socioeconomic level, poor adult and peer models, and many other factors.

The research literature underscores the importance of studying the complex interaction among the many factors. Although any of the above variables may be involved for given individuals, there is no one factor that can be assigned causal status in isolation. Delinquent behavior develops out of a complex network of biological, psychological, and environmental variables, each contributing in various ways and in varying degrees for individual delinquents. Hence identifying major causal factors for an individual, or identifying conditions that maintain the delinquent behavior, constitutes a formidable challenge.

The factors most frequently considered to be of potential etiological significance are included in the following paragraphs.

BIOLOGICAL FACTORS

Some researchers have noted that institutionalized offenders, whether in penal or mental health institutions, have an extra Y chromosome (Erickson, 1978). Others have suggested that delinquents have a high incidence of abnormal EEGs, and disturbances of behavior most likely to be associated with EEG abnormalities are of the aggressive type (Solomon, 1967). However, there is still no clear evidence of a direct causal relationship between such characteristics and delinquency.

Moreover, even when individuals with such chromosomal features show antisocial behavior, it does not follow necessarily that the behavior is genetic: it may be a result of stress arising from other characteristics associated with those abnormalities (Schwartz and Johnson, 1981).

SOCIOECONOMIC LEVEL

The oft-reported association between socioeconomic standing and delinquency is unclear and appears to be a very complex variable.

Short and Strodtbeck (1965), for instance, found that lower-class adolescents demonstrate more tolerance of behaviors which are considered deviant by the middle class. Also, both because they cannot plan ahead as well and because they are more often subject to unemployment layoffs and other misfortunes, lower-class adolescents have a less predictable and less controllable future than middle-class individuals; consequently they develop different orientations toward risk and short-run versus long-run decisions (Short and Strodtbeck, 1965). Discrepancies between goals and opportunities for attaining those goals are very important in the development of delinquent subcultures (Cloward and Ohlin, 1960).

However, some studies indicate that the suggested correlation of lower socioeconomic status with delinquency is misleading if not inaccurate; some data directly contradict such a relationship (Haney and Gold, 1973). There is evidence, for example, that adolescents from various socioeconomic levels do not differ significantly in *number* of offenses, particularly minor offenses (Clark and Wenninger, 1962; Empey and Erickson, 1966), though upper-class adolescents do commit somewhat fewer (Empey and Erickson, 1966; Erickson and Empey, 1965). Findings on the differences in the *seriousness* of the offenses are contradictory. Empey and Erickson (1966), using self-reports of fifteen- to seventeen-year-olds rather than official records, found that the middle-class adolescent respondents had committed the most serious offenses. On the other hand, Clark and Wenninger (1962) found serious offenses committed more frequently by lower-class adolescents.

Various explanations have been offered for socioeconomic differences. Erickson and Empey (1965) concluded that social class is less predictive of delinquency than a child's commitment to peers or to delinquent associates. Their upper-class group seemed the least committed to peer expectations, and the middle-class individuals the most committed. Clark and Wenninger (1962) reported that there was a relationship in specific "status areas" where one socioeconomic class predominated and where there seemed to be communitywide norms which influenced individuals from all social classes. Alternatively, Elkind (1967) explained delinquency among middle-class adolescents as a call for help from adolescents who are victims of exploitation by their parents. That is, the adolescents are vicariously satisfying parental needs, and their delinquency is a symptom of *parental* pathology, in which case the delinquency is "antifamilial" rather than antisocial (Elkind, 1967, p. 84).

Sometimes socioeconomic level is not sufficiently separated from other family characteristics. For example, in one study (Robins, 1966) the father's psychiatric status was found to correlate more highly than his socioeconomic level with the development of a sociopathic personality in the child. Robins concluded that social class may have contributed, but far less than the psychiatric status. In another study of institutionalized offenders (Kahn and McFarland, 1973), subjects were reported to be largely from disrupted families at the lower socioeconomic level, but it was not clear how much of the problem could be attributed to the disruption and how much to socioeconomic level. Obviously, such factors as severity of offense, peer association, and community standards interact with socioeconomic level in complex ways which are not yet clearly understood.

TV AND MOVIES

The notion that violence on TV and in movies leads to increased aggressive behavior in the real world has generated considerable controversy. The general trend of the research seems to be in the direction of implicating TV violence as a contributing factor to violent behavior. Several researchers have reported a positive relationship between viewing TV violence and increased aggressive behavior (Eron et al., 1972; Murray, 1973). Although early viewing of TV violence was not the only factor in one study, the TV effect was relatively independent and accounted for more of the variance than any other single factor studied, including socioeconomic level, parental dissension, IQ, ethnicity, and aspirations for mobility (Eron et al., 1972). A ten-year fol-

312

low-up of children first studied in grade three, when preference for violent programs was related to aggression in school, revealed that that preference was even more highly related to aggressive behavior after ten years (Eron et al., 1972).

PERSONALITY DIFFERENCES

Delinquent tendencies have been attributed to differences in inborn temperament or personality characteristics. Robins (1966), for example, not surprisingly found that children with antisocial behavior demonstrate coldness, hostility, and low motivation. He also found antisocial behavior in children to be a good predictor of later sociopathic personality and adult antisocial behavior in other diagnostic categories. Hetherington and her colleagues (1971) found an association between maternal dominance and neurotic delinquency for both sexes; those children of both sexes who were nondelinquent were relatively passive in interaction with their families. Psychopathic and socially delinquent girls were disruptive and inappropriately assertive with parents, whereas psychopathic and socially delinquent boys disagreed with their fathers but engaged in little overt conflict (Hetherington, Stouwie, and Ridberg, 1971).

Achenbach's (1966) factor analytic study of six hundred child psychiatric patients yielded internalization and externalization factors which reflected socialization differences. Aggression and delinquency factors were seen as subtypes within the externalization category. Such externalization symptoms are not exhibited by most children; children who do show them, according to Achenbach, were not adequately socialized and thus did not eliminate antisocial behavior.

There is also evidence to suggest that antisocial behavior may be a function of stimulus-seeking (Quay, 1965; Whitehill, DeMyer-Gapin, and Scott, 1976). The result of either less reactivity or faster adaptation/habituation, it may be intended to alleviate the unpleasant sensations the child experiences, which are similar to those associated with stimulus deprivation in normals (Quay, 1965).

Copel's (1973) explanation is a more psychoanalytic one. He suggested that in the background of many delinquents there is significant loss or frequent separation during the early years, which means unfulfilled dependency needs and a "depressive core." Thus, relationships are avoided because they always involve a risk of loss, and there is increased narcissism and hyperactivity. Moreover, the lack of constancy in early years leads, according to Copel, to poor or deficient superego development. The aggression serves to ward off feelings of helplessness, and the individual turns his or her anger on the outside world through projection. Finally, because of a limited ability to tolerate frustration, tensions build which require immediate discharge, resulting in hyperactivity, restlessness, and thrill-seeking behavior (Copel, 1973).

In their 1950 book, *Unraveling Juvenile Delinquency*, Glueck and Glueck described delinquents as less friendly than nondelinquents, more truant, and more involved in persistent or serious misbehavior, which occurred at an earlier age. They also found more academic retardation, marked dislike of school, resentment of restrictions, and eagerness to drop out. However, Glueck and Glueck later reported that children respond differently to environmental stress and pressure and that family backgrounds, as well as combinations of other factors and conditions, are important (Glueck and Glueck, 1968).

FAMILY ENVIRONMENT AND BACKGROUND

Associations have been reported between delinquency and instability in the family, whether because of death, divorce, separation, psychiatric disturbances, or other factors. Bakwin and Bakwin (1972), for example found that delinquents' families were more disturbed than those of nondelinquents at the same socioeconomic level, although psychiatric problems were no more common among juvenile offenders than among normals. According to Knopf (1979), family instability may be more damaging during the early years, and Quay (1965) noted the presence of early emotional trauma in the histories of delinquents. Reid and Hendricks (1973) found low levels of interaction, both positive and negative, in the families of children who steal. Some have found, however, that whether or not an individual has delinquent friends may be more important in predicting delinquency for both sexes than whether the home was broken or intact (Haney and Gold, 1973).

As aggressive behavior is often reinforced by the environment, it is important to find the antecedent conditions for the development of antisocial behavior in general, not just that of the small group that lands in court (Achenbach, 1974). There is also a need to determine what factors affecting that small, rather extreme group are not present in other children who commit antisocial acts.

One of the main reasons for the increase in juvenile delinquency may be a relaxation of deterrent factors, manifested in increased irresponsibility, decreased respect for authority, cynicism, diminished regard for history and tradition, and unemployment (Bakwin and Bakwin, 1972). The role of modeling and imitation of undesirable adult behavior should not be underemphasized either:

> A society in which young people are led to believe that to have fun is the primary aim of life, in which moral restraint and personal responsibility are minimized, in which authority—parental, religious, community—is flaunted breeds delinquency. (Bakwin and Bakwin, 1972, p. 582)

SUMMARY

It appears that the ways in which highly varied patterns of characteristics and experiences are associated with delinquent behavior are far from clear. Antisocial behavior occurs as a result of the interaction of physiological, psychological, sociological, environmental, and cultural factors and events which are interrelated in highly complex ways.

The following two case studies reflect the many different personality, family, and environmental characteristics which can be involved in complex interactions in the development of delinquent behavior. They also demonstrate how very diverse backgrounds can be associated with similar delinquent offenses. Two of the subtypes discussed above are represented in these case studies.

CASE STUDY: DAN
Dan was referred to a treatment center at the age of fourteen because of a wide range of behavior and academic problems, including stealing, depression, and reading retardation. He had become unpredictable and unmanageable at home and at school. He had no friends, spent much time watching TV, and had fallen seriously behind in school. His parents noted that some of his delinquent behavior involved taking the family car when he obviously had no license or taking things that belonged to family members. His behavior had not yet resulted in court appearances, however.

Dan was the third of four children but had become alienated from the other members of the family. His father was away from home a good deal, and his relationship with his mother

315

was very poor. Dan's mother felt totally inadequate to deal with Dan's problems and received very little support from her husband, as he was rarely around when various problems arose. She worried about Dan's academic problems and became exasperated and angry over his behavioral problems. She also resented the considerable unsolicited advice that she received from Dan's paternal grandparents on how she should handle Dan's increasing deviance.

At times he felt very depressed and sad, and could barely do his schoolwork. These times, during which his self-esteem was very low and he had little energy, alternated with times when he became involved in delinquent behavior. Relationships with peers were almost nonexistent.

Dan impressed the psychologist as a good-looking, intelligent, and very verbal boy who smiled and talked easily. Although his intellectual potential was average, his academic skills were poor. He was reading at a second-grade level and his math skills were at a third-grade level. Although his verbal and communication skills were good, his perceptual skills were far behind, causing him great difficulty in processing written information. He exhibited poor visual and auditory perception, partly because of attentional problems. His hastiness on some of the tasks initially seemed to indicate low motivation, but later seemed to reflect a more generalized impulsive and ineffective approach to problems.

During the course of treatment, Dan had an opportunity to talk over his feelings of alienation from his family. He felt that he was being treated unfairly, and was able to recognize that his deviant behavior was both an expression of anger and an attention-getting device. The negative attention it brought him, which was better than no attention, reinforced his behavior. His perceptual problems, impulsivity, and poor problem-attack skills resulted in underachievement in school and additional frustration. His parents were seen for counseling and were helped to work out a program in which they reinforced Dan for positive rather than negative behavior. They were able to discuss problems with him rather than simply punishing him. Eventually, Dan came to feel more accepted in the family, and some of the deviant behavior disappeared. As the deviance decreased, the family responded even more positively, and a positive cycle was established. Dan continued to show improvement; at discharge he was near grade level in school, and his deviant behavior had disappeared. There were never any court appearances, charges, or records.

CASE STUDY: JIM

Jim was fifteen when he was referred and had been in court many times. He had been referred to a treatment center as an alternative to incarceration in the correctional system, but was very hostile toward everyone. He was seriously behind in academic work, had few friends except for some delinquent associates, and engaged in many antisocial activities. Some of his delinquent behavior was directed against strangers and their property, and he had many breaking-and-entering offenses. Others were directed against familiar people in his environment and frequently involved bullying and intimidation.

Jim's background had been a very disrupted and disturbed one. He was the eighth child of nine and received little warmth or attention as an infant. In addition, he was frequently moved from his natural home to a string of foster homes, all of which eventually returned him to the Children's Aid Society because of their inability to handle or tolerate his hostile outbursts and his inability to delay gratification of his needs. School provided no satisfaction either. Undetected perceptual difficulties had caused him early difficulties in school, and school had become increasingly aversive.

When Jim came into the treatment clinic, he had resolved not to cooperate in any way. He resisted psychological testing, provoked countless "incidents" with others around him, and was consistently disruptive in the classroom. Infrequently, he cooperated with others in his group on specific tasks. Such incidents, though superficial and brief, served as a dramatic counterpoint to his otherwise unrelenting hostility.

Because of his frequent displays of hostility, he was in almost constant conflict. Occasionally his behavior led to conflicts with bigger peers and allowed a glimpse of a more vulnerable and frightened individual. However, these characteristics were very well covered most of the time, and he rarely showed remorse or misgivings of any kind about his behavior.

During his course of therapy at the clinic, he was able to develop some controls over his behavior as independence and privileges were contingent on such control. He developed some relationships with other patients and staff, but they remained fairly superficial. He was able to relax and enjoy things more, but when stress levels rose beyond his tolerance level, which had improved, he once again became aggressive. Much time was spent helping him to develop work and work-related skills, by reinforcing his progress and his appropriate handling of stress. At the end of treatment, he was able to live independently, but had sporadic police contacts and occasional aggressive encounters, though they were far less frequent than before.

Treatment

The type of approach one takes with delinquent children and adolescents is related to one's view of causal factors (Glueck and Glueck, 1970) and subtypes (Genshaft, 1980), one's theoretical perspective, and the demonstrated effectiveness of various procedures with specific problems. Juvenile delinquents have traditionally been considered very difficult to treat and discouragingly intractable. Rates of recidivism (repeat arrests or incarceration) are high; delinquent behavior may even increase after apprehension (Haney and Gold, 1973).

The location of treatment programs varies according to the type of offense, community resources, age of the offender, and family characteristics. Some of the many types and locations of treatment will be discussed in the following paragraphs, along with some research findings regarding their effectiveness.

Psychotherapy

Despite varied efforts, psychotherapy has a generally poor record of effectiveness in bringing about change among most delinquents (Erickson, 1978; Sobel, 1979; Stuart, 1969). Some behaviors even appear to get worse after psychiatric approaches (Stuart, 1969), although there are problems in assessing the behaviors.

The limited effectiveness of psychotherapy with the delinquent juvenile population seems attributable in part to the fact that some of the most central aspects of psychotherapy, such as motivation to change, ability to verbalize, reflective thought, and capacity for a meaningful relationship, are exactly those which, in their absence, are central to the delinquent problem, at least among unsocialized or psychopathic delinquents. Perhaps insight-oriented psychotherapy would be appropriate for a neurotic subgroup, whereas more environmentally oriented controls might be better for psychopathic types (Genshaft, 1980); but delinquents also need to develop tangible skills—in social, educational, and vocational areas—which can be

318

marketed. The effectiveness of psychotherapeutic techniques generally (as discussed in Chapter 7) must also be taken into account.

An unusual technique that produced results in adolescents otherwise considered untreatable was a collaborative effort between a psychiatric clinic and the court (Nir and Cutler, 1973). As two major problems in the treatment of delinquents are their resistance to treatment and their tendency to act out, Nir and Cutler used psychotherapy as a condition for probation for those adolescents for whom psychotherapy seemed potentially useful. Not coming to therapy constituted a violation of probation. They acknowledged that such an arrangement requires skillful handling and constitutes a new kind of relationship, but felt that such a combination of court authority and psychotherapy fit the current developmental stage of the individuals involved.

Behavioral Techniques

Behavioral techniques in a variety of forms seem to have been somewhat effective with juvenile delinquents, though more long-term data are required to assess the permanence of their effects. Such techniques have a number of advantages for delinquent youths, including objectivity, potential for defusing often volatile relationships with authority figures, specificity, and orientation toward the development of definite, practical skills from which the child or adolescent can derive satisfaction.

Operant conditioning has been used alone or in combination with other techniques, including psychotherapy. Staub and Conn (1970), for example, combined group psychotherapy with operant conditioning in their work with fourteen- to sixteen-year-old boys. Once a system of reinforcement was introduced to the group, the boys' behavior changed markedly. They were, in effect, paid for discussing problems and appropriate behavior, which made such discussion "acceptable" to their subculture peers. Tyler and Brown (1968) found that giving tokens for good academic performance was more effective than noncontingent reinforcement with thirteen- to fifteen-year-old boys; and the gains were maintained over a twelve-week period. They suggested that such tangible reinforcers were more important to the disadvantaged and delinquent youths than to middle-class adolescents who normally received many tangibles and who were successful in their own class culture. Such an approach may also be helpful with adolescents who are antagonistic toward academic work or who are uninterested (Tyler and Brown, 1968).

Cohen and Filipczak (1971) used an operant contingency system in their CASE II–MODEL Project with forty-one incarcerated adolescent delinquents who had committed serious crimes. They claimed that the specific procedures, models, and consequences they used resulted in increased academic progress, improved attitudes, and higher IQ scores, all of which would open other educational and vocational doors. Schwitzgebel (1967) found that positive reinforcement (verbal or small gifts) increased the frequency of such desirable behaviors as punctuality at work, general employability, and positive statements, though negative responses did not decrease hostile statements of the subjects.

Modeling and assertiveness training are also important behavioral tools. Staub and Conn (1970) used assertiveness training to increase appropriate assertive behavior and decrease inappropriately aggressive behavior. Sarason (1968, 1978) noted the potential for using the strong influence of modeling and observational learning to train social skills; he suggested that the best models would perhaps be those who were closest to being peers of the delinquent boys. In another study (Sarason and Ganzer, 1973), modeling or discussions of roles without modeling both resulted in less recidivism and more positive attitudes and behavior change than was seen in a control group, even three years after treatment. The modeling appeared to be better for those with high anxiety; interactions among such personality characteristics and various treatments need to be clarified. There is also a need to sort out which aspects of the modeling, reinforcement, rehearsal, and role-playing are most effective (Sarason, 1978).

Training of significant others in the child's environment may have a measurable effect; operant techniques have been used by teachers in the schools as well as by parents. When Patterson (1974) reinforced nondisruptive behavior with rewards that were shared with peers, such as movies and recess, he found marked changes which persisted in follow-ups up to six months later. An interesting twist to the use of behavioral techniques was a study (Gray, Graubard, and Rosenberg, 1974) in which twelve- to fifteen-year-olds in classes for children considered incorrigible were trained to change teacher behavior. They learned to recognize and respond to positive behavior of the teachers. Gray and colleagues noted that children can also shape their parents' behavior and that of their friends in the same manner.

320

After reviewing the literature on behavioral techniques and their effectiveness in modifying delinquent behavior, Burchard and Harig (1976) concluded that evidence suggests that concrete, material reinforcers are more effective than such social consequences as praise and that once the token reinforcement is withdrawn, behavior again deteriorates. They noted that behavioral approaches have been particularly successful in changing behaviors where there is maximum environmental control, as in institutions. They cautioned, however, that one cannot assume with any great confidence that behavior modified in a special situation will generalize to the natural environment and be maintained there. Modification of the child's behavior alone, without changes in others in the environment, is likely to be of little help. Two major trends they observed include an increasing focus on environmental conditions which maintain behavior and a growing emphasis on teaching behavior modification techniques to youths so that they can obtain their objectives in more acceptable and effective ways (Burchard and Harig, 1976), an approach that was demonstrated in the work of Gray and his colleagues described above.

Readers interested in pursuing the many facets of behavior therapy with delinquents, both within institutions and within the community, are referred to Stumphauzer (1973).

Parent Education and Training

Behavioral intervention with the families of delinquent adolescents and behavioral contracting with predelinquent adolescents (Stuart et al., 1976) can be very effective. For example, Patterson (1974) trained parents using programmed learning; defining, monitoring, and recording of behaviors; role-playing of appropriate techniques; and contracting. He found marked changes in the home which persisted in follow-ups up to six months later. Alexander and Parsons (1973), in a well-controlled study, tried to change the maladaptive interactions of some families and increase the use of clear communication, contingency contracting, and negotiation in their interactions. They found that a behavioral program led to significant changes in three measures of family interaction and rates of recidivism below those of families receiving other family therapy and families receiving no therapy.

Such work with families is particularly important in light of some evidence of parental apathy or inaction in the face of their children's delinquent behavior. Haney and Gold (1973), for example, reported

321

that 40 percent of the children in their study said that their parents had done nothing when they became involved in delinquent behavior—they felt that their parents didn't care. Clearly, such families need help to increase communication and to improve the quality of the parenting their children receive.

Institutionalization

There has been a gradual decrease in institutionalization of delinquent youth because the strategy has proved to be of little value either in reducing recidivism or in effectively teaching socially appropriate skills. The orientation in most institutions has been primarily custodial, with only token vocational, educational, or therapeutic programs (Achenbach, 1974). Worse, some feel that adolescents who are institutionalized with adults and hardened offenders develop poorer attitudes and learn more deviant techniques than they had when they entered. At best, imprisonment is expensive; and since it is likely to result in continued deviance (Stuart, 1969), it should be used only as long as it is required for society's protection (Phelps, 1976).

For all of these reasons, alternative programs have been developed to deal with delinquent adolescents. They are generally designed to place the offenders in a highly supervised living environment, usually within the community, while at the same time attempting to teach them more acceptable and marketable skills and to modify inappropriate behavior.

Group Homes

One of the earliest alternative programs was that of Redl and Wineman (1952), in which the importance of a "treatment climate" or "therapeutic milieu" was emphasized. In their approach, everything in the environment, including physical equipment, rules, adult behavior, and selection of situations to which residents are exposed, is an essential part of the treatment, in addition to any individual treatment efforts. It is assumed that the total climate has a significant therapeutic impact.

Group homes provide living arrangements which are between institutionalization and probation. The youths are not incarcerated, but neither do they live in their own homes, where supervision might be

322

inadequate. Although group homes have not reduced recidivism, they have not increased it, apparently; and they are far less expensive than institutionalization (Achenbach, 1974).

If a child must be removed from the home, community-based programs are best, as greater distances prevent the child from trying to improve the problem relationships which have been experienced within the community (Burchard and Harig, 1976).

Achievement Place has often been cited as a model for programs in which a wide variety of behaviors are altered through the use of a token economy in a controlled environment. Achievement Place (Phillips, 1968; Phillips et al., 1971), a home-style rehabilitation setting for "predelinquent" boys, used token reinforcement procedures. Residents were awarded points for appropriate behavior and lost points for inappropriate behavior. They could earn points for many specific behaviors and exchange them for a wide variety of privileges, from TV to home visits. The privileges could only be earned or bought a week at a time, so they could be used repeatedly as reinforcers. Inappropriate behavior decreased, and there was significant improvement in such appropriate behaviors as promptness, room-cleaning, saving money, and interest in news. For some behaviors, the point consequences were still effective six months later, even when they were given on only 8 percent of the days. Phillips and colleagues concluded that it was an economical and effective way to deal with and modify many social, academic, and self-care behaviors.

Kahn and McFarland's (1973) treatment program resulted in improvement in reading level and social behavior as well as in self-control and responsibility. Their program involved a cottage living arrangement, with counselors available for individual and group counseling, case workers, and a good recreation program. The workers created situations as similar as possible to those with which the residents had had trouble in the community in order to prepare them to cope with regular societal demands.

However, others have reported that intervention did not prevent delinquency or criminal behavior in adulthood. The Cambridge-Sommerville study showed that despite academic tutoring, contact with community resources, and counseling for boys and their families, the treated individuals were not significantly different from the untreated in number or type of crimes in adulthood (McCord, McCord, and Zola, 1959). Treatment was similarly ineffective regardless of personality characteristics, intelligence, parental discipline, family background, and neighborhood, though there was a decrease in criminal behavior with age (after twenty-two) in both treated and control groups. A thirty-year follow-up of that program indicated that although the subjective impression of the individuals who had been in the treatment program for five years was positive, objective comparisons with the control group revealed that the treatment group was no better off and in some respects worse off (McCord, 1978). McCord suggested that intervention may actually have produced negative effects by generating dependency, conflict, or unrealistic expectations.

Clearly, more research is needed to determine precisely what the critical facts are in the success or lack of success of such programs and to assess how long-lasting any observable effects or changes are.

Vocational and Educational Programs

It is generally agreed that delinquent adolescents need considerable help in developing socially acceptable and marketable skills. They also need to continue their education as far as they are able. Motivation, however, is often a very difficult problem. Jeffrey and Jeffrey (1970), for example, were unable to motivate delinquent dropouts to finish a remedial program by paying them—three-fourths of the youths dropped out. Although those who completed the program were achieving at the high school level in basic subjects and made an educational gain of three to six grades, the rate of delinquency was not decreased by participation. On the other hand, Shore and Massimo's (1969, 1973) use of a combination of job placement, psychotherapy, and remedial education in the treatment of delinquents resulted in better overall adjustment than was shown by a control group. Work is incompatible with delinquent behavior and can therefore help to prevent it, as well as providing such positive reinforcers as pay and personal satisfaction (Mills and Walter, 1979). Moreover, modeling in addition to job training may make a significant difference in the future of potential dropouts (Sarason, 1978).

The nature of the relationship between education and delinquency is unclear. Jeffrey and Jeffrey concluded that behavior cannot be controlled with one contingency if other responses can earn the same reward. That is, an educational program will not be successful as long as illegal opportunities are available for attaining the same objectives.

324

Therefore, the rewards accruing to delinquent behavior should be reduced (Jeffrey and Jeffrey, 1970). Perhaps the success of such programs as Achievement Place is largely due to the fact that the controlled environment, as well as rewarding correct behavior, ensured the unavailability of alternative routes to obtaining the same returns.

Positive and negative reinforcment have been found to be differentially effective for delinquents and nondelinquents. Schlichter and Ratliff (1971) reported that nondelinquents learned better when incorrect responses were punished, whereas delinquents learned better with reward for correct responses. Neither group learned under conditions of reward *and* punishment. The reinforcement most effective for each group was the one that was most uncommon for them and therefore increased their attention to the task (Schlichter and Ratliff, 1971).

Phelps (1976), cognizant of the problems children may have returning to school, suggested that a return to school—and the experience of success once there—is an excellent way for children to indicate that they want to change their behavior and avoid further delinquency. When children do go back, the emphasis should be on corrective help for academic deficiencies rather than labeling (Fakouri and Jerse, 1976).

Other Programs

Outward Bound is a program that emphasizes severe physical challenge and survival to demonstrate to youths that they are more capable than they thought. It provides risk and excitement and requires strength and stamina (Kelly, 1971). Kelly reported that sixty delinquent adolescents who participated in the program had a lower recidivism rate one year after parole than a comparison group and showed improvement as well in personality and self-concept measures.

Many communities offer diversion programs in which youthful offenders are streamed into specific activities in lieu of probation or incarceration and contingent on their maintaining appropriate behavior. For many offenders, the programs appear to increase their involvement in appropriate activities and decrease the likelihood of reinvolvement with delinquent behavior, providing a constructive second chance.

Evaluation and Prevention

Although some of the literature regarding the effectiveness of specific approaches has been discussed previously, some general evaluative comments are in order.

Despite the heterogeneity of the delinquent population in number and kinds of offenses, personality characteristics, and etiological background, only a few attempts have been made to match interventions with type of delinquent, though such distinctions would be helpful (Achenbach, 1974; Phelps, 1976). False assumptions and inaccurate images of "the Delinquent" need to be dispelled (Haney and Gold, 1973). In addition, more longitudinal studies are necessary, as cross-sectional ones do not demonstrate long-term effects (Sobel, 1979), which may even be negative (McCord, 1978).

Although some of the conditions that have been associated with juvenile delinquency are easier to modify than others, preventive efforts can be made on many fronts with individuals, families, and communities. They can focus on potential delinquents (Bakwin and Bakwin, 1972; Glueck and Glueck, 1968), aiming at early detection of emotional and character problems and deviations in order to deal with problems before they reach court (Glueck and Glueck, 1968).

Families should be included in any preventive effort because of the important relationship between parent and delinquent behavior (Fakouri and Jerse, 1976). Families may need help developing various relationship skills *before* programs aimed at reducing undesirable behavior are started (Reid and Hendricks, 1978). Good marriage preparation and parent education regarding child-rearing may also be useful in improving family life (Glueck and Glueck, 1968).

Many writers (Bakwin and Bakwin, 1972; Glueck and Glueck, 1970; Phelps, 1976; Stuart, 1969) have emphasized the critical role that community services and community integration play in the prevention of delinquency. Thirty years ago Powers and Witmer (1951) suggested that the term juvenile delinquency be dropped altogether and replaced with "delinquent communities" or "delinquent parents." Recreational and educational facilities should be good, and efforts should be directed specifically toward conditions that have been shown to increase the risk of delinquent behavior (Glueck and Glueck, 1970). The school system should provide varied curricula and good teachers (Glueck and Glueck, 1968). Preventive programs should aim

326

for an improved standard of living, better use of TV, learning centers with self-instructional material, and neighborhood centers that provide a number of services, as well as changes in the schools, courts, and mental hospitals (Stuart, 1969). Area programs in a community might involve discussion groups and educational and recreational programs carried out by the residents themselves (Bakwin and Bakwin, 1972). In addition, multidisciplinary programs based on psychological principles may facilitate efforts to better understand and prevent delinquency (Sobel, 1979).

Finally, although one can determine the risk of delinquency on the basis of the number of criminogenic factors in the backgrounds of children and adolescents, such as personality characteristics and family or environmental situations (Glueck and Glueck, 1970), care must be taken to avoid erroneous identification and self-fulfilling hypotheses (Fakouri and Jerse, 1976).

Discussion Questions

1. Discuss the delinquent behavior described in the two case studies in terms of the classifications they seem to exemplify most closely. Give reasons for your choices. What treatment(s) would you recommend?
2. Explain the possible reasons for the apparent success of behavioral techniques with delinquent populations. Which type of delinquent do you think would respond best to such techniques?
3. Design an ideal community aimed at prevention of delinquency among its members. What kinds of programs, resources, activities, and facilities would you consider to be essential?

PART V

Prevention and Advocacy

CHAPTER 15 # Prevention

In one sense, this whole book has been concerned with prevention issues. To the extent that various disorders in children are understood, steps can be taken to prevent their development. Hence many of the previous discussions related to causal issues are relevant to any discussion of prevention. Moreover, specific preventive programs have been described in relation to particular disorders such as mental retardation and juvenile delinquency. But there are other preventive approaches and considerations which need separate attention.

Forms of Prevention

In most discussions of prevention, the three major classifications of preventive work that emerge are primary, secondary, and tertiary. There is, of course, some overlap among the types (Wonderly et al., 1979).

Primary Prevention

Primary prevention refers to programs or changes that seek to decrease the incidence of problems and also to facilitate mental health in the general population. Such programs may be medical, psychological, or social. They are intended to prevent disease in high-risk populations; they also seek to promote good health practices and specific protection such as immunization (Eisenberg and Gruenberg, 1961). The focus is frequently on parents and schools because of their early and significant influence on a child's development. There are three interrelated basic components of primary prevention: healthy birth, wholesome family experiences, and a successful school experience (Bower, 1970). According to Roen (1967), primary prevention " ... either fortifies the risk group in such a manner as to enable it to ward off affliction or rearranges an environment so as to expel the harmful features" (p. 253). Such preventive efforts, concentrated on meeting the basic needs of children during the first decade of life, have been ignored too long (Bazelon, 1975).

Goldston's definition is most comprehensive:

Primary prevention encompasses activities directed toward specifically identified vulnerable high-risk groups within the community who have not been labeled psychiatrically ill and for whom measures can be undertaken to avoid the onset of emotional disturbance and/or to enhance their level of positive mental health. Programs for the promotion of mental health are primarily educational rather than clinical in conception and operation, their ultimate goal being to increase people's capacities for dealing with crises and for taking steps to improve their own lives. (Goldston, 1977, p. 20)

Primary prevention requires that strategies to improve programs which foster health and learning be implemented *before* disorders appear (Wonderly et al., 1979). These include such diverse programs as those dealing with prenatal education, medical care and immunization, educational facilities, and recreational activities. However, such programs have very often not been evaluated carefully, so their effectiveness in preventing later problems has not been clearly demonstrated (Robins, 1979; Schwartz and Johnson, 1981).

One of the problems in primary prevention is our limited ability to predict which factors or variables are critical in the development of psychological disorders, and hence which areas most need our attention. Assuming that critical areas can be identified, we still lack adequate knowledge about the kinds of interventions that work best to prevent problems (Schwartz and Johnson, 1981).

A relatively recent phenomenon described by Wright (1979) is the emergence of the health care psychologist and the pediatric psychologist. They differ from the traditional child psychologist in many ways, one of which is in their emphasis on " . . . primary health care" as opposed to the secondary and tertiary forms provided by many practitioners (Wright, 1979, p. 1002). Such primary care, according to Wright, allows less time with each person but affords contact with many more individuals with less debilitating problems. It is rooted in the basic social system (Cowen and Zax, 1967).

Kessler and Albee (1977), trying to order the considerable literature in this area, discussed the number of models that could be used. One can, for instance, discuss preventive programs aimed at various developmental levels (for example, childhood, adolescence), programs aimed at various kinds of problems (organic, psychological, social), programs aimed at specific disorders (autism, schizophrenia), or programs designed to change the emphasis from preventing disorders to promoting competence and mental health. All of these lead to different areas of study. Albee and Joffe's (1977) book, in which Kessler and Albee's article appears, is devoted entirely to issues of primary prevention; this important text gives an idea of the complexity of the area and of the number of ways it can be approached.

333

Secondary Prevention

Secondary prevention usually refers to efforts that are made to intervene soon after problems have appeared, in order to prevent those problems from becoming more serious or to prevent additional ones from developing. Such secondary prevention is closely related to early detection and intervention programs, which will be discussed later in this chapter.

Secondary preventive efforts are designed to shorten the " . . . duration, impact, and negative after-effects of disorder through heavy emphasis on early detection and treatment" (Cowen and Zax, 1967, p. 18). This can be either early in the person's life or early in the course of a problem (Cowen and Zax, 1967).

In a sense, secondary prevention is "treatment" of one problem to prevent another. Although it is not necessary to fully understand etiology to successfully intervene, such knowledge may lead to more efficient and less expensive programs of intervention (Erickson, 1978). For example, a secondary prevention strategy that has been highly effective in preventing serious problems is the routine and wide-scale screening of infants for phenylketonuria (PKU), discussed in Chapter 9. When the presence of PKU is discovered early, dietary intervention can prevent the further problems associated with it, including mental retardation.

Other secondary prevention programs include such interventions as infant stimulation programs and preschool educational programs for culturally disadvantaged children. In both cases, inadequate parenting or insufficient stimulation already exists, and intervention is made early to prevent those problems from becoming worse and interfering even more seriously with the child's development.

Tertiary Prevention

Tertiary strategies refer to treatment and rehabilitative efforts undertaken after a problem has become so severe as to be beyond a person's capacity to cope (Wonderly et al., 1979). They are intended to minimize discomfort and to help individuals to function as well as possible in spite of their handicap or problem. Used with disorders that are essentially irreversible, they are aimed primarily at minimizing impairment (Cowen and Zax, 1967). Tertiary efforts are an essential

334

part of a humane and caring society, and so encounter little resistance. In fact, they are not, strictly speaking, "preventive," though research into the most effective way to intervene is imperative. Many of the intervention strategies that fall into this category have already been discussed in earlier chapters dealing with specific problems.

Wonderly and his colleagues (1979) use an analogy from dentistry to illustrate the differences among the three kinds of prevention. Cleaning, flossing, drinking fluoridated water, and regular checkups are intended primarily to prevent or reduce decay in the general population; they are primary prevention strategies. Secondary prevention encompasses fillings, root canal work, and other treatment carried out to repair teeth where problems have already developed in order to prevent loss of teeth. Tertiary efforts might involve removal of a tooth and construction of a bridge to facilitate eating and minimize discomfort.

Perhaps Kanner (1972) summed up the view of many when he suggested that "prevention is practiced by doing things calmly in a way that has been found to produce and maintain a condition of well-being" (p. 247).

Problems in Prevention

At first glance, it would seem that the value of prevention is unarguable, that it is an unequivocally desirable undertaking which would be guaranteed support from all sides. However, there has been resistance to preventive efforts, and there have been problems associated with the implementation of preventive programs.

Wonderly and his colleagues (1979) discussed some of the problems that have been encountered. These include impatience regarding results, too few specialists trained in prevention, resistance to a preventive focus in clinics, and the notion that the costs of such programs are too high to warrant implementation. Other problems they noted included the limited number of successful models and the long time required to evaluate results. To these, Bower (1970) added the possibility that invasion of privacy may be an issue, as the intervention is to occur *before* a person has been singled out as needing special help. There is also uncertainty as to the definitions of "prevention" and "goals," and reliable indices of health and illness are necessary (Bower, 1970).

In one survey reported by Wonderly et al., (Van Antwerp, 1971), 90 percent of mental health administrators believed that primary prevention should be part of the mental health program in the community. At the same time, they gave three reasons why such programs have been resisted. One was that very comprehensive planning is required before such a program can be introduced, and few have the proper training for such a task. Second, they noted apprehension on the one hand about programs that require organized community social action, combined with the conviction on the other that the program will fail *unless* there is major social change, a problem noted by Bower as well. Third, they observed a lack of conviction that primary preventive programs would in fact cost less in the long run than secondary and tertiary programs.

There is no doubt that good preventive programs would require major planning efforts and considerable expenditures. However, it seems apparent that improvement in community and family resources, such as might follow a program of primary prevention, would benefit everyone and would improve the quality of life for all children. Early intervention, or secondary prevention, can decrease greatly the pain and suffering of individuals and their families. In addition, there can be little doubt that treating a single or simpler problem early is far less expensive than remediation of more extensive and more complex problems later.

The specific nature and direction of primary and secondary programs is a matter that requires very careful planning. Evaluative data regarding the relative effectiveness of such programs is necessary.

Early Identification

If one cannot prevent disorders and problems from developing in the first place, perhaps the next best option is to identify them early and intervene early; that is, embark on a program of secondary prevention. Programs of early identification often involve wide-scale screening, designed to monitor the physical, cognitive, social, and emotional development of children, particularly high-risk children. They often involve highly varied techniques, including neurological and physical examinations, vision and hearing tests, behavioral checklists, rating scales, and observational data, as well as various kinds of psychological tests.

Eagle and Brazelton (1977) have pointed out the need to determine in infancy which children are at risk, because such children cope less well than normals in disorganized environments and hence their problems are compounded. They also observed that children who were admitted for abuse, accidents, neglect, or failure to thrive often had parents who had successfully raised other children; in most cases these parents had noted from the beginning that their problem child was different. Early intervention with such families in the form of instruction in improved handling of difficult children and supportive counseling for the parents might be quite effective in preventing more serious problems from developing.

According to Eagle and Brazelton (1977), some of the assessment indices used immediately after delivery, such as the Apgar score (1960), do not correlate very well with mild central nervous system dysfunction or predict later problems unless they are used with other more sensitive tests. Early testing of the neonate may include checking reflexes, posture, and vision, as well as behavioral and social responsiveness. They reported that neurological examination had a high "false-alarm rate"—80 percent of infants reported as "suspect/abnormal" were later found to be normal. They suggest that use of the Brazelton scale, with which they report a false-alarm rate of only 24 percent, would help to decrease mislabeling and self-fulfilling hypotheses as well as other problems which such labeling might cause.

The number of "false positives," or children who are positively identified as having problems and then are later classified as normal, is an important consideration in early identification programs. If children are wrongly identified, the consequent responses to them, and the changes in environmental reactivity to them, may have many far-reaching and largely unforeseen ramifications. For example, parents' reactions might include anxiety, depression, anger, rejection, hostility, and pessimism, which in turn would affect the child's feelings and behavior. The child's feelings and behavior would then further influence those of the parents, and an intricate network of subtle messages could be set up. Such patterns of communication and associated attitudes may be difficult to change later on, even when the child is found to be "normal" or only suffering a maturational lag.

Stuart (1970) warned that diagnostic labels are not sufficiently reliable or likely to evoke good treatment decisions, and the risks involved in their use may well outweigh any possible benefits. He noted further that, once given a negative label, the individual is a victim of negative reactions solely because of a diagnosis of deviance, regardless of the behavior which led to the diagnosis or of subsequent behavior. According to Stuart, the individuals involved may then expect less of themselves and more of others or may become involved in deviant behavior consistent with the label they have been given. As predictions about future performance are so problematic, Lindsay and Wedell (1982) advocate instead using a series of educational objectives to help children with current problems without making assumptions about their future performance. They argue that this approach allows for ongoing evaluation and monitoring rather than prediction based on an assessment at a specific time.

Although early identification can be valuable and can help to prevent considerable suffering of children and families, it must be carefully researched and carried out in such a way as to minimize the possibility of early misdiagnosis.

Role of the Schools

Wonderly and his colleagues (1979) maintain that the school is an appropriate setting for prevention and that the school psychologist can implement such a program. They consider the school a more desirable place to intervene than the home for a number of reasons: it is the first institution to service all children in a community; it has those children during their formative years; and it has them for a long enough time to realize some benefit from preventive work. Also, schools are convenient geographically and are amenable to a systematic introduction of programs (Cowen et al., 1973). Parents can assist the teachers by helping their children in specific areas, thereby enhancing feelings of effectiveness and competence in the children and in themselves (Berlin and Berlin, 1975).

One problem with early identification programs in the school may be reluctance on the part of teachers to identify children at risk for emotional disorders because they feel inadequate to make such judgments or because they feel that there are too few resources to help children so identified (Hambley and Freeman, 1977).

Zax and Cowen's (1967) work serves as one example of how such resistance might be met. Zax and Cowen found that children who were likely to have problems later could be detected as early as grade one. By third grade, those children were doing less well in achievement, adjustment, anxiety level, and peer relationship areas. Therefore, their program emphasized early identification of problems and secondary preventive interventions. It involved early detection, through a psychological battery and parent interviews, of first-graders who were exhibiting problems or the potential for problems. They then followed that step with the recruitment of teachers' aides and volunteers for an after-school activities program. Hambley and Freeman also developed a program that involved consultation with teachers and the employment of volunteers for direct service to the children, in order to help teachers cope with such children within the classroom.

Cowen and his colleagues (1973) urged the development of more practical approaches, including techniques to identify school maladaptation early. Such programs can familiarize teachers with diagnostic issues and improve the teachers' ability to recognize problems, thus increasing their confidence in their ability to identify such children. Once the problems are identified, the teachers can receive help in working with the children and thus become a very important helping resource as well.

Morse (1967) emphasized that resource people helping in the school should focus on facilitating the staff's ability to cope within their own setting and with their own resources. They should help to alleviate the teachers' burden by assisting them with day-to-day problems, involving them in a problem-solving process as co-equals. The psychological view, according to Morse, must be relevant to the school situation, rather than divorced from it, as traditional psychological practice has been.

New Directions

Many new programs have been developed to try to overcome some of the problems discussed in this chapter.

One approach is a very comprehensive early identification and developmental program which spans the whole range of primary, secondary, and tertiary concerns. Brown and Perkins (1977) instituted the program based on what they call a "successive sieves" model. It consists of the series of program steps illustrated in Figure 15.1.

In this model, there is first a consideration of all children in a classroom or school, through the use of observation, group tests, and information from teachers regarding their cognitive, social, perceptual, expressive, sensory, and emotional development. Particular children are then selected for additional investigation or assessment. The nature of such further study depends, of course, on the reason for their selection; it usually involves more observation, interviews with parents and teachers, and tests to clarify the children's needs. Suggestions may then be made regarding classroom management or remedial activities, or referrals may be made to community resources. The next

FIGURE 15.1   *Successive sieves model of screening employed in the Early Identification and Developmental Programme. Source:* A. E. Brown and M. J. Perkins, "The Toronto Early Identification and Developmental Programme: Evolution and Expansion," *The Ontario Psychologist* 9 (1977), pp. 39–44. Reprinted with the permission of *The Ontario Psychologist.*

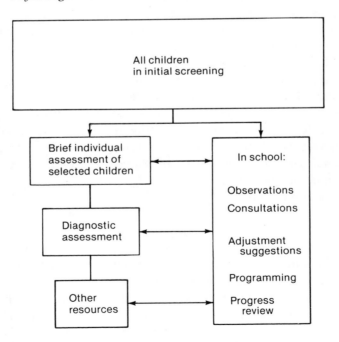

step is to single out children from that smaller group who may need more intensive evaluation or "third level" assessment (p. 41). It is at this juncture that the usual diagnostic referral begins. In this model, however, it comes early for the child, before more serious problems have developed and before the child's self-esteem has suffered. According to Brown and Perkins, this model is more economical than others, and it keeps teachers more involved. It serves a preventive function by providing service for many children, not just those identified as at risk. Such a model offers various degrees of psychological assistance to the whole classroom, to small groups, and to individual children. The degree and type of service depends on the child's needs, but more emphasis is placed on developing suitable programs and curricula than on identifying high-risk children.

Another direction that is receiving increased attention is the multidisciplinary approach to problems. Salk (1974) noted the important role of pediatricians not only in identifying problems early but also in influencing the child-rearing techniques parents use. Salk advocates the involvement of psychological consultants with pediatricians, as pediatricians have typically had little training in the behavioral sciences. Such consultants could provide the pediatrician with invaluable information and guidance in such areas as normal development, behavioral disorders, and learning. They would also facilitate the early diagnosis of developmental, emotional, and learning problems and sensitize the medical staff to the children's emotional needs (Salk, 1974).

Wright (1979) observed the new differentiations being made among developmental psychology, clinical child psychology, pediatric psychology, and behavioral medicine, specialties which encompass many problems not included in traditional psychopathology. Sobel (1979) suggested that psychology can make its greatest contribution to the well-being of children through increased use of psychological theories, research data, evaluation data, and service delivery techniques in developing public policies.

Garmezy's (1977) emphasis on the need to study the adaptation techniques of "invulnerable children" is relevant here. The invulnerable children are those who resist or avoid psychiatric problems despite very disordered and disturbed backgrounds. Garmezy, noting a shift from an emphasis on maladaptation to one on adaptation and competence, suggested that we may ultimately be able to intervene

341

more effectively against disturbances if we have a better understanding of how positive adaptation to crises develops.

There is still much to be learned. Knowledge of critical variables and their interactions is essential if we are to develop the more accurate predictive ability needed for meaningful and effective screening, early identification, and intervention programs. The future of preventive work is a challenging and important one. It is also an exciting one. It is to be hoped that innovative thinking and rigorous experimentation and evaluation will eventually lead to a greatly reduced incidence of psychological disorders as well as a better quality of life for all children.

Discussion Questions

1. Discuss the advantages and disadvantages of implementing large-scale primary prevention programs. How would you justify the deployment of resources—financial and professional—into such a program?

2. Drawing on information in this chapter and in previous chapters, examine the kinds of physical, personality, and family characteristics which might indicate that a child was "at risk." How could an early intervention program forestall the development of disorders in such children? What do you think would be essential elements in a program to meet the needs of those children?

3. Ask your instructor for an APA directory, membership application, or other APA literature which lists all of the divisions of APA. List the different specialities that might be directly involved or relevant in a primary prevention program as discussed in this chapter.

CHAPTER 16   Child Advocacy

Background for Advocacy

Because children as a group are virtually powerless to change events and situations that affect them, they need others to make interventions on their behalf. Such efforts have come to be known as "child advocacy." The area of child advocacy is an exciting and relatively new one. It developed in response to a number of factors which were beginning to highlight the frequency with which very basic rights of children were being denied or basic needs were not being met.

In one section of their report, the Joint Commission on Mental Health of Children stated:

> We believe that the child deserves an advocate to represent him and his needs to the society in which he lives, an advocate who will insist that programs and services based on sound child development knowledge be available to every child as a public utility." (Joint Commission, 1970, p. 9)

In its report, the Joint Commission recommended the appointment by the President of the United States of an Advisory Council on Children in order to provide to child advocates the strength, support, and commitment of that high office. It also stressed the importance of a broad and developmental view of mental health, with strong emphasis on the prevention of problems and on the facilitation of optimal mental health. To this end, the Commission delineated seven rights which must be upheld for all infants, but which of course would be true for children of any age. These include the right to be wanted, to be born healthy, to live in a healthy environment, to receive satisfaction of basic needs, to receive continuous loving care, to acquire the necessary intellectual and emotional skills to achieve individual goals and to cope effectively in society, and to receive care and treatment in facilities that are appropriate for them and that resemble as closely as possible their normal social environment (Joint Commission, 1970, pp. 3–4). To these Berlin (1975) added, in his Bill of Rights, the right to engage in meaningful employment, the right to racial and ethnic identity and self-determination, equal opportunity, and the right to informed political participation (p. 5).

Shore (1979) noted that the judicial clarification of rights goes back to a 1948 court decision. In *Haley v. Ohio* the court ruled that rights guaranteed to adults apply to children as well. There has been, over this century, steady and gradual progress in improving the environ-

344

ment of and protecting developing children. The report of the Joint Commission has given further impetus to this movement.

How did we arrive at a stage where a statement of the rights of children was necessary? What forces led society to the point where such rights had to be legislated into the programs of people who care for children? Various attitudes, assumptions, findings, and trends gave impetus to this movement, some of which are discussed in the following sections.

Child Abuse

The greatly increased activity and research in the area of child abuse was partly stimulated by and has contributed to the stepped-up interest in child advocacy. Many books and articles have been written on the subject of child abuse, and since 1977 an entire journal has been devoted to that specific topic *(Child Abuse and Neglect)*. An in-depth discussion of the subject and all of the related literature is quite beyond the scope of this chapter. However, in the context of this discussion, some brief comments are in order about the nature of child abuse and why it prompted a greater interest in child advocacy.

Child abuse takes many forms—physical, emotional, verbal, sexual—some of which are easier to define and to prove than others. X-rays, for instance, can provide very objective evidence of past injuries and likely abuse. On the other hand, evidence or proof of verbal or emotional abuse, which may be even more destructive for the child, is very difficult to obtain, and there is less consensus among professionals regarding these subtler forms of abuse (Starr, 1979).

Incidence figures vary, but they are underestimates, as the majority of cases are not reported (Starr, 1979). Until relatively recently, there was even greater underreporting of abuse and neglect. People who did not want "to get involved," physicians who were wary of possible lawsuits, a "spare the rod" approach to child-rearing, and other attitudes worked to prevent reporting in many cases. Today, however, everyone is required by law to report suspected cases of abuse to the appropriate authorities. Thus the decision to report has become a social policy matter (Paulsen, 1974).

In some cases it is difficult to draw the line between severe physical punishment and actual abuse. Sometimes parents who use corporal punishment cross that line without having originally intended to inflict serious injury. Despite the many associated problems and consequences, physical punishment is still widely condoned and accepted—by parents, schools, and correctional institutions (Gil, 1973). Gelles (1978), in a discussion of violence in the U.S., sampled 2143 families and found violence to be " . . . an extensive and patterned phenomenon in parent-child relations" (pp. 590–91), which went beyond regular physical punishment. The largest share of the reported incidents in his study involved milder forms of violence. However, if one extrapolates from the smaller percentage of more serious ones, according to Gelles, one finds that millions of children were kicked, punched, or beaten. Seventy-three percent of the respondents reported at least one violent incident while raising a child, and 63 percent reported at least one during the year of the survey (1975).

The causes of child abuse are still being actively studied and debated. Many explanations have been advanced, including the parents' own experience of abuse as children, their low self-esteem, their low socioeconomic level (Pelton, 1978), and their excessive demands on infants incapable of meeting them (Steele and Pollock, 1974). There is not, however, unanimity about the relative importance of these various factors. Garmezy (1977), for example, noted that although some abusive parents were abused as children, there are many abused children who do not later become abusing parents. Pelton's (1978) finding of a higher incidence of abuse and neglect in the lower socioeconomic level prompted him to conclude that not only is there a correlation, but the problems which poverty presents are causal in abusive and negligent behavior.

In examining the causes of child abuse, one needs to study not only the psychological and sociological factors but the reciprocal influences of all of these, as well as others such as the parents' own child-rearing (Starr, 1979). The interaction of characteristics of parents and children may also be crucial; research has begun to focus on the stimulus the child provides in the family constellation (Garmezy, 1977) and how the child can unwittingly contribute to or trigger an attack (Steele and Pollock, 1974).

There are some difficult questions involved in determining the way abusive or neglectful behavior should be handled or responded to. Starr (1979) stressed the need to be careful about undesirable effects of labeling, possible invasions of privacy, and issues of freedom and control. Helfer and Kempe (1974) noted that once child abuse prob-

346

lems are brought to a lawyer's attention, he or she is in a difficult situation. The lawyer must uphold the clients' rights, but could "win" a case without the child's having "won." Therefore, the parents' lawyer must consider the child's welfare also, according to Helfer and Kempe, to avoid, for instance, reuniting a child with battering parents too soon. Newberger and Bourne (1978) emphasized that only children should win in custody disputes—for example, where there are allegations of neglect or abuse. Helfer and Kempe suggested that the judge, parents, lawyers, physicians, and welfare representatives meet to discuss all aspects of a situation in order to ensure that decisions are in the best possible interests of the child.

Underlying Assumptions

Underlying the child advocacy movement are some important assumptions which have been described and discussed by Knitzer (1976). Advocacy assumes that individuals have certain rights and that they are enforceable. The enforceability, according to Knitzer, is a necessary condition if advocacy is to be effective, especially with children, who are particularly vulnerable because they " . . . are not fully competent to determine and safeguard their interests" (Goldstein, Freud, and Solnit, 1973). Another assumption Knitzer points out is that the focus of efforts should be on institutional failures which produce or exacerbate problems. These "institutional barriers" which hinder access to needed help include such problems as violation of rights, denial of due process, administrative difficulties, and statutory and budgetary constraints. Advocacy also assumes inequities and tries to give more power to those who have little. As children cannot vote, advocates need to ensure that their needs get adequate attention from persons in administrative and policy-making positions. (Knitzer, 1976). Finally, she notes that advocacy is most effective when it focuses on specific issues, but is different from the provision of direct service.

Current Findings

Compiled more than a decade after the Joint Commission's urgent call to action on behalf of children, Edelman's (1981) statistics regarding children in the United States are shocking. Her findings include the following: (1) 17 percent of children are poor; (2) 70 percent of mothers under fifteen receive no prenatal care in the first trimester of pregnancy; (3) an estimated half million children are born to teenagers every year; (4) 10 million children get no health care at all; (5) day-care facilities are woefully inadequate, and a two-thirds increase over present requirements is predicted for the next decade; and (6) a half million or more children live out of the home, 20 percent of whom have been in care for six years or more. Moreover, access to service is uneven, and minority children are more likely to receive less adequate help. She predicted that the needs of children will increase during the 1980s, at the same time that, unless policies change, there will be pressure *not* to provide needed supports for children and families.

Such statistics, as well as others on violence and socioeconomic level to be reported later in this chapter, underscore the need for some agency or force to take the child's position, to make sure that the child has adequate protection, and to ensure that the child's most basic needs are met.

Forms of Advocacy

There are many forms and definitions of advocacy. The term can refer to efforts on behalf of children in general, groups of children, or individual children with special needs. Although it usually means action, advocacy is just as strongly attitudinal, according to Suran and Rizzo (1979). There are so many kinds of advocacy that the Department of Health, Education, and Welfare organized a National Center for Child Advocacy in 1971. The Center limits the term "child advocacy" to interventions where the chief focus is on secondary institutions such as agencies, schools, and courts rather than on families (Suran and Rizzo, 1979).

Basically, one can discuss advocacy in terms of social action, family and community advocacy, and individual advocacy taken on behalf of individual children, frequently children with problems of one kind or another.

Social Action

Included in social advocacy are all of the efforts extended on behalf of children in general, efforts directed toward providing a better life for all children. In this context, advocacy is very closely related to or is a

348

form of primary prevention. Psychologists have not traditionally been socially active, but recently they have become increasingly involved politically and legislatively in order to effect greater social change. Several writers (Edelman, 1981; Lourie, 1975a; Shore, 1979; Sobel, 1979; Suran and Rizzo, 1979; Williams, 1970) have stressed the need for psychologists to get involved politically. Williams, for instance, suggested that "child advocacy *in vivo* means changing the odds against the powerless child by actively challenging and remaking diabolical structures within our society" (p. 48).

Edelman (1981) claimed that there are millions of children in the United States whose health and mental needs are not being met. She urged psychologists to challenge some of the myths that affect how families are "helped," and to get involved in the development and evaluation of programs. Advocacy can bring pressure to bear on the social structure in order to reverse social inequities and injustices (Lourie, 1975a). It can also bring out developmental issues, such as what special protections for children need to be built in because of the ways in which children differ from adults (Shore, 1979). The law recognizes more and more the basic "entitlement" of all citizens, which includes a good start in life for children (Bazelon, 1975).

An outgrowth of the changing legal view of children was the establishment in 1977 of an organization to improve the effectiveness of legal representation for children, the National Association of Counsel for Children (Bross, 1980). The three major goals of the new organization are self-training, setting standards, and involvement in special cases of general importance to children. It aims to provide training and education to those who are acting as children's advocates, to help to ensure good-quality representation, and to support the general position of children through consultation, briefs, and other means. Although nonlawyers as well as lawyers can join, the emphasis is on legal advocacy. The hope is that the organization can develop children's law to provide a system that protects children from cruelty and allows for healthy development (Bross, 1980).

Family and Community Advocacy

A somewhat more narrowly focused kind of advocacy is that practiced by and within the family and the community on behalf of specific children or specific groups of children. Parents, for example, can become very active in the schools and in the community on behalf of their own children and others in the community. This may begin as a special interest when parents feel that their own children are not getting a "fair deal" and may then expand and set in motion action for all of the children in the community, as in the area of educational practices, for example. Parents may also bring pressure to bear on policy makers in their community for improved recreational facilities, remedial and treatment resources, or any other programs which would better meet the needs of the children in their care and in the wider community.

Lourie (1975b) discussed the need for "operational advocacy," which increases the accessibility of services. The current delivery systems, according to Lourie, are so fragmented that they can offer no guarantee that the services available are accessible to those who need them or who are at risk. Sometimes the word "advocate" in this context refers specifically to a representative or person within the community who helps families to obtain necessary services. (Suran and Rizzo, 1979).

Individual Advocacy

Individual advocacy is the area in which clinical psychologists have, in the past, been most active. They have always been, and continue to be, deeply committed to obtaining the best possible treatment for disturbed children, and to developing the most growth-producing environment for children who are referred to them for help. Clinicians have traditionally carried on their work with the best interests of the child at heart; their efforts, however, have been largely restricted to their day-to-day practice or work situation, with relatively less involvement in legislative and social policy decision making. Recently, Polier (1976) extended an urgent plea for a stronger stance, an insistence on whatever is necessary to overcome obstacles and extend service delivery. He urged an end to the prevailing apathy, hostility, and alienation toward those children who most need services and protection of their rights. Some of the important rights issues Polier focused on included the " . . . right of a child or adult deprived of freedom in the name of treatment [institutionalized] to receive appropriate treatment" (p. 80); the right to protection from cruel and unusual punishment under the guise of treatment or rehabilitation; the right to receive help in the least restrictive environment; and, finally, the right to equal treatment and protection, without regard to race, sex, religion, or other factors. He also pointed out the rights of children to an education and to independent and adequate counsel by persons who can serve as their advocates.

Ross (1980) raises the issue of one important area of advocacy that is rarely discussed: protection of a child in psychotherapy. It is generally assumed that the adults involved in psychotherapy are acting in the child's interest. However, as the child has relatively little to say about entering, refusing, or terminating treatment, or about the goals of treatment, Ross suggests introducing an independent advocate into the treatment picture to ensure that the treatment is actually in the child's best interest and that basic human rights are protected (patterned after the system followed in institutions regarding research projects).

Ethical Issues

Much of what constitutes advocacy overlaps with, and can also be discussed in terms of, ethical issues or ethical behavior on the part of professionals working with children. If one is truly interested in safeguarding the rights of children, one is by definition interested in treating them ethically. This means that they cannot be exploited or manipulated in either treatment or research situations. They cannot be taken advantage of because of their age or naïveté. They cannot be placed in situations in which they might suffer psychological or physical harm. They cannot be put into environments that are not optimally beneficial for their development in the interest of testing certain hypotheses. Their confidential statements and their trust cannot be betrayed through loose or careless discussions of their feelings or problems or personalities. Privacy must be maintained. It is necessary to treat children as persons regardless of age or degree of impairment or disturbance, to take them seriously, to be honest, and to involve them in decision making as fully as is possible and appropriate to their level of maturity (Ross, 1980).

All practicing psychologists are child advocates when they work to ensure that these principles are upheld and when they act on a child's behalf when contraventions occur. Such action on the part of psychologists is called for ethically, whether or not the requirement is formalized in legislative statutes. It is part of their professional responsibility in their day-to-day dealings with children and their families and with schools, courts, and other community agencies. They must, however, also work for legislative and social change that will protect children legally. All of these considerations are, of course, also relevant to the work of psychologists with adults, but they are underscored in work with children because of the greater vulnerability of children.

Problems with Advocacy

As Edelman (1981) stated, it is hard to imagine anyone being *against* children, but not enough people are *for* them on important issues. Despite the strong case that can be made for child advocacy and the need to protect children because of their vulnerability and relative powerlessness, there have been blocks to an easy advocate role. Lourie (1975b) cited the problems of overspecialization of services, a proliferation of new programs, competition for funds, limited evaluation, and selective servicing of problem types. Lourie and Berlin (1975) claimed that the approximately 1000 human service programs in the United States are inadequately coordinated and integrated and that none of them has ever received sufficient resources to satisfactorily meet the needs of children. Therefore, according to Lourie (1975a), even when advocacy issues are resolved, needs will still be unmet until adequate systems of service delivery are devised. There is much research data available concerning the means by which many disorders might be prevented or alleviated, and even legislation regarding children's right to treatment or better environments; but the legislation of itself cannot provide either money or change (Lourie and Berlin, 1975). Besides, there is a considerable difference of opinion as to whether everyone even has a *right* to adequate services (Lourie, 1975a). Advocacy as a principle cannot solve all the problems or bring needed policy changes; but, if properly implemented, it can help to build checks and balances into various systems which now frequently fail to meet the needs of children and their families (Knitzer, 1976).

Complicating the advocacy issue are the rights of parents to bring up children without government interference, protection of which can result in very knotty judicial decisions (Goldstein, Freud, and Solnit, 1973). When parental rights conflict with those of children, resolv-

352

ing the conflict in the children's best interests can be extremely difficult (Shore, 1979). New legislation needs to be monitored and coordinated so that it does not conflict with existing laws or lead to unforeseen and undesirable consequences (Shore, 1979). For example, in some cases Shore found that separation of children from their families, carried out by professionals eager to protect the children from harm, was actually destructive of their growth and development.

Future Directions

Many suggestions and recommendations have been made as to how best to accomplish the difficult task of meeting the needs of children and adolescents and reversing some of the injustices which have existed in the past. Two recommendations have been that efforts be directed against specific undesirable policies or programs and that emotionally charged and hard-to-define labels be avoided (Edelman, 1981). Shore (1979) suggested that the President outline each year's progress regarding children and families, with specific proposals for more legislation, in an annual message to Congress and to the country, and that all legislation be reviewed systematically with regard to its effect or impact on children and families.

Lourie and Berlin (1975) predicted that if the right course is followed, in the next century there will be significant gains in social knowledge and technology and an integration of health, education, and welfare programs into one human services system; that is, " . . . a full national commitment for human well-being" (p. 328). The question, according to Lourie and Berlin, is not whether we *can* reduce many of the disorders of children or improve their environments and hence facilitate and enhance their learning and development, but whether we *will*. Their paraphrase of a Chinese proverb correlates with the three kinds of prevention discussed in the previous chapter:

The superior "professional effort" prevents human disease and disorder and suffering.
The mediocre "professional effort" tries for early cure.
The inferior "professional effort" concentrates only on curing fully developed conditions. (Lourie and Berlin, 1975, p. 328)

The Joint Commission recommended several priorities to be considered equally in allocating funds. These included comprehensive services to ensure the health of all children and adolescents; a broad range of remedial services for children with problems or handicaps, and for their families; and the development of a system of advocacy at all levels of government to ensure that these goals are met. If these priorities are in fact followed, all children will have a higher quality of life and the incidence of psychological disorders will be drastically reduced. As Lourie and Berlin said, it is not a question of whether we *can* but whether we *will*.

Discussion Questions

1. Discuss some of the practical problems involved in the child advocacy movement. Who should be most centrally involved in such activity?
2. What are some possible ways of reconciling conflicts which arise between parents' rights and children's rights? What issues or factors need to be considered in such conflicts?
3. What is the minimum age at which you feel children could be centrally involved in decisions regarding their lives and circumstances, as might occur in custody disputes, for example? What kinds of cognitive, emotional, and personal qualities or characteristics would they need to have acquired?

References

Abramowitz, C. V. The effectiveness of group psychotherapy with children. *Arch. Gen. Psychiat.*, 1976, 33, 320–326.

Achenbach, T. M. The classification of children's psychiatric symptoms: A factor-analytic study. *Psych. Monog.*, 1966, 80 (7).

Achenbach, T. M. *Developmental psychopathology.* New York: Ronald Press, 1974.

Achenbach, T. M. Developmental aspects of psychopathology in children and adolescents. In M. E. Lamb (Ed.), *Social and personality development.* New York: Holt, Rinehart and Winston, 1978a, pp. 272–303.

Achenbach, T. M. The Child Behavior Profile: I. Boys aged 6–11. *J. Consult. Clin. Psych.*, 1978b, 46, 478–488.

Achenbach, T. M., and Edelbrock, C. S. The Child Behavior Profile: II. Boys aged 12–16 and girls aged 6–11 and 12–16. *J. Consult. Clin.*, 1979, 47, 223–233.

Ackerman, N. W. *The psychodynamics of family life.* New York: Basic Books, 1958.

Ackerman, N. *Family therapy in transition.* Boston: Little, Brown and Co., 1970.

Adams, P. L. *A primer of child psychotherapy.* Boston: Little, Brown and Co., 1974.

Adams, P. L. Dynamic, here-and-now focused psychotherapy with obsessive children. In C. E. Schaefer and H. L. Millman, *Therapies for children.* San Francisco: Jossey-Bass, 1978, pp. 27–31.

Ader, R., and Cohen, N. Behaviorally conditioned immunosuppression. *Psychosom. Med.*, 1975, 37, 333–340.

Albee, G. W., and Joffe, J. M. (Eds.). *Primary prevention of psychopathology.* Vol. 1: *The issues.* Hanover, N. H.: Univ. Press of New England, 1977.

Alderton, H. R. Psychoses in childhood and adolescence. In P. D. Steinhauer and Q. Rae-Grant (Eds.), *Psychological problems of the child and his family.* Toronto: Macmillan of Canada, 1977.

Alexander, A. B. Systematic relaxation and flow rates in asthmatic children: Relationship to emotional precipitants and anxiety. *J. Psychosom. Res.*, 1972, 16, 405–410.

Alexander, A. B.; Cropp, G. J. A.; and Chai, H. Effects of relaxation training on pulmonary mechanics in children with asthma. *J. Applied Behav. Anal.*, 1979, 12, 27–35.

Alexander, A. B., Miklich, D. R.; and Hershkoff, H. The immediate effects of systematic relaxation training on peak expiratory flow rates in asthmatic children. *Psychosom. Med.*, 1972, 34, 388–394.

Alexander, F. *Psychosomatic medicine*. New York: W. W. Norton and Co., 1950. Cited in H. I. Kaplan and H. S. Kaplan, Current theoretical concepts in psychosomatic medicine. *Amer. J. Psychiat.*, 1959, 115, 1091–1096.

Alexander, J. F., and Parsons, B. V. Short-term behavioral intervention with delinquent families: Impact on family process and recidivism. *J. Abn. Psych.*, 1973, 81, 219–225.

Alexander, T.; Roodin, P.; and Gorman, B. *Developmental psychology*. New York: Van Nostrand, 1980.

American Psychiatric Association. *Diagnostic and statistical manual of mental disorders*. 3rd ed. Washington, D.C., 1980.

Anastasi, A. *Psychological testing*. 4th ed. New York: Macmillan, 1976.

Anderson, H. H., and Anderson, G. L. *An introduction to projective techniques*. Englewood Cliffs, N.J.: Prentice-Hall, 1951.

Anderson, J. R. *Cognitive psychology and its implications*. San Francisco: W. H. Freeman and Co., 1980.

Anthony, E. J. Behavior disorders. In P. H. Mussen (Ed.), *Carmichael's manual of child psychology*. 3rd ed. Vol. 2. New York: John Wiley and Sons, 1970, pp. 667–764.

Anthony, J., and Scott, P. Manic-depressive psychosis in childhood. *J. Child Psychol. Psychiat.*, 1960, 1, 53–72.

Apgar, V. A. A proposal for a new method of evaluation of the newborn infant. *Current Researches in Anesthesia and Analgesia*, 1960, 32, 260. Cited in T. B. Brazelton, *Neonatal Behavioral Assessment Scale*. London: Spastics International Medical Publications, 1973.

Aragona, J.; Cassady, J.; and Drabman, R. S. Treating overweight children through parental training and contingency contracting. *J. Applied Behav. Anal.*, 1975, 8, 269–278.

Aries, P. *Centuries of childhood*. New York: Vintage Books, 1962.

Axline, V. M. *Play therapy*. Cambridge, Mass.: Riverside Press, 1947.

Axline, V. M. *Dibs in search of self*. New York: Ballantine Books, 1964.

Backman, J., and Firestone, P. A review of psychopharmacological and behavioral approaches to the treatment of hyperactive children. *Amer. J. Ortho.*, 1979, 500–504.

Baker, B. L. Symptom treatment and symptom substitution in enuresis. *J. Abn. Psych.*, 1969, 74, 42–49.

Baker, B. L., and Heifetz, L. J. Behavioral training for parents of mentally retarded children: One-year follow-up. *Amer. J. Ment. Defic.*, 1980, 85, 31–38.

Bakwin, H., and Bakwin, R. M. *Behavior disorders in children*. Philadelphia: W. B. Saunders Co., 1972.

Baldwin, A. L. A congitive theory of socialization. In D. A. Goslin (Ed.), *Handbook of socialization theory and research*. Chicago: Rand McNally, 1969, 325–345.

Bandura, A.. and Walters, R. H. *Social learning and personality development.* New York: Holt, Rinehart and Winston, 1963.

Barkley, R., and Cunningham, C. Do stimulant drugs improve the academic performance of hyperkinetic children? A review of outcome studies. *Clin. Pediat.,* 1979, 17, 85–92.

Barrett, B. H. Reduction in rate of multiple tics by free operant conditioning methods. *J. Nerv. Ment. Dis.,* 1962, 135, 187–195.

Barsch, R. H. *Achieving perceptual-motor efficiency.* Vol. 1. Seattle: Special Child Publications, 1967. Cited in J. Lerner, *Children with learning disabilities.* Boston: Houghton Mifflin, 1976.

Barten, H. H. (Ed.). *Brief therapies.* New York: Behavioral Publications, Inc., 1971.

Bateson, G.; Jackson, D. D.; Haley, J.; and Weakland, J. Toward a theory of schizophrenia. *Behavioral Science,* 1956, 1, 251–264.

Bayley, N. *Bayley Scales of Infant Development.* New York: Psych. Corp., 1969.

Bazelon, D. L., Courts and the rights of human beings, including children. In I. N. Berlin (Ed.), *Advocacy for child mental health.* New York: Brunner/ Mazel, 1975.

Beck, A. T. *Cognitive therapy and the emotional disorders.* New York: International Univ. Press, 1976.

Beck, A. T.; Rush, A. J.; Shaw, B.; and Emery, G. *Cognitive therapy of depression.* New York: The Guilford Press, 1979.

Bedell, J. R.; Giordani, B.; Amour, J. L.; Tavormina, J.; and Boll, T. Life stress and the psychological and medical adjustment of chronically ill children. *J. Psychosom. Res.,* 1977, 21, 237–242.

Beers, C. W. *A mind that found itself.* New York: Longmans, Green and Co., 1908.

Beery, K. E. *Developmental Test of Visual-Motor Integration.* Chicago: Follett Educ. Corp., 1967.

Bellak, L. *The Thematic Apperception Test and the Children's Apperception Test in clinical use.* New York: Grune and Stratton, 1971.

Bellak, L., and Adelman, C. The Children's Apperception Test (CAT). In A. I. Rabin and M. R. Haworth (Eds.), *Projective techniques with children.* New York: Grune and Stratton, 1960, pp. 62–94.

Belmont, H. S. Theoretical considerations in child psychotherapy. In S. L. Copel (Ed.), *Behavior pathology of childhood and adolescence.* New York: Basic Books, 1973.

Bemis, K. Current approaches to the etiology and treatment of anorexia nervosa. *Psych. Bull.,* 1978, 85, 593–617.

Bender, L. *Bender Motor Gestalt Test.* New York: American Orthopsychiatric Ass'n., 1946.

Bender, L. Childhood schizophrenia. *Amer. J. Ortho.,* 1947, 17, 40–56.

Bender, L. Childhood schizophrenia. *Psychiat. Quart.,* 1953, 663–681.

Bender, L. Schizophrenia in childhood—Its recognition, description and treatment, Childhood Schizophrenia Symposium, 1955. *Amer. J. Ortho.*, 1956, 26, 499–506.

Bereiter, C., and Engelmann, S. *Teaching disadvantaged children in the preschool.* Englewood Cliffs, N.J.: Prentice-Hall, 1966.

Bergin, A. E. Some implications of psychotherapy research for therapeutic practice. *J. Abn. Psych.*, 1966, 71, 235–246.

Bergin, A. E. The evaluation of therapeutic outcomes. In A. E. Bergin and S. L. Garfield (Eds.), *Handbook of psychotherapy and behavior change.* New York: John Wiley and Sons, 1971.

Berlin, I. N. We advocate this bill of rights. In I. N. Berlin (Ed.), *Advocacy for child mental health.* New York: Brunner/Mazel, 1975, pp. 1–10.

Berlin, I. N. Psychotherapeutic work with parents of psychotic children. In M. Rutter and E. Schopler (Eds.), *Autism.* New York: Plenum Press, 1978, pp. 303–312.

Berlin, R. B., and Berlin, I. N. Parents' advocate role in education as primary prevention. In I. N. Berlin (Ed.), *Advocacy for child mental health.* New York: Brunner/Mazel, 1975, pp. 145–157.

Bersoff, D. N. Silk purses into sow's ears. *Amer. Psychol.*, 1973, 28, 892–899.

Bettelheim, B. *The empty fortress.* New York: Free Press, 1967.

Binet, A., and Simon, T. *The development of intelligence in children.* Vineland, N.J.: Vineland Training School, 1916.

Birch, H. G.; Richardson, S. A.; Baird, D.; Horobin, G.; and Illsley, R. *Mental subnormality in the community: A clinical and epidemiologic study.* Baltimore: Williams and Wilkins, 1970.

Black, S.; Humphrey, J. H.; and Niven, J. S. Inhibition of Mantoux reaction by direct suggestion under hypnosis. *Brit. Med. J.*, 1963, 6, 1649–1652. Cited in M. P. Rogers, D. Dubey, and P. Reich, The influence of the psyche and the brain on immunity and disease susceptibility: A critical review. *Psychosom. Med.*, 1979, 41, 147–164.

Blackman, D. *Operant conditioning.* London: Methuen and Co., 1974.

Blackman, S., and Goldstein, K. M. Cognitive styles and learning disabilities. *J. Lear. Dis.*, 1982, 15(2), 106–115.

Blinder, B. J.; Freeman, D. M. A.; and Stunkard, A. J. Behavior therapy of anorexia nervosa: Effectiveness of activity as a reinforcer of weight gain. *Amer. J. Psychiat.*, 1970, 126, 1093–1098.

Bliss, E. L., and Branch, C. H. H. *Anorexia nervosa: Its history, psychology and biology.* New York: Paul Hoeber, 1960.

Block, J.; Jennings, P. H.; Harvey, E.; and Simpson, E. Interaction between allergic potential and psychopathology in childhood asthma. *Psychosom. Med.*, 1964, 26, 307–320.

Blom, G. E. A psychoanalytic viewpoint of behavior modification in clinical and educational settings. In J. F. McDermott, Jr., and S. I. Harrison (Eds.), *Psychiatric treatment of the child.* New York: Jason Aronson, Inc.. 1977.

Blum, G. S. The Blacky Pictures with children. In A. I. Rabin and M. R.

Haworth (Eds.), *Projective techniques with children.* New York: Grune and Stratton, 1960, pp. 95–104.

Bornstein, P. H., and Quevillon, R. P. The effects of a self-instructional package on overactive preschool boys. *J. Applied Behav. Anal.,* 1976, 9, 179–188.

Boverman, H., and French, A. P. Treatment of the depressed child. In A. P. French and I. N. Berlin (Eds.), *Depression in children and adolescents.* New York: Human Sciences Press, 1979, pp. 129–139.

Bower, E. M. Primary prevention of mental and emotional disorders: A conceptual framework and action possibilities. In L. A. Fass (Ed.), *The emotionally disturbed child.* Springfield, Ill.: Charles C. Thomas, 1970.

Bower, G. H. Mood and memory. In H. E. Fitzgerald and T. H. Carr (Eds.), *Human development, 82/83.* Guilford, Conn.: Dushkin Pub. Co. 1982, pp. 116–120.

Bower, T. G. R. *Human development.* San Francisco: W. H. Freeman, 1979.

Bowlby, J. Grief and mourning in infancy and early childhood. *Psychoanal. Stud. Child.,* 1960, 15, 9–52.

Brazelton, T. B. *Neonatal Behavioral Assessment Scale.* London: Spastics International Medical Publications, 1973.

Bross, D. C. An organization to improve legal representation of children—The National Association of Counsel for Children. *Child Abuse and Neglect,* 1980, 4, 115–117.

Brown, A. E., and Perkins, M. J. The Toronto Early Identification and Developmental Programme: Evolution and expansion. *Ontario Psychologist,* 1977, 9, 39–44.

Brown, J., and Hepler, R. Stimulation. A corollary to physical care. *Amer. J. Nursing,* 1976, 76, 578–581.

Brown, L. K. Familial dialectics in a clinical context. *Human Development,* 1975, 18, 223–238.

Brown, L. K. Psychology and mental retardation. In W. M. Cruickshank (Ed.), *Psychology of exceptional children and youth.* Englewood Cliffs, N.J., Prentice-Hall, 1980.

Bruch, H. Conceptual confusion in eating disorders. *J. Nerv. Ment. Dis.,* 1961, 133, 46–54.

Bruch, H. Family background in eating disorders. In E. J. Anthony and C. Koupernik (Eds.), *The child in his family.* Vol. 1. New York: Wiley-Interscience, 1970, 285–309.

Bruch, H. *The Golden cage. The enigma of anorexia nervosa.* Cambridge, Mass.: Harvard Univ. Press, 1978.

Brumback, R. A., and Weinberg, W. A. Childhood depression: An explanation of a behavior disorder of children. *Percep. and Motor Skills,* 1977, 44, 911–916.

Bryan, T. H., and Bryan, J. H. *Understanding learning disabilities.* 2nd ed. Sherman Oaks, Calif.: Alfred Pub. Co., 1978.

Bryant, N. D. Some principles of remedial instruction for dyslexia. In E. C.

Frierson and W. B. Barbe (Eds.), *Educating children with learning disabilities: Selected readings.* New York: Appleton-Century-Crofts, 1967, pp. 414–420.

Bucher, B., and Lovaas, O. O. In M. R. Jones (Ed.), *Miami symposium on the prediction of behavior. 1967: Aversive stimulation.* Coral Gables, Fl.: Univ. of Miami Press, 1968.

Buck, J. N. The H-T-P technique—A qualitative and quantitative scoring manual. *J. Clin. Psych.,* 1948, Monograph supplement 5. Brandon, Vermont: Clinical Psychology Pub. Co., Inc.

Burbeck, T. W. An empirical investigation of the psychosomatogenic family model. *J. Psychosom. Res.,* 1979, 23, 327–337.

Burchard, J. D., and Harig, P. T. Behavior modification and juvenile delinquency. In H. Leitenberg (Ed.), *Handbook of behavior modification and behavior therapy.* Englewood Cliffs, N.J.: Prentice-Hall, 1976.

Burns, R. C., and Kaufman, S. H. *Kinetic family drawings (K-F-D).* New York: Brunner/Mazel, 1970.

Buros, O. K. (Ed.). *The eighth mental measurements yearbook.* Vols. I and II. Highland Park, N.J.: Gryphon Press, 1978.

Caccioppo, J. T. and Petty, R. E. Electromyograms as measures of extent and affectivity of information processing. *Amer. Psychol.,* 1981, 36, 441–456.

Camp, B. W.; Blom, G. E.; Hebert, F.; and van Doornick, W. J. "Think aloud": A program for developing self-control in young aggressive boys. *J. Abn. Child Psych.,* 1977, 5 (2), 157–169.

Campbell, M. Biological interventions in psychoses of childhood. In E. Schopler and R. J. Reichler, *Psychopathology and child development.* New York: Plenum Press, 1976.

Campbell, M. Pharmacotherapy. In M. Rutter and E. Schopler (Eds.), *Autism.* New York: Plenum Press, 1978, pp. 337–355.

Campbell, M., and Small, A. M. Chemotherapy. In B. B. Wolman, J. Egan, and A. O. Ross (Eds.), *Handbook of treatment of mental disorders in childhood and adolescence.* Englewood Cliffs, N.J.: Prentice-Hall, 1978.

Campbell, S. B.; Endman, M. W.; and Bernfeld, G. A. three-year followup of hyperactive preschoolers into elementary school. *J. Child Psychol. Psychiat.,* 1977a, 18, 243–249.

Campbell, S.; Schleifer, M.; Weiss, G.; and Perlman, T. A two-year follow-up of hyperactive preschoolers. *Amer. J. Ortho.,* 1977b, 47, 149–162.

Cantwell, D. P.; Mattison, R.; Russell, A. T.; and Will, L. A comparison of DSM-II and DSM-III in the diagnosis of childhood psychiatric disorders. IV. Difficulties in use, global comparisons, and conclusions. *Arch. Gen. Psychiat.,* 1979, 36, 1227–1228.

Carlberg, C., and Kavale, K. The efficacy of special versus regular class placements for exceptional children: A meta-analysis. *J. Spec. Educ.,* 1980, 14, 295–309.

Carlson, G. A., and Cantwell, D. P. A survey of depressive symptoms, syndrome and disorder in a child psychiatric population. *J. Child Psychol. Psychiat.,* 1980, 21, 19–25.

References

Carter, C. H. *Handbook of mental retardation syndromes.* Springfield, Ill.: Charles C Thomas, 1970.

Cattell, P. *The measurement of intelligence in infants and young children.* New York: Psych. Corp., 1960.

Cattell, R. B. *The scientific analysis of personality.* Baltimore, Md.: Penguin Books, Inc., 1965.

Cermak, L. S.; Goldberg-Warter, J.; De Luca, D.; Cermak, S.; and Drake, C. The role of interference in the verbal retention ability of learning disabled children. *J. Lear. Dis.*, 1981, 14(5), 291–295.

Chapel, J. L.; Brown, N.; and Jenkins, R. L. Tourette's disease: Symptomatic relief with haloperidol. *Amer. J. psychiat.*, 1964, 121, 608–610.

Chess, S., and Hassibi, M. *Principles and practices of child psychiatry.* New York: Plenum Press, 1978.

Chinese proverb. Quoted by Irwin Emanuel in "New leader stresses problem solving at CDMRC." *Health Science Review*, 1974, 3(3), 3. Cited in N. V. Lourie and I. N. Berlin, Child advocacy: Political and legislative implications. In I. N. Berlin (Ed.), *Advocacy for child mental health.* New York, Brunner/Mazel, 1975, pp. 311–333.

Clarizio, H. F., and McCoy, G. F. *Behavior disorders in children.* 2nd Ed. New York: Thomas Y. Crowell Co., 1976.

Clark, G. R., and Rosen, M. Mental retardation. In S. L. Copel (Ed.), *Behavior pathology of childhood and adolescence.* New York: Basic Books, 1973, pp. 240–269.

Clark, J. P., and Wenninger, E. P. Socio-economic class and area as correlates of illegal behavior among juveniles. *Amer. Sociol. Rev.*, 1962, 27, 826–834.

Clawson, A. *The Bender Visual Motor Gestalt Test for Children: A Manual.* Los Angeles: Western Psychological Services, 1962.

Clement, P. W.; Fazzone, R. A.; and Goldstein, B. Tangible reinforcers and child group therapy. *Amer. Acad. Child Psychiat.*, 1970, 9, 409–427.

Clement, P. W., and Milne, D. C. Group play therapy and tangible reinforcers used to modify the behavior of 8-year-old boys. *Behavior Res. and Ther.*, 1967, 5, 301–312.

Cloward, R. A., and Ohlin, L. E. *Delinquency and opportunity. A theory of delinquent gangs.* New York: Free Press of Glencoe, 1960.

Cobb, J. A., and Ray, R. S. The classroom behavior observation code. In E. Mash and L. G. Terdal (Eds.), *Behavior-therapy assessment.* New York: Springer Pub., 1976.

Cobb, S. Social support as a moderator of life stress. *Psychosom. Med.*, 1976, 38, 300–314.

Cohen, D. J.; Caparulo, B.; and Shaywitz, B. Primary childhood aphasia and childhood autism; clinical, biological, and conceptual observations. *J. Amer. Acad. Child Psychiatry*, 1976, 15(4), 604–645.

Cohen, E. L. Psychosomatic aspects of acne vulgaris. In J. Hambling and P. Hopkins (Eds.), *Psychosomatic disorders in adolescents and young adults.* Oxford: Pergamon Press, 1965, pp. 107–115.

References

Cohen, H. L., and Filipczak, J. *A new learning environment*. San Francisco: Jossey-Bass, Inc., 1971.

Coles, G. S. Evaluation of genetic explanations of reading and learning problems. *J. Spec. Educ.*, 1980, 14, 365–383.

Conners, C. K. A Teacher Rating Scale for use in drug studies with children. *Amer. J. Psychiat.*, 1969, 126, 884–888.

Conners, C. K. Drugs in the management of children with learning disabilities. In L. Tarnapol (Ed.), *Learning disorders in children: Diagnosis, medication, and education*. Boston: Little, Brown and Co., 1971, pp. 253–301.

Conners, C. K.; Goyette, C. H.; and Newman, E. B. Dose-time effect of artificial colors in hyperactive children. *J. Lear. Dis.*, 1980, 13, 512–516.

Coolidge, J. C.; Hahn, P. B.; and Peck, A. School phobia: Neurotic crisis or way of life. *Amer. J. Ortho.*, 1957, 27, 296–306.

Coolidge, J. C.; Miller, M.; Tessman, E.; and Waldfogel, S. School phobia in adolescence: A manifestation of severe character disturbance. *Amer. J. Ortho.*, 1960, 30, 599–608.

Copel, S. L. Juvenile delinquency. In S. L. Copel (Ed.), *Behavior pathology of childhood and adolescence*. New York: Basic Books, 1973.

Cowen, E. L.; Door, D.; Clarfield, S.; Kreling, B.; McWilliams, S. A.; Pokracki, F.; Pratt, D. M.; Terrell, D.; and Wilson, A. The AML: A quick-screening device for early identification of school maladaptation. *Amer. J. Commun. Psych.*, 1973, 1, 12–35.

Cowen, E. L., and Zax, M. The mental health field today: Issues and problems. In E. L. Cowen, E. A. Gardner, and M. Zax (Eds.), *Emergent approaches to mental health problems*. New York: Appleton-Century-Crofts, 1967, pp. 3–29.

Craig, G. J. *Child development*. Englewood Cliffs, N.J.: Prentice-Hall, 1979.

Craighead, W. E.; Kazdin, A. E.; and Mahoney, M. J. *Behavior modification: principles, issues and applications*. Boston: Houghton Mifflin, 1976.

Cratty, B. J. *Active learning: Games to enhance academic abilities*. Englewood Cliffs, N.J.: Prentice-Hall, 1971.

Creak, M. and Ini, S. Families of psychotic children. *J. Child Psychol. Psychiat.*, 1960, 1, 156–175.

Crisp, T., and Coll, P. Modification of self-injurious behavior in a profoundly retarded child by differentially reinforcing incompatible behavior. *Brit. J. Mental Subnormality*, 1980, 26, 81–85.

Critchley, D. L., and Berlin, I. N. Parent participation in milieu treatment of young psychotic children. *Amer. J. Ortho.*, 1981, 51, 149–155.

Dalton, P., and Hardcastle, W. J. *Disorders of fluency and their effects on communication*. London: Edward Arnold, 1977.

Daniels, L. K. *The management of childhood behavior problems in school and at home*. Springfield, Ill.: Charles C Thomas, 1974.

Darwin, C. A biographical sketch of an infant. *Mind*, 1877, 2, 286–294.

David, O. J.; Hoffman, S. P.; Sverd, J.; and Clark, J. Lead and hyperactivity: Lead levels among hyperactive children. *J. Abn. Child Psych.*, 1977, 5, 405–416.

References

Davidson, P. O. Thumbsucking. In C. G. Costello (Ed.), *Symptoms of psychopathology. A handbook.* New York: John Wiley and Sons, 1970, 320–335.

De Hirsch, K. Language deficits in children. *Psychoanal. Stud. Child.*, 1975, 30, 95–123.

De Leon, G., and Mandell, W. A comparison of conditioning and psychotherapy in the treatment of functional enuresis. *J. Clin. Psych.*, 1966, 22, 326–330.

De Silva, P., and Rachman, S. Is exposure a necessary condition for fear-reduction? *Behav. Res. and Ther.*, 1981, 19, 227–232.

Dekker, E.; Pelser, H. D.; and Groen, J. Conditioning as a cause of asthmatic attacks. *J. Psychosom. Res.*, 1957, 2, 97–108.

Delacato, C. H. *The treatment and prevention of reading problems: The neurological approach.* Springfield, Ill.: Charles C Thomas, 1959.

Delacato, C. H. *The diagnosis and treatment of speech and reading problems.* Springfield, Ill.: Charles C Thomas, 1963.

Delacato, C. H. *Neurological organization and reading.* Springfield, Ill.: Charles C Thomas, 1966.

Dennis, W. Historical beginnings of child psychology. *Psych. Bull.*, 1949, 46, 224–235.

Denny, D. R. Modeling effects upon conceptual styles and cognitive tempos. *Child Devel.*, 1972, 43, 105–119.

DesLauriers, A. M., and Carlson, C. F. *Your child is asleep.* Homewood, Ill.: Dorsey Press, 1969.

Despert, J. L. Psychosomatic study of fifty stuttering children. *Amer. J. Ortho.*, 1946, 16, 100–113.

Despert, J. L. Differential diagnosis between obsessive-compulsive neurosis and schizophrenia in children. In P. H. Hoch and J. Zobin (Eds.), *Psychopathology of childhood.* New York: Grune and Stratton, 1955, pp. 240–253. Cited in T. M. Achenbach, *Developmental psychopathology,* New York: Ronald Press, 1974.

Despert, J. L. *Schizophrenia in children.* New York: Brunner/Mazel, 1968.

Doll, E. A. *Vineland Social Maturity Scale.* Minneapolis, Minn.: Education Test Bureau, 1947.

Dollard, J., and Miller, N. E. *Personality and psychotherapy.* New York: McGraw-Hill, 1950.

Doman, R. J.; Spitz,E. B.; Zucman, E.; Delacato, C. H.; and Doman, G. Children with severe brain injuries: Neurological organization in terms of mobility. In E. C. Frierson and W. B. Barbe (Eds.), *Educating children with learning disabilities: Selected readings.* New York: Appleton-Century-Crofts, Educational Div., Meredith Pub. Co., 1967, p. 363–372.

Dowling, A. S. Psychosomatic disorders of childhood. In S. L. Copel (Ed.), *Behavior pathology of childhood and adolescence.* New York: Basic Books, 1973, 203–239.

Dunn, L. M. *Expanded manual for the Peabody Picture Vocabulary Test.* Circle Pines, Minn.: American Guidance Services, 1965.

References

Dunn, L. M., and Dunn, L. M. *Peabody Picture Vocabulary Test–Revised.* Circle Pines, Minn.: American Guidance Services, 1981.

Eagle, D. B., and Brazelton, T. B. The infant at risk—Assessment and implications for intervention. In M. F. McMillan and S. Henao (Eds.), *Child psychiatry: Treatment and research.* New York: Brunner/Mazel, 1977, p. 37–50.

Eastman, C. Behavioral formulations of depression. *Psych. Review,* 1976, 83, 277–291.

Eaton, L., and Menolascino, F. J. Psychotic reactions of childhood: A follow-up study. *Amer. J. Ortho.,* 1967, 37, 521–529.

Edelman, M. W. Who is for children? *Amer. Psychol.,* 1981, 36, 109–116.

Egel, A. L.; Richman, G. S.; and Koegel, R. L. Normal peer models and autistic children's learning. *J. Applied Beh. Anal.* 1981, 14, 3–12.

Eisenberg, L. The autistic child in adolescence. *Amer. J. Psychiat.,* 1956, 112, 607–612.

Eisenberg, L. School phobia: A study of communication of anxiety. *Amer. J. Psychiat.,* 1958, 114, 712–718.

Eisenberg, L. The classification of the psychotic disorders in childhood. In L. D. Eron (Ed.), *The classification of behavior disorders.* Chicago: Aldine Pub. Co. 1966, pp. 87–114.

Eisenberg, L. Child psychiatry: The past quarter century. *Amer. J. Ortho.,* 1969, 39, 389–401.

Eisenberg, L. the classification of childhood psychosis reconsidered. *J. Autism Childhood Schiz.,* 1972, 2, 338–342.

Eisenberg, L., and Gruenberg, E. M. The current status of secondary prevention in child psychiatry. *Amer. J. Ortho.,* 1961, 31, 355–367.

Eisenberg, L., and Kanner, L. Childhood schizophrenia: Early infantile autism. *Amer. J. Ortho.,* 1956, 26, 556–566.

Elkind, D. Middle-class delinquency. *Mental Hygiene,* 1967, 51, 80–84.

Elkind, D. Cognitive development and psychopathology: Observations on egocentrism and ego defense. In E. Schopler and R. J. Reichler (Eds.), *Psychopathology and child development.* New York: Plenum Press, 1976.

Empey, L. T., and Erickson, M. L. Hidden delinquency and social status. *J. Soc. Forces,* 1966, 44, 546–554.

Engel, G. L. Studies of ulcerative colitis. *Psychosom. Med.,* 1954, 16, 496–501.

Erickson, M. L., and Empey, L. T. Class position, peers, and delinquency. *Social and Soc. Research,* 1965, 49, 268–282.

Erickson, M. T. *Child psychopathology. Assessment, etiology, and treatment.* Englewood Cliffs, N.J.: Prentice-Hall, 1978.

Erikson, E. H. *Childhood and society.* New York: W. W. Norton, 1963.

Eron, L. D.; Lefkowitz, M. M.; Huesmann, L. R.; and Walder, L. C. Does television violence cause aggression? *Amer. Psychol.,* 1972, 27, 253–263.

Etemad, J. G.; Szurek, S. A.; Yeager, C. L.; and Schulkin, F. R. Evaluation of EEG findings in a group of psychotic children. In S. A. Szurek and I. N. Berlin (Eds.), *Clinical studies in childhood psychoses.* New York: Brunner/Mazel, 1973.

References

Eysenck, H. J. The effects of psychotherapy: An evaluation. *J. Consult. Psych.*, 1952, 16, 319–324.

Eysenck, H. J. The effects of psychotherapy. In H. J. Eysenck (Ed.), *Handbook of abnormal psychology*. New York: Basic Books, 1961, 697–725.

Eysenck, H. J. The effects of psychotherapy. *Int. J. of Psychiat.*, 1965, 1, 99–142.

Fakouri, M. E., and Jerse, F. W. Unobtrusive detection of signs of potential delinquency. *Psych. Reports*, 1976, 39, 551–558.

Fay, G.; Trupin, E.; and Townes, B. D. The young disabled reader: Acquisition strategies and associated deficits. *J. Lear. Dis.*, 1981, 14, 32–35.

Feingold, B. *Why your child is hyperactive*. New York: Random House, 1975.

Feingold, B. R. Hyperkinesis and learning disabilities linked to the ingestion of artificial food colors and flavors. *J. Lear. Dis.*, 1976, 9. Cited in *Readings in hyperactivity*. Guilford, Conn.: Special Learning Corp. 1980, pp. 54–58.

Feinstein, S. C., and Wolpert, E. A. Juvenile manic-depressive illness. *J. Amer. Acad. Child Psychiat.*, 1973, 2, 123–136.

Feldman, G. M. The effect of biofeedback training on respiratory resistance in asthmatic children. *Psychosom. Med.*, 1976, 38, 27–34.

Ferguson, L. R. *Personality development*. Belmont, Calif.: Brooks/Cole Pub., 1970.

Fernald, G. *Remedial techniques in basic school subjects*. New York: McGraw-Hill, 1943.

Ferster, C. B. Positive reinforcement and behavioral deficits of autistic children. *Child Devel.*, 1961, 32, 437–456.

Feuerstein, M.; Ward, M. M.; and LeBaron, S. W. M. Neuropsychological and neurophysiological assessment of children with learning and behavior problems: A critical appraisal. In B. B. Lahey and A. E. Kazdin (Eds.), *Advances in clinical child psychology*, Vol 2. New York: Plenum Press, 1979, pp. 241–278.

Finch, S. M. Psychophysiologic disorders in children and adolescents. In Z. J. Lipowski, D. R. Lipsitt, and P. C. Whybrow (Eds.), *Psychosomatic medicine*. New York: Oxford Univ. Press, 1977, 497–509.

Finch, S. M., and Hess, J. H. Ulcerative colitis in children. *Amer. J. Psychiat.*, 1962, 118, 819–826.

Fine, S. Family therapy and a behavioral approach to childhood obsessive-compulsive neurosis. *Arch. Gen. Psychiat.*, 1973, 28, 695–697.

Finucci, J. M. Genetic considerations in dyslexia. In H. Myklebust (Ed.), *Progress in learning disabilities*. Vol. 4. New York: Grune and Stratton, 1978, pp. 41–63.

Fiss, H. Current dream research: A psychobiological perspective. In B. B. Wolman (Ed.), *Handbood of dreams. Research, theories, and applications*. New York: Van Nostrand, 1979, pp. 20–75.

Flavell, J. H. *Cognitive development*. Englewood Cliffs, N.J.: Prentice-Hall, 1977.

Foa, E. B.; Steketee, G.; and Milby, J. B. Differential effects of exposure and prevention in obsessive-compulsive washers. *J. Consult. Clin. Psych.*, 1980, 48, 71–79.

References

Folstein, S., and Rutter, M. A twin-study of individuals with infantile autism. In M. Rutter and E. Schopler (Eds.), *Autism.* New York: Plenum Press, 1978.

Foulkes, D. Children's dreams, In B. B. Wolman (Ed.), *Handbook of dreams. Research, theories, and applications.* New York: Van Nostrand. 1979, pp. 131–167.

Fowler, S. A., and Baer, D. M. "Do I have to be good all day?" The timing of delayed reinforcement as a factor in generalization. *J. Applied Behav. Anal.,* 1981, 14, 13–24.

Frankenburg, W. K.; Dodds, J. B.; Fandal, A. W.; Kazuk, E.; and Cohrs, M. *Denver Developmental Screening Test* (Rev. ed.). Denver: Ladoca Project and Publishing Foundation, 1975.

Franks, C. M. Behavior therapy, psychology and the psychiatrist: Contributions, evaluation and overview. *Amer. J. Ortho.,* 1965, 35, 145–151.

Franks, C. M., and Leigh, D. The theoretical and experimental application of a conditioning model to a consideration of bronchial asthma in man. *J. Psychosom. Res.,* 1959, 4, 88–98.

Freedman, A. M.; Kaplan, H. I.; and Sadock, B. J. (Eds.), *Comprehensive textbook of psychiatry—II.* 2nd ed. Vol. 1. Baltimore: Williams and Wilkins Co., 1975.

Freeman, B. J.; Ritvo, E. R.; Schroth, P. C.; Tonick, I.; Guthrie, D.; and Wake, L. Behavioral characteristics of high- and low-IQ autistic children. *Amer. J. Psychiat.,* 1981, 138 (1), 25–29.

Freud, A. *Psychoanalytic treatment of children.* New York: Schocken Books, 1946.

Freud, S. *A general introduction to psychoanalysis.* Trans. by Joan Riviere. New York: Washington Square Press, 1935.

Freud, S. *Psychopathology of everyday life.* New York: New American Library, 1952.

Froeschels, E. Pathology and therapy of stuttering. *Nerv. Child,* 1943, 2, 148–161.

Frommer, E. A. Treatment of a childhood depression with antidepressant drugs. *Brit. Med. J.,* 1967, 1, 729–732. Cited in W. I. Halpern and S. Kissel, *Human resources for troubled children.* New York: John Wiley and Sons, 1976, Ch. 11.

Frostig, M.; Maslow, P.; Lefever, D. W.; and Whittlesey, J. R. B. *The Marianne Frosting Developmental Test of Visual Perception, 1963 standardization.* Missoula, Mont.: Southern Univ. Press, 1964.

Furer, M. Observations on the treatment of the symbiotic syndrome of infantile psychosis—reality, reconstruction, and drive maturation. In J. B. McDevitt and C. F. Settlage (Eds.), *Separation-individuation.* New York: International Univ. Press, 1971.

Garber, H., and Heber, R. The Milwaukee project: Early intervention as a technique to prevent mental retardation. Storrs, Conn.: Univ. of Conn. Unpublished paper, 1973. Cited in D. P. Hallahan and J. M. Kauffman, *Exceptional children: Introduction to special education.* Englewood Cliffs, N.J.: Prentice-Hall, 1978.

References

Gardner, H. Children's art: Nadia's challenge. *Psychology Today.* 1979, 13(4), 18.

Garfield, S. L. Psychotherapy: A 40-year appraisal. *Amer. Psychol.,* 1981, 36, 174–183.

Garfinkel, B., and Golombek, H. Suicide and depression in childhood and adolescence. In P. D. Steinhauer and Q. Rae-Grant (Eds.), *Psychological problems of the child and his family.* Toronto: Macmillan, 1977.

Garmezy, N. Observations on research with children at risk for child and adult psychopathology. In M. F. McMillan and S. Henao (Eds.), *Child psychiatry: Treatment and research.* New York: Brunner/Mazel, 1977, pp. 51–70.

Garmezy, N. The year of the child: What does the child need? Paper presented to Ontario Psychological Association, Feb. 1979.

Gelfand, D. M., and Hartmann, D. P. Behavior therapy with children: A review and evaluation of research methodology. In A. M. Graziano (Ed.), *Behavior therapy with children.* Chicago: Aldine Pub. Co., 1971.

Gelfand, D. M., and Hartmann, D. P. *Child behavior analysis and therapy.* New York: Pergamon Press, 1975.

Gelles, R. J. Violence toward children in the United States. *Amer. J. Ortho.,* 1978, 48, 580–592.

Genshaft, J. L. Personality characteristics of delinquent subtypes. *J. Abn. Child Psych.,* 1980, 8, 279–283.

Gesell, A., and Amatruda, C. S. *Developmental diagnosis.* 2nd ed. New York: Harper and Row, 1947.

Getman, G. N. The visuomotor complex in the acquisition of learning skills. In J. Hellmuth (Ed.), *Learning disorders.* Vol. 1. Seattle: Special Child Publications, 1965, pp. 49–76.

Gil, D. G. *Violence against children.* Cambridge, Mass.: Harvard Univ. Press, 1973.

Giles, D. K., and Wolf, M. W. Toilet training institutionalized, severe retardates: An application of operant behavior modification techniques. *Amer. J. Ment. Defic.,* 1966, 70, 766–780.

Gillingham, A., and Stillman, B. *Remedial training for children with disability in reading, spelling, and penmanship.* Cambridge, Mass.: Educators Pub. Service, 1960, 1968.

Girardeau, F. L. Cultural-familial retardation. In N. R. Ellis (Ed.), *International review of research in mental retardation.* New York: Academic Press, 1971, 303–348.

Gittleman-Klein, R.; Klein, D. F.; Abikoff, H.; Katz, S.; Gloisten, A. C.; and Kates, W. Relative efficacy of methylphenidate and behavior modification in hyperkinetic children: An interim report. In B. B. Lahey, *Behavior therapy with hyperactive and learning disabled children.* New York: Oxford Univ. Press, 1979.

Glaser, K. Masked depression in children and adolescents. *Amer. J. Psychother.,* 1967, 21, 565–574.

Glaser, K. Suicidal children—management. *Amer. J. Psychother.,* 1971, 25, 27–36.

References

Glueck, S., and Glueck, E. *Unraveling juvenile delinquency.* New York: Commonwealth Fund, 1950.

Glueck, S., and Glueck, E. *Delinquents and nondelinquents in perspective.* Cambridge, Mass.: Harvard Univ. Press, 1968.

Glueck, S., and Glueck, E. *Toward a typology of juvenile offenders. Implications for therapy and prevention.* New York: Grune and Stratton, 1970.

Goldberg, B. Management of hyperkinetic behavior in the classroom: A diagnostic approach. Paper read at the 23rd Annual Convention, Council for Exceptional Children, Hamilton, Ontario, 1979.

Goldfarb, W. An investigation of childhood schizophrenia. *Arch. Gen. Psychiat.,* 1964, 11, 620–634.

Goldfarb, W.; Braunstein, M. A.; and Lorge, I. Childhood schizophrenia: A study of speech patterns in a group of schizophrenic children. *Amer. J. Ortho.,* 1956, 26, 544–555.

Goldfarb, W.; Mintz, I.; and Stroock, K. W. *A time to heal.* New York: International Univ. Press, 1969.

Goldfried, M. R., and Sprafkin, J. N. *Behavioral personality assessment.* Morristown, N.J.: General Learning Press, 1974.

Goldfried, M. R.; Stricker, G.; and Weiner, I. B. *Rorschach handbook of clinical and research applications.* Englewood Cliffs, N.J.: Prentice-Hall, 1971.

Goldstein, J.; Freud, A.; and Solnit, A. J. *Beyond the best interests of the child.* New York: The Free Press, 1973.

Goldston, S. E. Defining primary prevention. In G. W. Albee and J. M. Joffe (Eds.), *Primary prevention of psychopathology.* Vol. 1: *The issues.* Hanover, N.H.: Univ. Press of New England, 1977, pp. 18–23.

Golick, M. *Deal me in: The use of playing cards in teaching and learning.* Guilford, Conn.: Special Learning Corp., 1973.

Golick, M. She thought I was dumb, but I told her I had a learning disability. *CBC Learning Systems 1973,* © Canadian Broadcasting Corp., 1969. Reprinted in *Readings in learning disabilities.* Guilford, Conn.: Special Learning Corp., 1978, 196–207.

Goodenough, F. L. *Measurement of intelligence by drawings.* New York: World Book Co., 1926.

Gordon, D. A., and Young, R. D. School phobia: A discussion of etiology, treatment, and evaluation. In S. Chess and A. Thomas (Eds.), *Annual progress in child psychiatry and child development.* New York: Brunner/Mazel. 1977, pp. 409–433.

Gould, J. L., and Gould, C. G. The instinct to learn. *Science 81,* May 1981. Reprinted in H. E. Fitzgerald and T. H. Carr (Eds.), *Annual editions human development 82/83.* Guilford, Conn.: Dushkin Pub. Group, 1982, pp. 7–11.

Gray, F.; Graubard, P. S.; and Rosenberg, H. Little brother is changing you. *Psychology Today,* 1974, 8, 42–45.

Graziano, A. M. (Ed.) *Behavior therapy with children.* Chicago: Aldine Pub. Co., 1971.

Graziano, A. M. Behavior therapy. In B. B. Wolman, J. Egan, and A. O. Ross

References

(Eds.), *Handbook of treatment of mental disorders in childhood and adolescence.* Englewood Cliffs, N.J.: Prentice-Hall, 1978.

Graziano, A. M.; De Giovanni, I. S.; and Garcia, K. A. Behavioral treatment of children's fears: A review. *Psych. Bull.,* 1979, 86, 804–830.

Greenberg, N. H. Atypical behavior during infancy: Infant development in relation to the behavior and personality of the mother. In E. J. Anthony and C. Koupernik (Eds.), *The child in his family.* Vol. 1. New York: Wiley-Interscience, 1970, pp. 87–120.

Greene, W. A., and Miller, G. Psychological factors and reticuloendothelial disease. IV. Observations on a group of children and adolescents with leukemias: An interpretation of disease development in terms of mother-child unit. *Psychosom. Med.,* 1958, 20, 124–144.

Grossman, F. K. *Brothers and sisters of retarded children. An exploratory study.* New York: Syracuse Univ. Press, 1972.

Grossman, H. J. (Ed.). *Manual on terminology and classification in mental retardation: 1973 revision.* Special publication of the American Association on Mental Deficiency, 1973.

Grossman, H. J. (Ed.). *Manual on terminology and classification in mental retardation: 1977 revision.* Washington, D.C.: American Association on Mental Deficiency, 1977.

Group for the Advancement of Psychiatry. *Psychopathological disorders in childhood. Theoretical considerations and a proposed classification.* New York: Jason Aronson, 1974, 1966.

Gualtieri, C. T., and Hawk, B. Clinical guidelines for psychopharmacologic and nutritional approaches in behavioral and emotional problems of childhood. In S. Gabel (Ed.), *Behavioral problems in childhood. A primary care approach.* New York: Grune and Stratton, 1981, pp. 409–424.

Guerin, P. J. *Family therapy.* New York: Gardner Press, 1976.

Guerney, B. Filial therapy: Description and rationale. *J. Consult. Psych.,* 1964, 28, 304–310.

Guerney, L. F. Play therapy with learning disabled children. *J. Clin. Child Psychol.,* 1979, 8, 242–244.

Gutelius, M. F.; Millican, F. K.; Layman, E. M.; Cohen, G. J.; and Dublin, C. C. Nutritional studies of children with pica. *Pediatrics,* 1962, 29, 1012–1023.

Guthrie, J. T., and Siefert, M. Education for children with learning disabilities. In H. R. Myklebust (Ed.), *Progress in learning disabilities.* Vol. IV. New York: Grune and Stratton, 1978, pp. 223–255.

Haley vs. Ohio, 332, U.S. 596 (1948). Cited in M. F. Shore, Legislation, advocacy, and the rights of children and youth. *Amer. Psychol.,* 1979, 34, 1017–1019.

Haley, J. Approaches to family therapy. In J. Haley (Ed.), *Changing families.* New York: Grune and Stratton, 1971, pp. 227–236.

Haley, J. *Problem-solving therapy.* San Francisco: Jossey-Bass, 1976.

Haley, J., and Hoffman, L. *Techniques of family therapy.* New York: Basic Books, 1967.

References

Hall, M. B. Our present knowledge about manic-depressive states in childhood. *Nerv. Child.* 1952, 9, 319–325.

Hallahan, D. P., and Cruickshank, W. M. *Psychoeducational foundations of learning disabilities.* Englewood Cliffs, N.J.: Prentice-Hall, 1973.

Hallahan, D. P., and Kauffman, J. M. *Introduction to learning disabilities: A psychobehavioral approach.* Englewood Cliffs, N.J.: Prentice-Hall, 1976.

Hallahan, D. P., and Kauffman, J. M. *Exceptional children. Introduction to special education.* Englewood Cliffs, N.J.: Prentice-Hall, 1978.

Halpern, F. The Rorschach Test with children. In A. I. Rabin and M. R. Haworth (Eds.), *Projective techniques with children.* New York: Grune and Stratton, 1960.

Halpern, W. I., and Kissel, S. *Human resources for troubled children.* New York: John Wiley and Sons, 1976.

Hambley, W. D., and Freeman, G. Mental health in schools: A programme for early identification. *Ontario Psychologist, 1977, 9,* 21–28.

Hammill, D. D., and Bartel, N. R. *Teaching children with learning and behavior problems.* Boston: Allyn and Bacon, 1975.

Haney, B., and Gold, M. The juvenile delinquent nobody knows. *Psychology Today, 1973, 7,* 49–55.

Harley, J.; Ray, R.; Tomasi, L.; Eichman, P.; Matthews, C.; Chun, R.; Cleeland, C.; and Traisman, E. Hyperkinesis and food additives: Testing the Feingold hypothesis. *Pediatrics, 1978, 61.* Reprinted in R. Piazza (Ed.), *Readings in hyperactivity.* Guilford, Conn.: Special Learning Corp., 1980, pp. 59–68.

Harris, D. B. *Children's drawings as measures of intellectual maturity.* New York: Harcourt, Brace and World, 1963.

Harrison, S. Reassessment of eclecticism in child psychiatric treatment. In M. F. McMillan and S. Henao (Eds.), *Child psychiatry: Treatment and research.* New York: Brunner/Mazel, 1977.

Hartmann, E. The strangest sleep disorder. *Psychology Today, 1981, 15 (4),* 14–18.

Hastings, J. E., and Barkley, R. A. A review of psychophysiological research with hyperkinetic children. *J. Abn. Child Psych., 1978, 6,* 413–447.

Hathaway, S. R., and McKinley, J. C. *The Minnesota Multiphasic Personality Inventory Manual* (rev.). New York: Psych. Corp., 1967.

Havelkova, M. Follow-up study of 71 children diagnosed as psychotic in preschool age. *Amer. J. Ortho., 1968, 38,* 846–857.

Heisel, J. S. Life changes as etiological factors in juvenile rheumatoid arthritis. *J. Psychosom. Res., 1972, 16,* 411–420.

Heisel, J. S.; Ream, S.; Raite, R.; Rapport, M.; and Coddington, R. D. The significance of life events as contributing factors in the diseases of children. III. A study of pediatric patients. *J. Pediat., 1975, 83,* 119.

Helfer, R. E., and Kempe, C. H. (Eds.). *The battered child.* 2nd ed. Chicago: Univ. of Chicago Press, 1974.

Hersen, M., and Eisler, R. M. Social skills training. In W. E. Craighead, A. E. Kazdin, and M. J. Mahoney, *Behavior modification: Principles, issues and applications.* Boston: Houghton Mifflin, 1976, pp. 361–375.

References

Hersov, L. A. Refusal to go to school. *J. Child Psychol. Psychiat.*, 1960, 1, 137–145.

Hertz, M. R. The Rorschach in adolescence. In A. I. Rabin and M. R. Haworth, *Projective techniques with children.* New York: Grune and Stratton, 1960.

Hetherington, E. M., and Martin, B. Family interaction and psychopathology in children. In H. C. Quay and J. S. Werry (Eds.), *Psychopathological disorders of childhood.* New York: John Wiley and Sons, 1972.

Hetherington, E. M., and Martin, B. Family interaction. In H. C. Quay and J. S. Werry (Eds.), *Psychopathological disorders of childhood.* 2nd ed. New York: John Wiley and Sons, 1979, pp. 247–302.

Hetherington, E. M.; Stouwie, R. J.; and Ridberg, E. H. Patterns of family interaction and child-rearing attitudes related to three dimensions of juvenile delinquency. *J. Abn. Psych.*, 1971, 78, 160–176.

Hewett, F. M. Teaching speech to an autistic child through operant conditioning. *Amer. J. Ortho.*, 1965, 35, 927–936.

Hobbs, S. A.; Moguin, L. E.; Tyroler, M.; and Lahey, B. B. Cognitive behavior therapy with children: Has clinical utility been demonstrated? *Psych. Bull.*, 1980, 87, 147–165.

Hollingsworth, C. E.; Tanguay, P. E.; Grossman, L.; and Pabst, P. Long-term outcome of obsessive-compulsive disorder in childhood. *J. Amer. Acad. Child Psychiat.*, 1980, 19, 134–144.

Hollon, T. H. Poor school performance as a symptom of masked depression in children and adolescents. *Amer. J. Psychother.*, 1970, 24, 258–263.

Hoy, E.; Weiss, G.; Minde, K.; and Cohen, N. The hyperactive child at adolescence: Cognitive, emotional, and social functioning. *J. Abn. Child Psych.*, 1978, 6, 311–324.

Hunt, J. McV. *Intelligence and experience.* New York: Ronald Press, 1961.

Hutt, S. J.; Hutt, C.; Lee, D.; and Ounsted, C. A behavioral and electroencephalographic study of autistic children. *J. Psychiat. Res.*, 1965, 3, 181–197.

Itard, J. *The wild boy of Aveyron.* New York: Appleton-Century-Crofts, Meredith Pub. Co., 1962.

Jacobs, T. J., and Charles, E. Life events and the occurrence of cancer in children. *Psychosom. Med.*, 1980, 42, 11–24.

Jastak, J. F., and Jastak, S. R. *The Wide Range Acheivement Test* (rev. ed.). Wilmington, Del.: Guidance Associates, 1965.

Jeffrey, C. R., and Jeffrey, I. A. Delinquents and dropouts: An experimental program in behavior change. *Can. J. Corrections*, 1970, 12, 47–58.

Jensen, A. R. How much can we boost IQ and scholastic achievement? *Harvard Educ. Rev.*, 1969, 39, 1–123.

Jensen, A. R. IQs of identical twins reared apart. *B. Genetics*, 1970, 1, 133–148.

Johnson, A. M.; Falstein, E.; Szurek, S.; and Svendson, M. School phobia. *Amer. J. Ortho.*, 1941, 11, 702–711.

Joint Commission on Mental Health of Children. *Crisis in child mental health: Challenge to the 1970's.* New York: Harper and Row, 1969, 1970.

Jones, H. G. Stuttering. In C. G. Costello (Ed.), *Symptoms of psychopathology. A handbook.* New York: John Wiley and Sons, 1970. pp. 336–358.

Jones, R. L.; Gottlieb, J.; Guskin, S.; and Yoshida, R. K. Evaluating mainstreaming programs: Models, caveats, considerations, and guidelines. *Excep. Chil.*, 1978, 44, 588–601.

Kagan, J. Reflection-impulsivity: The generality and dynamics of conceptual tempo. *J. Abn. Psych.*, 1966, 71, 17–24.

Kahn, M. W., and McFarland, J. A demographic and treatment evaluation study of institutionalized juvenile offenders. *J. Commun. Psych.*, 1973, 1, 282–284.

Kales, A., and Berger, R. J. Psychopathology of sleep. In C. G. Costello (Eds.), *Symptoms of psychopathology. A handbook.* New York: John Wiley and Sons, 1970, 418–447.

Kales, A.; Jacobson, A.; Paulson, M. J.; Kales, J. D.; and Walter, R. D. Somnambulism: Psychophysiological correlates. I. All-night EEG studies. *Arch. Gen. Psychiat.*, 1966a, 14, 586–594.

Kales, A.; Paulson, M. J.; Jacobson, A.; and Kales, J. Somnambulism: Psychophysiological correlates. *Arch. Gen. Psychiat.*, 1966b, 14, 595–604.

Kanfer, F. H., and Grimm, L. G. The future of behavior modification. In W. E. Craighead, A. E. Kazdin, and M. J. Mahoney, *Behavior modification. Principles, issues, and applications.* Boston: Houghton Mifflin, 1976, pp. 447–462.

Kanfer, F. H.; Karoly, P.; and Newman, A. Reduction of children's fear of the dark by competence-related and situational threat-related verbal cues. *J. Consult. Clin. Psych.*, 1975, 43 (2), 251–258.

Kanner, L. *Child psychiatry.* Springfield, Ill.: Charles C Thomas, 1935.

Kanner, L. Autistic disturbances of affective contact. *Nerv. Child*, 1943, 2, 217–250.

Kanner, L. Do behavioral symptoms always indicate psychopathology? *J. Child Psychol. Psychiat.*, 1960, 1, 17–25.

Kanner, L. Childhood psychosis: A historical review. *J. Autism Childhood Schiz.*, 1971a, 1, 14–19.

Kanner, L. Follow-up study of eleven autistic children originally reported in 1943. *J. Autism Childhood Schiz.*, 1971b, 1, 119–145.

Kanner, L. *Child psychiatry.* 4th ed. Springfield, Ill.: Charles C Thomas, 1972.

Kanner, L. Historical perspective on developmental deviations. In E. Schopler and R. J. Reichler (Eds.), *Psychopathology and child development.* New York: Plenum Press, 1976, pp. 7–17.

Kanner, L.; Rodriguez, A.; and Ashenden, B. How far can autistic children go in matters of social adaptation? *J. Autism Childhood Schiz.*, 1972, 2, 9–33.

Kaplan, H. I., and Kaplan, H. S. Current theoretical concepts in psychosomatic medicine. *Amer. J. Psychiat.*, 1959, 115, 1091–1096.

Karasu, T. B., and Plutchik, R. Research problems in psychosomatic medicine and psychotherapy of somatic disorders. In T. B. Karasu and R. I. Steinmuller (Eds.), *Psychotherapeutics in medicine.* New York: Grune and Stratton, 1978.

Kauffman, J. M. Behavior modification. In W. M. Cruickshank and D. P. Hallahan (Eds.), *Perception and learning disabilities in children.* Vol. 2: *Research and theory.* Syracuse: Syracuse Univ. Press, 1975, pp. 395–344.

References

Kavale, K. The relationship between auditory perceptual skills and reading ability. A meta-analysis. *J. Lear. Dis.*, 1981, 14(9), 539–546.

Kazdin, A. E. Assessing the clinical or applied importance of behavior change through social validation. In C. M. Franks and G. T. Wilson, *Annual review of behavior therapy theory and practice.* New York: Brunner/Mazel, 1978, pp. 193–213.

Kazdin, A. E.; Matson, J. L.; and Esveldt-Dawson, K. Social skill performance among normal and psychiatric inpatient children as a function of assessment conditions. *Behav. Res. Ther.*, 1981, 19, 145–152.

Kellerman, J. Anorexia nervosa: The efficacy of behavior therapy. *J. Behav. Ther. and Exp. Psychiat.*, 1977, 8, 387–390.

Kellerman, J. Rapid treatment of nocturnal anxiety in children. *J. Behav. Ther. and Exp. Psychiat.*, 1980, 11, 9–11.

Kelly, F. J. The effectiveness of survival camp training with delinquents. *Amer. J. Ortho.*, 1971, 41, 305–306.

Kelly, J. A. Using puppets for behavior rehearsal in social skills training sessions with young children. *Child Behav. Ther.*, 1981, 3 (1), 61–64.

Kelman, D. H. Gilles de la Tourette's disease in children: A review of the literature. *J. Child Psychol. Psychiat.*, 1965, 6, 219–226.

Kendall, P. C., and Finch, A. J. A cognitive-behavioral treatment for impulsivity: A group comparison study. *J. Consult. Clin. Psych.*, 1978, 46 (1), 110–118.

Kendall, P. C., and Hollon, S. D. (Eds.), *Cognitive-behavioral interventions. Theory, research, and procedures.* New York: Academic Press, 1979.

Kennedy, W. A. School phobia: Rapid treatment of fifty cases. *J. Abn. Psych.*, 1965, 70, 285–289.

Kent, R. N., and O'Leary, K. D. A controlled evaluation of behavior modification with conduct problem children. *J. Consult. Clin. Psych.*, 1976, 44, 586–596.

Kephart, N. C. *The slow learner in the classroom.* Columbus, Ohio: Charles E. Merrill, 1960.

Kephart, N. C. Perceptual-motor aspects of learning disabilities. In E. C. Frierson and W. E. Barbe (Eds.), *Educating children with learning disabilities: Selected readings.* New York: Appleton-Century-Crofts, 1967, pp. 405–413.

Kessler, J. *Psychopathology of childhood.* Englewood Cliffs, N.J.: Prentice-Hall, 1966.

Kessler, M., and Albee, G. W. An overview of the literature of primary prevention. In G. W. Albee and J. M. Joffe (Eds.), *Primary prevention of psychopathology.* Vol. 1: *The issues.* Hanover, N.H.: Univ. Press of New England, 1977, pp. 351–399.

Kimmel, H. D., and Kimmel, E. An instrumental conditioning method for the treatment of enuresis. *J. Behav. Ther. and Exp. Psychiat.*, 1970, 1, 121–123.

Kinsbourne, M. Perceptual learning determines beginning reading. Paper presented at the meeting of the Eastern Psychological Association, Philadelphia, 1973. Cited in T. H. Bryan and J. H. Bryan, *Understanding learning disabilities.* 2nd ed. Sherman Oaks, Calif.: Alfred Pub. Co., 1978.

Kirk, S. A., *Educating exceptional children.* Boston: Houghton Mifflin, 1962.

Kirk, S. A., and Kirk, W. D. *Psycholinguistic learning disabilities: Diagnosis and remediation.* Urbana, Ill.: Univ. of Illinois Press, 1971.

Kirk, S. A.; Kliebhan, J. M.; and Lerner, J. W. *Teaching reading to slow and disabled learners.* Boston: Houghton Mifflin, 1978.

Kirk, S. A.; McCarthy, J. J.; and Kirk, W. D. *Illinois Test of Psycholinguistic Abilities* (rev. ed.). Urbana, Ill.: Univ. of Illinois Press, 1968.

Kirkland, K. D., and Thelen, M. H. Uses of modeling in child treatment. In B. B. Lahey and A. E. Kazdin (Eds.), *Advances in clinical child psychology.* Vol. 1. New York: Plenum Press, 1977, pp. 307–328.

Kirschenbaum, H. *On becoming a person.* New York: Van Nostrand, 1968.

Klein, M. *The psychoanalysis of children.* London: Hogarth Press, 1932.

Klein, M. *Narrative of a child analysis.* New York: Basic Books, 1961.

Kleiser, J. R. Milieu therapy. In S. Copel (Ed.), *Behavior pathology of childhood and adolescence.* New York: Basic Books, 1973.

Klerman, G. L. Depression and adaptation. In R. J. Friedman and M. M. Katz (Eds.), *The psychology of depression: Contemporary theory and research.* New York: John Wiley and Sons, Hemisphere Publishing, 1974.

Knitzer, J. E. Child advocacy: A perspective. *Amer. J. Ortho.,* 1976, 46, 200–216.

Knopf, I. J. *Childhood psychopathology.* Englewood Cliffs, N.J.: Prentice-Hall, 1979.

Koegel, R. L., and Covert, A. The relationship of self-stimulation to learning in autistic children. *J. Applied Behav. Anal.,* 1972, 5, 381–387.

Kohlberg, L. Stage and sequence: The cognitive-developmental approach to socialization. In D. A. Goslin (Ed.), *Handbook of socialization theory and research.* Chicago: Rand McNally, 1969, pp. 347–380.

Kolansky, H. An overview of child psychiatry. In S. L. Copel (Ed.), *Behavior pathology of childhood and adolescence.* New York: Basic Books, 1973.

Kratochwill, T. R. *Selective mutism: Implications for research and treatment.* Hillsdale, N.J.: Lawrence Erlbaum Assoc., 1981.

Kratochwill, T. R.; Brody, G. H.; and Piersel, W. C. Elective mutism in children. In B. B. Lahey and A. E. Kazdin (Eds.), *Advances in clinical child psychology.* Vol. 2. New York: Plenum Press, 1979, pp. 193–240.

Lachman, S. J. *Psychosomatic disorders: A behavioristic interpretation.* New York: John Wiley and Sons, 1972.

Lally, M. Computer-assisted teaching of sight-word recognition for mentally-retarded school children. *Amer. J. Ment. Defic.,* 1981, 85, 383–388.

Lambert, N. M.; Sandoval, J.; and Sassone, D. Prevalence of treatment regimens for children considered to be hyperactive. *Amer. J. Ortho.,* 1979, 49, 482–490.

Langford, W. S. Anxiety attacks in children. *Amer. J. Ortho.,* 1937, 7, 210–218.

LaPouse, R., and Monk, M. A. Behavior deviations in a representative sample of children: Variation by sex, age, race, social class, and family size. *Amer. J. Ortho.,* 1964, 34, 436–446.

References

Lazarus, A. A. *Behavior therapy and beyond.* New York: McGraw-Hill, 1971.

Lazarus, A. A. Multimodal behavior therapy: Treating the "BASIC ID." *J. Nerv. Ment. Dis.,* 1973, 156, 404–411.

Lazarus, A. A.; Davison, G. C.; and Polefka, D. A. Classical and operant factors in the treatment of a school phobia. In A. M. Graziano (Ed.), *Behavior therapy with children.* Chicago: Aldine Pub. Co., 1971.

Leff, R. Behavior modification and the psychoses of childhood. *Psych. Bull.,* 1968, 69, 396–409.

Lefkowitz, M. M., and Burton, N. Childhood depression: A critique of the concept. *Psych. Bull.,* 1978, 85, 716–726.

Lerner, J. *Children with learning disabilities.* 2nd ed. Boston: Houghton Mifflin, 1976.

Lerner, J. W. *Learning disabilities. Theories, diagnosis, and teaching strategies.* 3rd ed. Boston: Houghton Mifflin, 1981.

Levis, D. J., and Hare, N. A review of the theoretical rationale and empirical support for the extinction approach of implosive (flooding) therapy. In M. Hersen, R. M. Eisler, and P. M. Miller (Eds.), *Progress in behavior modification.* Vol. 4. New York: Academic Press, 1977, pp. 299–376.

Leviton, H., and Kiraly, J. Different views of the elephant: Conceptual models of the behavior disordered and learning disabled child. *Child Study Journal,* 1976, 6, 127–137.

Levitt, E. E. The results of psychotherapy with children: An evaluation. *J. Consult. Psych.,* 1957, 21, 189–196.

Levitt, E. E. Research on psychotherapy with children. In A. E. Bergin and S. L. Garfield (Eds.), *Handbook of psychotherapy and behavior change.* New York: John Wiley and Sons, 1971.

Levitt, E. E.; Beiser, H. R.; and Robertson, R. E. A follow-up evaluation of cases treated at a community child guidance clinic. *Amer. J. Ortho.,* 1959, 29, 337–347.

Levitt, E. E., and Lubin, B. *Depression. Concepts, controversies, and some new facts.* New York: Springer Pub. Co., 1975.

Levy, D. *Maternal overprotection.* New York: Columbia Univ. Press, 1943.

Levy, D. M. On the problems of movement restraint. Tics, stereotyped movements, hyperactivity. *Amer. J. Ortho.,* 1944, 14, 644–671.

Levy H. *Square pegs, round holes: The learning-disabled child in the classroom and at home.* Boston: Little Brown and Co. 1973.

Lewin, M. *Understanding psychological research.* New York: John Wiley and Sons, 1979.

Lewis, M., and Lewis, D. O. A psychobiological view of depression in childhood. In A. P. French and I. N. Berlin (Eds.), *Depression in children and adolescents.* New York: Human Sciences Press, 1979, pp. 29–45.

Lezak, M. D. *Neuropsychological assessment.* New York: Oxford Univ. Press, 1976.

Liberman, R. Behavioral approaches to family and couple therapy. *Amer. J. Ortho.,* 1970, 40 (1) 106–118.

References

Lidz, T., and Rubenstein, R. Psychology of gastrointestinal disorders. In S. Arieti (Ed.), *American handbook of psychiatry*. New York: Basic Books, 1959, pp. 678–689.

Liebman, R.; Minuchin, S.; and Baker, L. The use of structural family therapy in the treatment of intractable asthma. *Amer. J. psychiat.*, 1974, 131, 535–540.

Lindsay, G. A., and Wedell, K. The early identification of educationally "at risk" children revisited. *J. Lear. Dis.*, 1982, 15 (4), 212–217.

Lipton, E. L.; Steinschneider, A.; and Richmond, J. B. Psychophysiolologic disorders in children. In L. W. Hoffman and M. L. Hoffman (Eds.), *Review of child development research*. Vol. 2. New York: Russell Sage, 1966, 169–220.

Loney, J. Hyperkinesis comes of age: What do we know and where should we go? *Amer. J. Ortho.*, 1980, 50, 28–42.

Long, R. T.; Lamont, J. H.; Whipple, B.; Bandler, L.; Blom G. E.; Burgin, L.; and Jessner, L. A psychosomatic study of allergic and emotional factors in children with asthma. *Amer. J. Psychiat.*, 1958, 114, 890–899.

Lotter, V. Epidemiology of autistic conditions in young children. *Soc. Psychiat.*, 1966, 1, 124–137.

Lourie, N. V. The many faces of advocacy. In I. N. Berlin (Ed.), *Advocacy for child mental health*. New York: Brunner/Mazel, 1975,a, pp. 68–80.

Lourie, N. V. Operational advocacy: Objectives and obstacles. In I. N. Berlin (Ed.), *Advocacy for child mental health*. New York: Brunner/Mazel, 1975b, pp. 81–91.

Lourie, N. V., and Berlin, I. N. Child advocacy: Political and legislative implications. In I. N. Berlin (Ed.), *Advocacy for child mental health*. New York: Brunner/Mazel, 1975, pp. 311–333.

Lovaas, O. I. A program for the establishment of speech in psychotic children. In J. K. Wing (Ed.), *Early childhood autism*. New York: Pergamon Press, 1966.

Lovaas, O. I. Parents as therapists. In M. Rutter and E. Schopler (Eds.), *Autism*. New York: Plenum Press, 1978, pp. 369–378.

Lovaas, O. I.; Freitas, L.; Nelson, K.; and Whalen, C. The establishment of imitation and its use for the development of complex behavior in schizophrenic children. *Behav. Res. and Ther.*, 1967, 5, 171–181.

Lovaas, O. I.; Koegel, R.; Simmons, J. Q.; and Long, J. S. Some generalization and follow-up measures on autistic children in behavior therapy. *J. Applied Behav. Anal.*, 1973, 6, 131–136.

Lovaas, O. I.; Schaeffer, B.; and Simmons, J. Q. Building social behavior in autistic children by use of electric shock. *J. Exper. Res. in Pers.*, 1965, 1, 99–109.

Lovaas, O. I.; Schreibman, L.; Koegel, R. L. A behavior modification approach to the treatment of autistic children. In E. Schopler and R. J. Reichler (Eds.), *Psychopathology and child development*. New York: Plenum Press, 1976.

Lovaas, O. I.; Schreibman, L.; Koegel, R.; and Rehm, R. Selective responding by autistic children to multiple sensory input. *J. Abn. Psych.*, 1971, 77, 211–222.

Love, H. D. *The mentally-retarded child and his family.* Springfield, Ill.: Charles C Thomas, 1973.

Love, L. R.; Kaswan, J.; and Bugenthal, D. B. Differential effectiveness of three clinical interventions for different socioeconomic groupings. *J. Consult. Clin. Psych.*, 1972, 39, 347–360.

Lovibond, S. H., and Coote, M. A. Enuresis. In C. G. Costello (Ed.), *Symptoms of psychopathology. A handbook.* New York: John Wiley and Sons, 1970, pp. 373–396.

Lowe, L. Families of children with early childhood schizophrenia. *Arch. Gen. Psychiat.*, 1966, 14, 26–30.

Lugo, J. O., and Hershey, G. L. *Human development. A psychological, biological, and sociological approach to the life span.* 2nd ed. New York: Macmillan, 1979.

Lustman, S. Mental health research and the university. Paper prepared for Task Force IV, Joint Commission on Mental Health of Children, 1968. Cited in *Crisis in child mental health: Challenge for the 1970's.* Report of the Joint Commission on Mental Health of Children. New York: Harper and Row, 1970.

Lutey, C. *Individual intelligence testing: A manual and sourcebook.* Greeley, Colo.: Carol J. Lutey Pub., 1977.

Lykken, D. T. A study of anxiety in the sociopathic personality. *J. Abn. Soc. Psych.*, 1957, 55, 6–10.

Lyle, J. G., and Goyen, J. D. Visual recognition, developmental lag, and strephosymbolia in reading retardation. *J. Abn. Psych.*, 1968, 73, 25–29.

Lyon, R., and Watson, B. Empirically-derived subgroups of learning disabled readers: Diagnostic characteristics. *J. Lear. Dis.*, 1981, 14(5), 256–261.

Machover, K. *Personality projection in the drawing of the human figure.* Springfield, Ill.: Charles C Thomas, 1949.

MacKeith, R. A frequent factor in the origins of primary nocturnal enuresis: Anxiety in the third year of life. *Devel. Med. Child Neurol.*, 1968, 10, 465–470.

MacKenzie, J. N. The production of the so-called "rose cold" by means of an artificial rose. *Amer. J. Med. Sciences*, 1886, 91, 45–57. Cited in N. J. Yorkston, Behavior therapy in the treatment of bronchial asthma. In T. Thompson and W. S. Dockens, III. (Eds.). *Applications of behavior modification.* New York: Academic Press, 1975.

Mahler, M. S. On child psychosis and schizophrenia. *Psychoanal. Stud. Child,* 1952, 7, 286–305.

Mahler, M. S. *On human symbiosis and the vicissitudes of individuation.* Vol. 1. London: Hogarth Press, 1969.

Mahler, M. S., and Gosliner, B. J. On symbiotic child psychosis. *Psychoanal. Stud. Child,* 1955, 10, 195–212.

Mahler, M. S.; Pine, F.; and Bergman, A. *The psychological birth of the human infant.* New York: Basic Books, 1975.

References

Mahoney, M. J. *Cognition and behavior modification.* Cambridge, Mass.: Ballinger Pub., 1974.

Mahoney, M. J., and Mahoney, K. Treatment of obesity: A clinical exploration. In B. J. Williams, S. Martin, and J. P. Foreyt (Eds.), *Obesity: Behavioral approaches to dietary management.* New York: Brunner/Mazel, 1976.

Marks, I. M. Review of behavioral therapy. I: Obsessive-compulsive disorders. *Amer. J. Psychiat.,* 1981, 138, 584–592.

Mash, E. J., and Terdal, L. G. (Eds.). *Behavior-therapy assessment.* New York: Springer Pub., 1976.

Maslow, A. *Toward a psychology of being.* New York: Van Nostrand, 1968.

Matarazzo, J. D. Behavioral health and behavioral medicine: Frontiers for a new health psychology. *Amer. Psychol.,* 1980, 35, 807–817.

Matson, J. L.; Kazdin, A. E.; and Esveldt-Dawson, K. Training interpersonal skills among mentally retarded and socially dysfunctional children. *Behav. Res. Ther.,* 1980, 18, 419–427.

Mattison, R.; Cantwell, D. P.; Russell, A. T.; and Will, L. A comparison of DSM-II and DSM-III in the diagnosis of childhood psychiatric disorders. II. Interrater agreement. *Arch. Gen. Psychiat..* 1979, 36, 1217–1222.

Matus, I. Assessing the nature and clinical significance of psychological contributions to childhood asthma. *Amer. J. Ortho.,* 1981, 51, 327–341.

Maudsley, H. *The physiology and pathology of the mind.* New York: Appleton and Co., 1867.

McCandless, B. R. The socialization of the individual. In E. Schopler and R. J. Reichler (Eds.), *Psychopathology and child development.* New York: Plenum Press, 1976.

McCarthy, J. J., and McCarthy, J. F. *Learning disabilities.* Boston: Allyn and Bacon, 1969.

McCord, J. A thirty-year follow-up of treatment effects. *Amer. Psychol.,* 1978, 33, 284–289.

McCord, W., and McCord, J., with Zola, I. K. *The origins of crime. A new evaluation of the Cambridge-Somerville youth study.* New York: Columbia Univ. Press, 1959.

McMahon, R. C. Genetic etiology in the hyperactive child syndrome: A critical review. *Amer. J. Ortho.,* 1980, 50, 145–150.

Meichenbaum, D. *Cognitive behavior modification.* Morristown, N.J.: General Learning Press, 1974.

Meichenbaum, D. H. *Cognitive-behavior modification: An integrative approach.* New York: Plenum Press, 1977.

Meichenbaum, D. Teaching children self-control. In B. B. Lahey and A. E. Kazdin (Eds.), *Advances in clinical child psychology.* Vol. 2. New York: Plenum Press, 1979, pp. 1–33.

Meichenbaum, D., and Asarnow, J. Cognitive-behavioral modification and metacognitive development: Implications for the classroom. In P. C. Kendall and S. D. Hollon (Eds.), *Cognitive-behavioral interventions.* New York: Academic Press, 1979. pp. 11–35.

References

Meichenbaum, D. H., and Goodman, J. Training impulsive children to talk to themselves: A means of developing self-control. *J. Abn. Psych.*, 1971, 77, 115–126.

Mendelson, M.; Hirsch, S.; and Webber, C. S. A critical examination of some recent theoretical models in psychosomatic medicine. *Psychosom. Med.*, 1956, 18, 363–373.

Menyuk, P. *Sentences children use.* Cambridge, Mass.: MIT Press, 1969.

Messer, S. B., and Winokur, M. Some limits to the integration of psychoanalytic and behavior therapy. *Amer. Psychol.*, 1980, 35, 818–827.

Metz, J. R. Conditioning generalized imitation in autistic children. *J. Exper. Child Psych.*, 1965, 2, 389–399.

Metz, J. R. Stimulation level preferences of autistic children. *J. Abn. Psych.*, 1967, 72, 529–535.

Meyer, A. Objective psychology, or psychobiology with subordination of the medically useless contrast of mental and physical. *J.A.M.A.*, 1915, 65, 860.

Miller, L. C.; Barrett, C. L.; and Hampe, E. Phobias of childhood in a prescientific era. In A. Davids (Ed.), *Child personality and psychopathology: Current topics.* Vol. 1. New York: John Wiley and Sons, 1974, pp. 89–134.

Miller, L. C.; Barrett, C. L.; Hampe, E.; and Noble, H. Comparison of reciprocal inhibition, psychotherapy, and waiting list control for phobic children. *J. Abn. Psych.*, 1972, 79, 269–279.

Millican, F. K., and Lourie, R. S. The child with pica and his family. In E. J. Anthony and C. Koupernik (Eds.), *The child in his family.* Vol. 1. New York: Wiley-Interscience, 1970, 333–348.

Mills, C. M., and Walter, T. L. Reducing juvenile delinquency: A Behavioral-Employment Intervention Program. In J. S. Stumphauzer (Ed.), *Progress in behavior therapy with delinquents.* Springfield, Ill.: Charles C Thomas, 1979.

Minde, K. The role of drugs in the treatment of disturbed children. In P. D. Steinhauer and Q. Rae-Grant, *Psychological problems of the child and his family.* Toronto: Macmillan, 1977.

Minkin, N.; Braukmann, C. J.; Minkin, B. L.; Timbers, G. D.; Timbers, B. J.; Fixsen, D. L.; Phillips, E. L.; and Wolf, M. M. The social validation and training of conversational skills. *J. Applied Behav. Anal.*, 1976, 9, 127–139.

Minuchin, S.; Baker, L.; Rosman, B. L.; Liebman, R.; Milman, L.; and Todd, T. C. A conceptual model of psychosomatic illness in children. *Arch. Gen. Psychiat.*, 1975, 32, 1031–1038.

Monaghan, J. H.; Robinson, J. O.; and Dodge, J. A. The Children's Life Events Inventory. *J. Psychosom. Res.*, 1979, 23, 63–68.

Moncur, J. P. Symptoms of maladjustment differentiating young stutterers from non-stutters. *Child Devel.*, 1955, 26, 91–96.

Moore, N. Behavior therapy in bronchial asthma: A controlled study. *J. Psychosom. Res.*, 1965, 9, 257–276.

References

Mordock, J. B. *The other children. An introduction to exceptionality.* New York: Harper and Row, 1975.

Morganstern, K. P. Implosive therapy and flooding procedures: A critical review. *Psych. Bull.,* 1973, 79, 318–334.

Morse, W. C. Enhancing the classroom teacher's mental health function. In E. L. Cowen, E. A. Gardner, and M. Zax, *Emergent approaches to mental health problems.* New York: Appleton-Century-Crofts, 1967, pp. 271–289.

Moustakas, C. *Father and children: The living relationship.* New York: Harper and Row, 1959a.

Moustakas, C. *Psychotherapy with children.* New York: Ballantine Books, 1959b.

Mowatt, M. H. Group therapy approach to emotional conflicts of the mentally retarded and their parents. In F. J. Menolascino (Ed.), *Psychiatric approaches to mental retardation.* New York: Basic Books, 1970.

Mowrer, O. H., and Mowrer, W. M. Enuresis: A method for its study and treatment. *Amer. J. Ortho.,* 1938, 8, 436–459.

Murray, H. A. *Thematic Apperception Test.* Cambridge, Mass.: Harvard Univ. Press, 1943.

Murray, J. P. Television and violence. Implications of the Surgeon General's research program. *Amer. Psychol..* 1973, 28, 472–478.

Mushin, D. N. General principles of treatment in child psychiatry. In P. D. Steinhauer and Q. Rae-Grant, *Psychological problems of the child and his family.* Toronto: Macmillan, 1977.

Myklebust, H. Learning disabilities: Definition and overview. In H. Myklebust (Ed.), *Progress in learning disabilities.* Vol. 1. New York: Grune and Stratton, 1968, pp. 1–15.

Myklebust, H. R. What is the future for learning disabilities? *J. Lear. Dis.,* 1980, 13, 468–471.

Nay, W. R. *Behavioral intervention.* New York: Gardner Press, 1976.

Neal, D. H. Behavior therapy and encopresis in children. *Behav. Res. and Ther.,* 1963, 1, 139–150.

Neilans, T. H., and Israel, A. C. Towards maintenance and generalization of behavior change: Teaching children self-regulation and self-instructional skills. *Cog. Ther. Res.,* 1981, 5 (2), 189–195.

Neuhaus, E. C. A personality study of asthmatic and cardiac children. *Psychosom. Med.,* 1958, 20, 181–186.

Newberger, E. H., and Bourne, R. The medicalization and legalization of child abuse. *Amer. J. Ortho.,* 1978, 48, 593–607.

Ney, P. Operant conditioning of schizophrenic children. *Can. Psychiat. Ass'n. J.,* 1967, 12, 9–13.

Nihira, K.; Foster, R.; Shellhaas, M.; and Leland, H. *AAMD Adaptive Behavior Scale* (1974 revision). Washington, D.C.: American Association on Mental Deficiency, 1974.

Nir, Y., and Cutler, R. The therapeutic utilization of the juvenile court. *Amer. J. Psychiat.,* 1973, 130, 1112–1117.

O'Leary, S. G., and Pelham, W. E. Behavior therapy and withdrawal of stimulant medication with hyperactive children. In B. B. Lahey, *Behavior therapy with hyperactive and learning disabled children.* New York: Oxford Univ. Press. 1979.

O'Malley, J. E.; Koocher, G.; Foster, D.; and Slavin, L. Psychiatric sequelae of surviving childhood cancer. *Amer. J. Ortho.,* 1979, 49, 608–616.

Ornitz, E. M., and Ritvo, E. R. Perceptual inconstancy in early infantile autism. *Arch. Gen. Psychiat.,* 1968, 18, 76–97.

Ornitz, E. M., and Ritvo, E. R. The syndrome of autism: A critical review. *Amer. J. Psychiat.,* 1976, 133, 609–621.

Orton, S. R. *Reading, writing, and speech problems in children.* New York: W. W. Norton, 1937.

Ott, J. N. Influence of fluorescent lights on hyperactivity and learning disabilities. *J. Lear. Dis.,* 1976, 9. Cited in *Readings in learning disabilities.* Guilford, Conn.: Special Learning Corp., 1978, 99–103.

Owen, F. W.; Adams, P. A.; Forrest, T.; Stolz, L. M.; and Fisher, S. Learning disorders in children: Sibling studies. *Monographs of the Society for Research in Child Development,* 1971 (4, Ser. No. 144), 36.

Padilla, E. R.; Rohsenow, J.; and Bergman, A. B. Predicting accident frequency in children. *Pediat.,* 1976, 58, 223. Cited in J. H. Monaghan, J. O. Robinson, and J. A. Dodge, The Children's Life Events Inventory. *J. Psychosom. Res.,* 1979, 23, 63–68.

Paluszny, M. J. Psychoactive drugs in the treatment of learning disabilities. In W. M. Cruickshank, *Learning disabilities in home, school, and community.* Syracuse, N.Y.: Syracuse Univ. Press, 1977, pp. 292–319.

Papalia, D. E., and Olds, S. W. *A child's world. Infancy through adolescence.* 3rd ed. New York: McGraw-Hill, 1982.

Papp, P. *Family therapy full length case studies.* New York: Gardner Press, 1977.

Parker, G., and Lipscombe, P. Parental overprotection and asthma. *J. Psychosom. Res.,* 1979, 23, 295–299.

Patterson, G. R. Interventions for boys with conduct problems: Multiple settings, treatments, and criteria. *J. Consult. Clin. Psych.,* 1974, 42, 471–481.

Patterson, G. R. Naturalistic observation in clinical assessment. *J. Abn. Child Psych.,* 1977, 5, 309–322.

Paul, G. L. *Insight vs. desensitization in psychotherapy.* Stanford, Calif.: Stanford Univ. Press, 1966.

Paul, G. L. Strategy of outcome research in psychotherapy. *J. Consult. Psych.,* 1967a, 31, 109–118.

Paul, G. L. Insight vs. desensitization in psychotherapy two years after termination. *J. Consult. Psych.,* 1967b, 31, 333–348.

Paul, G. L. Behavior modification research. In C. M. Franks (Ed.), *Behavior therapy: Appraisal and status.* New York: McGraw-Hill, 1969, 29–62.

Paulsen, M. G. The law and abused children. In Helfer, R. E., and Kempe, C. H. (Eds.), *The battered child.* 2nd ed. Chicago: Univ. of Chicago Press, 1974, pp. 153–178.

Pearce, J. Annotation. Depressive disorder in childhood. *J. Child Psychol. Psychiat.,* 1977, 18, 79–83.

References

Pearson, G. H. J. A survey of learning difficulties in children. *Psychoanal. Stud. Child*, 1952, 7, 322–386.

Peck, H. B.; Rabinovitch, R. D.; and Cramer, J. B. A treatment program for parents of schizophrenic children. *Amer. J. Ortho.*, 1949, 19, 592–598.

Pelton, L. H. Child abuse and neglect: The myth of classlessness. *Amer. J. Ortho.*, 1978, 48, 608–617.

Peshkin, M. M., and Abramson, H. A. Psychosomatic group therapy with parents of children having intractible asthma. *Ann. Allergy*, 1959, 17 (3), 344. Cited in P. Pinkerton, Correlating physiologic with psychodynamic data in the study and management of childhood asthma. *J. Psychosom. Res.*, 1967, 11, 11–25.

Peters, R. DeV., and Davies, K. Effects of self-instructional training on cognitive impulsivity of mentally retarded adolescents. *Amer. J. Ment. Defic.*, 1981, 85, 377–382.

Peterson, D. P.; Quay, H. C.; and Tiffany, T. L. Personality factors related to juvenile delinquency. *Child Devel.*, 1961, 32, 355–372.

Peterson, D. R. Behavior problems of middle childhood. *J. Consult. Psych.*, 1961, 25, 205–209.

Phelps, T. R. *Juvenile delinquency: A contemporary view.* Santa Monica, Calif.: Goodyear Pub. Co., 1976.

Phillips, E. L. Contributions to a learning theory account of childhood autism. *J. Psychol.*, 1957, 43, 117–125.

Phillips, E. L. Achievement Place: Token reinforcement procedures in a home-style rehabilitation setting for "predelinquent" boys. *J. Applied Behav. Anal.*, 1968, 1, 213–223.

Phillips, E. L.; Phillips, E. A.; Fixsen, D. L.; and Wolf, M. M. Achievement Place: Modification of the behaviors of pre-delinquent boys within a token economy. *J. Applied Behav. Anal.*, 1971, 4, 45–59.

Phillips, J. S., and Ray, R. S. Behavioral approaches to childhood disorders. *Behav. Modif.*, 1980, 4, 3–34.

Piaget, J., and Inhelder, B. *The psychology of the child.* New York: Basic Books, 1969.

Pines, M. In praise of "invulnerables." *Readings in human development—77/78.* Guilford, Conn.: Dushkin Pub., 1977.

Pinkerton, P. Correlating physiologic with psychodynamic data in the study and management of childhood asthma. *J. Psychosom. Res.*, 1967, 11, 11–25.

Pinneau, S. R. The infantile disorders of hospitalism and anaclitic depression. *Psych. Bull.*, 1955, 52, 429–452.

Pitfield, M., and Oppenheim, A. N. Child rearing attitudes of mothers of psychotic children. *J. Child Psychol. Psychiat.*, 1964, 5, 51–57

Polier, J. W. In defense of children. *Child Welfare*, 1976, 55, 75–84.

Powell, L. F. The effect of extra stimulation and maternal involvement on the development of low-birth-weight infants and on maternal behavior. *Child Devel.*, 1974, 45, 106–113.

Powers, E., and Witmer, H. *An experiment in the prevention of delinquency.* New York: Columbia Univ. Press, 1951.

Poznanski, E. O. Childhood depression: A psychodynamic approach to the etiology of depression in children. In A. P. French and I. N. Berlin (Eds.), *Depression in children and adolescents.* New York: Human Sciences Press, 1979, pp. 46–48.

Preyer, W. Die Seele des Kindes. Beobachtungen über die geistige Entwicklung des Menschen in den ersten Lebensjahren. Leipzig: T. Grieben, 1882. Cited in W. Dennis, Historical beginnings of child psychology. *Psych. Bull.,* 1949, 46, 224–235.

Prichard, A., and Taylor. J. A demonstration of the concept of "hyperlearning." *J. Lear. Dis.,* 1981, 14, 19–21.

Public Law 94–142. The Education for All Handicapped Children Act of 1975, and Rules and Regulations for the Education of the Handicapped Act, *Federal Register,* Aug. 23, 1977, 42, 42474–42518.

Purcell, K.; Brady, K.; Chai, H.; Muser, J.; Molk, L.; Gordon, N.; and Means, J. The effect on asthma in children of experimental separation from the family. *Psychosom. Med.,* 1969, 31, 144–164.

Purcell, K., and Weiss, J. H. Asthma. In C. G. Costello (Ed.). *Symptoms of psychopathology. A handbook.* New York: John Wiley and Sons, Inc., 1970, pp. 597–623.

Purcell, K.; Weiss, J.; and Hahn, W. Certain psychosomatic disorders. In B. B. Wolman (Ed.), *Manual of child psychopathology.* New York: McGraw-Hill, 1972, 706–740.

Pyke, D. Diabetes mellitus. In J. Hambling and P. Hopkins (Eds.), *Psychosomatic disorders in adolescents and young adults.* Oxford: Pergamon Press, 1965, pp. 101–106.

Quay, H. C. Psychopathic personality as pathological stimulation-seeking. *Amer. J. Psychiat.,* 1965, 122, 180–183.

Quay, H. C. Patterns of aggression, withdrawal, and immaturity. In H. C. Quay and J. S. Werry (Eds.), *Psychopathological disorders of childhood.* New York: John Wiley and Sons, 1972, pp. 1–29.

Quay, H. C. Measuring dimensions of deviant behavior: The Behavior Problem Checklist. *J. Abn. Child Psychol.,* 1977, 5, 277–287.

Quay, H. C. Classification. In H. C. Quay and J. S. Werry (Eds.), *Psychopathological disorders of childhood.* 2nd ed. New York: John Wiley and Sons, 1979, pp. 1–42.

Quay, H. C., and Quay, L. C. Behavior problems in early adolescence. *Child Devel.,* 1965, 36, 215–220.

Rabin, A. I., and Haworth, M. R. (Eds.). *Projective techniques with children.* New York: Grune and Stratton, 1960.

Rabinovitch, R. D. Reading and learning disabilities. In S. Arieti, *American handbook of psychiatry.* Vol. 1. New York: Basic Books, 1959.

Rachman, S. J. The effects of psychological treatment. In H. J. Eysenck (Ed.), *Handbook of abnormal psychology.* San Diego, Calif.: Robert R. Knapp, 1973, 805–861.

Rachman, S.; DeSilva, P.; and Roper, G. The spontaneous decay of compulsive urges. *B. Res. Ther.,* 1976, 14, 445–453. Cited in L. Stanley, Treatment of ritualistic behavior in an 8-year-old girl by response prevention: A case report. *J. Child Psychol. Psychiat.*, 1980, 21, 85–90.

Rapaport, D.; Gill, M. M.; and Schafer, R. Ed. by R. R. Holt. *Diagnostic psychological testing* (rev. ed.). New York: International Univ. Press, 1968.

Raven, J. C. *Progressive matrices*. London: Lewis, 1938.

Rawls, D. J.; Rawls, J. R.; and Harrison, C. W. An investigation of six- to eleven-year-old children with allergic disorders. *J. Consult. Clin. Psych.*, 1971, 36, 260–264.

Redl, F. *When we deal with children*. New York: Free Press, 1966.

Redl, F., and Wineman, D. *Controls from within. Techniques for the treatment of the aggressive child*. New York: Free Press, 1952.

Reed, G. F. Elective mutism in children: A reappraisal. *J. Child Psychol. Psychiat.*, 1963, 4, 99–107.

Rees, L. The importance of psychological, allergic, and infective factors in childhood asthma. *J. Psychosom. Res.*, 1964, 7, 253–262.

Reid, D. K., and Hresko, W. P. *A cognitive approach to learning disabilities*. New York: McGraw-Hill, 1981.

Reid, J. B., and Hendriks, A. F. C. J. Preliminary analysis of the effectiveness of direct home intervention for the treatment of predelinquent boys who steal. In L. A. Hamerlynck, L. C. Handy, and E. J. Mash (Eds.), *Behavior change: Methodology, concepts, and practice*. Champaign, Ill.: Research Press, 1973, pp. 209–219.

Reinhart, J.; Kenna, M.; and Succop, R. Anorexia nervosa in children: Outpatient management. *J. Child Psychiat.*, 1972, 11, 114–131.

Rhodes, W. C., and Paul, J. L. *Emotionally disturbed and deviant behavior*. Englewood Cliffs, N.J.: Prentice-Hall, 1978.

Ribordy, S. C.; Tracy, R. J.; and Bernotas, T. D. The effects of an attentional training procedure on the performance of high and low test-anxious children. *Cog. Ther. and Res.*, 1981, 5, 19–28.

Rickers-Ovsiankina, M. A. *Rorschach psychology*. New York: John Wiley and Sons, 1960.

Ridberg, E. H.; Parke, R. D.; and Hetherington, E. M. Modification of impulsive and reflective cognitive styles through observation of film-mediated models. *Devel. Psych.*, 1971, 5, 369–377.

Rimland, B. *Infantile autism*. New York: Appleton-Century-Crofts, Meredith Pub., 1964.

Risley, T. R. The effects and side effects of punishing the autistic behaviors of a deviant child. *J. Applied Behav. Anal.*, 1968, 1, 21–34.

Risley, T. R. Behavior modification: An experimental-therapeutic endeavor. In R. B. Stuart, T. R. Risley, and G. R. Patterson, *Behavior modification and ideal mental health services*. Calgary, Alberta: Univ. of Calgary, 1969.

Ritter, B. The group desensitization of children's snake phobias using vicarious and contact desensitization procedures. *Behav. Res. Ther.*, 1968, 6, 1–6.

Robins, L. N. *Deviant children grown up*. Baltimore: Williams and Wilkins, 1966.

Robins, L. N. Follow-up studies of behavior disorders in children. In H. C.

Quay and J. S. Werry (Eds.), *Psychopathological disorders of childhood.* New York: John Wiley and Sons, 1972, pp. 414–450.

Robins, L. N. Follow-up studies. In H. C. Quay and J. S. Werry (Eds.), *Psychopathological disorders of childhood.* New York: John Wiley and Sons, 1979, pp. 483–513.

Robinson, H. B., and Robinson, N. M. Mental retardation. In P. H. Mussen (Ed.), *Carmichael's manual of child psychology.* 3rd ed. Vol. 2. New York: John Wiley and Sons, 1970, pp. 615–666.

Rodin, J. Current status of the internal-external hypothesis for obesity: What went wrong? *Amer. Psychol.,* 1981, 36, 361–372.

Rodriguez, A.; Rodriguez, M.; and Eisenberg, L. The outcome of school phobia: A follow-up study based on 41 cases. *Amer. J. Psychiat.,* 1959, 116, 540–544.

Roen, S. R. Primary prevention in the classroom through a teaching program in the behavioral sciences. In E. L. Cowen, E. A. Gardner, and M. Zax, *Emergent approaches to mental health problems.* New York: Appleton-Century-Crofts, 1967, pp. 252–270.

Rogers, C. R. *Client-centered therapy: Its current practice, implications, and theory.* Boston: Houghton Mifflin, 1951.

Rogers, C. R. *On becoming a person: A therapist's view of psychotherapy.* Boston: Houghton Mifflin, 1961.

Rogers, M. P.; Dubey, D.; and Reich, P. the influence of the psyche and the brain on immunity and disease susceptibility: A critical review. *Psychosom. Med.,* 1979, 41, 147–164.

Rogers, M. P.; Reich, P.; Strom, T. B.; and Carpenter, C. B. Behaviorally conditioned immunosuppression. Replication of a recent study. *Psychosom. Med.,* 1976, 38, 447–451.

Rorschach, H. *Psychodiagnostics: A diagnostic test based on perception.* Trans. by B. Kronenberg and P. Lemkau. New York: Grune and Stratton, 1975.

Rose, S. D. *Treating children in groups.* San Francisco: Jossey-Bass, 1972.

Rosen, J. C., and Wiens, A. N. Changes in medical problems and use of medical services following psychological intervention. *Amer. Psychol.,* 1979, 34, 420–431.

Rosenthal, T. L., and Bandura, A. Psychological modeling: Theory and practice. In S. L. Garfield and A. E. Bergin (Eds.), *Handbook of psychotherapy and behavior change: An empirical analysis.* 2nd ed. New York: John Wiley and Sons, 1978, pp. 621–658.

Rosman, B. L.; Minuchin, S.; and Liebman, R. Family lunch session: An introduction to family therapy in anorexia nervosa. *Amer. J. ortho.,* 1975, 45, 846–853.

Rosner, J. Language arts and arithmetic achievement, and specifically related perceptual skills. *Amer. Educ. Res. J.,* 1973, 10, 59–68.

Ross, A. O. Behavior therapy. In H. C. Quay and J. S. Werry (Eds.), *Psychopathological disorders of childhood.* New York: John Wiley and Sons, 1972, pp. 273–315.

Ross, A. O. *Psychological disorders of children. A behavioral approach to theory, research, and therapy.* New York: McGraw-Hill, 1974.

References

Ross, A. O. *Psychological aspects of learning disabilities and reading disorders.* New York: McGraw-Hill, 1976.

Ross, A. O. *Learning disabilities: The unrealized potential.* New York: McGraw-Hill, 1977.

Ross, A. O. *Psychological disorders of children: A behavioral approach to theory, research, and therapy.* 2nd ed. New York: McGraw-Hill, 1980.

Rotter, J. B. *Incomplete Sentences Blank.* New York: Psych. Corp., 1950.

Rousseau, J. J. *Emile.* Trans. by A. Bloom. New York: Basic Books, 1979.

Routh, D. K., and Roberts, R. D. Minimal brain dysfunction in children: Failure to find evidence for a behavioral syndrome. *Psych. Reports,* 1972, 31, 307–314.

Rubinstein, E. A. Childhood mental disease in America. A review of the literature before 1900. *Amer. J. Ortho.,* 1948, 18, 314–321.

Rudolph, A. B. (Ed.). *Pediatrics.* 16th ed. New York: Appleton-Century-Crofts, 1977.

Rutter, M. The influence of organic and emotional factors on the origins, nature and outcome of childhood psychosis. *Develop. Med. Child Neurol.,* 1965, 7, 518–528.

Rutter, M. Concepts of autism: A review of research. *J. Child Psychol. Psychiat.,* 1968, 9, 1–25.

Rutter, M. Childhood schizophrenia reconsidered. *J. Autism Childhood Schiz.,* 1972a, 2, 315–337.

Rutter, M. Maternal deprivation reconsidered. *J. Psychosom. Res.,* 1972b, 6, 241–250.

Rutter, M. *Helping troubled children.* London: Penguin Books, 1975.

Rutter, M.; Lebovici, S.; Eisenberg, L.; Sneznevskij, A. V.; Sadoun, R.; Brooke, E.; and Tsung-Yi Lin. A tri-axial classification of mental disorders in childhood. An international study. *J. Child Psychol. Psychiat.,* 1969, 10, 41–61.

Safer, D. J., and Allen, R. P. *Hyperactive children. Diagnosis and management.* Baltimore: University Park Press, 1976.

Sajwaj, T.; McNees, M. P.; and Schnelle, J. F. Clinical and community interventions with children: A comparison of treatment strategies. In B. B. Lahey and A. E. Kazdin (Eds.), *Advances in clinical child psychology,* Vol. 2. New York: Plenum Press, 1979, pp. 173–191.

Salk, L. Psychologist and pediatrician: A mental health team in the prevention and early diagnosis of mental disorders. In G. J. Williams and S. Gordon (Eds.), *Clinical child psychology: Current practices and future perspectives.* New York: Behavioral Publications, 1974, pp. 110–115.

Salvia, J., and Ysseldyke, J. E. *Assessment in special and remedial education.* 2nd ed. Boston: Houghton Mifflin, 1981.

Sarason, I. G. Verbal learning, modeling, and juvenile delinquency. *Amer. Psychol.,* 1968, 23, 254–266.

Sarason, I. G. A cognitive social learning approach to juvenile delinquency. In R. D. Hare and D. Schalling (Eds.), *Psychopathic behavior: Approaches to research.* Chichester, N.Y.: John Wiley and Sons, 1978, pp. 299–317.

References

Sarason, I. G., and Ganzer, V. J. Modeling and group discussion in the rehabilitation of juvenile delinquents. *J. Couns. Psych.*, 1973, 20, 442–449.

Satir, V. *Conjoint family therapy.* Palo Alto, Calif.: Science and Behavioral Books, 1967.

Satterfield, J. M.; Cantwell, D. P.; and Satterfield, B. T. Pathophysiology of the hyperactive child syndrome. *Arch. Gen. Psychiat.*, 1974, 31, 839–844.

Sattler, J. M. *Assessment of children's intelligence.* Philadelphia: W. B. Saunders Co., 1974.

Sattler, J. M. *Assessment of children's intelligence and special abilities.* 2nd ed. Boston: Allyn and Bacon. 1982.

Satz, P., and Sparrow, S. S. Specific developmental dyslexia: A theoretical formulation. In D. J. Bakker and P. Satz (Eds.), *Specific reading disability. Advances in theory and method.* Amsterdam: Rotterdam University Press, 1970, pp. 17–40.

Satz, P., Rardin, D., and Ross, J. An evaluation of a theory of specific developmental dyslexia. *Child Devel.*, 1971, 42(6), 2009–2021.

Scarr-Salapatek, S., and Williams, M. L. The effects of early stimulation on low birth-weight infants. *Child devel.*, 1973, 44, 94–101.

Schaefer, C. E., and Millman, H. L. *Therapies for children.* San Francisco: Jossey-Bass, 1978.

Schlichter, K. J., and Ratliff, R. G. Discrimination learning in juvenile delinquents. *J. Abn. Psych.*, 1971, 77, 46–48.

Schofield, W. The role of psychology in the delivery of health services. *Amer. Psychol.*, 1969, 24, 565–584.

Schopler, E., and Loftin, J. Thought disorders in parents of psychotic children. *Arch. Gen. Psychiat.*, 1969, 20, 174–181.

Schwartz, G. E. Psychobiological foundations of psychotherapy and behavior change. In S. L. Garfield and A. E. Bergin (Eds.), *Handbook of psychotherapy and behavior change: An empirical analysis.* 2nd ed. New York: John Wiley and Sons, 1978, pp. 63–99.

Schwartz, S., and Johnson, J. H. *Psychopathology of childhood. A clinical-experimental approach.* New York: Pergamon Press, 1981.

Schwitzgebel, R. L. Short-term operant conditioning of adolescent offenders on socially relevant variables. *J. Abn. Psych.*, 1967, 72, 134–142.

Sears, R. R. A theoretical framework for personality and social behavior. *Amer. Psychol.*, 1951, 6, 476–483.

Seim, R. Development characteristics of mentally retarded children: Classification categories compared. From a lecture presented at the Institute for the Study of Learning Disabilities. St. Jerome's College, University of Waterloo, Waterloo, Ontario, 1980.

Seligman, M. E. P. Depression and learned helplessness. In R. J. Friedman and M. M. Katz (Eds.), *The psychology of depression: Contemporary theory and research.* Washington, D.C.: Winston Press, 1974.

Shapiro, D., and Surwit, R. S. Learned control of physiological function and disease. In H. Leitenberg (Ed.), *Handbook of behavior modification and behavior therapy.* Englewood Cliffs, N.J.: Prentice-Hall, 1976, pp. 74–123.

References

Shapiro, S. H. Disturbances in development and childhood neurosis. In S. L. Copel (Ed.), *Behavior pathology of childhood and adolescence.* New York: Basic Books, 1973, pp. 21–59.

Shapiro, T. Therapy with autistic children. In M. Rutter and E. Schopler (Eds.), *Autism.* New York: Plenum Press, 1978, pp. 357–368.

Shepherd, M.; Oppenheim, A. N.; and Mitchell, S. Childhood behaviour disorders and the child guidance clinic: An epidemiological study. *J. Child. Psychol. Psychiat.*, 1966, 7, 39–52.

Shepherd, M.; Oppenheim, B.; and Mitchell, S. *Childhood behavior and mental health.* New York: Grune and Stratton, 1971.

Sherman, J. A., and Baer, D. M. Appraisal of operant therapy techniques with children and adults. In C. M. Franks (Ed.), *Behavior therapy: Appraisal and status.* New York: McGraw-Hill, 1969, pp. 192–219.

Shneidman, E. S. The MAPS test with children. In A. I. Rabin and M. R. Haworth (Eds.), *Projective techniques with children.* New York: Grune and Stratton, 1960.

Shore, M. F. Legislation, advocacy, and the rights of children and youth. *Amer. Psychol.*, 1979, 34, 1017–1019.

Shore, M. F., and Massimo, J. L. Five years later: A followup study of comprehensive vocationally oriented psychotherapy. *Amer. J. Ortho.*, 1969, 39, 769–773.

Shore, M. F., and Massimo, J. L. After ten years: A follow-up study of comprehensive vocationally oriented psychotherapy. *Amer. J. Ortho.*, 1973, 43, 128–132.

Short, J. F., and Strodtbeck, F. L. *Group process and gang delinquency.* Chicago: Univ. of Chicago Press, 1965.

Simmons, R. Psychophysiological disorders in childhood and adolescence. In P. D. Steinhauer and Q. Rae-Grant (Eds.), *Psychological problems of the child and his family.* Toronto: Macmillan, 1977, pp. 191–207.

Skeels, H. M. Adult status of children with contrasting early life experiences. *Monograph of Society for Research in Child Development.*, Ser. 105, 1966, 31 (3).

Skinner, B. F. *Walden two.* New York: Macmillan, 1948.

Skinner, B. F. *Beyond freedom and dignity.* New York: Bantam/Vintage Books, 1971.

Skodak, M., and Skeels, H. M. A final follow-up study of one hundred adopted children. *J. Genetic Psych.*, 1949, 75, 85–125.

Skynner, A. C. R. School phobia: A reappraisal. *Brit. J. Med. Psych.*, 1974, 47, 1–6.

Smith, D. W., and Wilson, A. A. *The child with Down's syndrome (monogolism).* Philadelphia: W. B. Saunders Co., 1973.

Smith, M. L., and Glass, G. V. Meta-analysis of psychotherapy outcome studies. *Amer. Psychol.*, 1977, 32, 752–760.

Sobel, S. B. Throwing the baby out with the bathwater: The hazards of follow-up research. *Amer. Psychol.*, 1978, 33, 290–291.

References

Sobel, S. B. Psychology and the juvenile justice system. *Amer. Psychol.,* 1979, 34, 1020–1023.

Solomon, S. The neurological evaluation. In A. M. Freedman and H. I. Kaplan (Eds.), *Comprehensive textbook of psychiatry.* Baltimore: Williams and Wilkins Co., 1967, pp. 420–443.

Spitz, R. A. Hospitalism: An inquiry into the genesis of psychiatric conditions in early childhood. *Psychoanal. Stud. Child,* 1945, 1, 53–74.

Spitz, R., and Wolf, K. M. Anaclitic depression. *Psychoanal. Stud. Child,* 1946, 2, 313–342.

Spivack, G., and Swift, M. *Devereux Elementary School Behavior Rating Scale.* Devon, Pa.: The Devereux Foundation, 1967.

Spivack, G., and Swift, M. The Hahnemann High School Behavior (HHSB) Rating Scale. *J. Abn. Child Psychol.,* 1977, 5, 299–307.

Spock, B. *Baby and child care.* Montreal: Pocket Books of Canada, 1957.

Sprague, R. L., Psychopharmacotherapy in children. In M. F. McMillan and S. Henao (Eds.), *Child psychiatry: Treatment and research.* New York: Brunner/Mazel, 1977, pp. 130–149.

Stampfl, T. G., and Levis, D. J. Essentials of implosive therapy: A learning-theory-based psychodynamic behavioral therapy. *J. Abn. Psych.,* 1967, 72 (6), 496–503.

Stanley, L. Treatment of ritualistic behavior in an 8-year-old girl by response prevention: A case report. *J. Child Psychol. Psychiat.,* 1980, 21, 85–90.

Starr, R. J. Child abuse. *Amer. Psychol.,* 1979, 34, 872–878.

Staub, E., and Conn, L. K. Aggression. In C. G. Costello (Ed.), *Symptoms of psychopathology. A handbook.* New York: John Wiley and Sons, 1970, pp. 481–510.

Steele, B. F., and Pollock, C. B. A psychiatric study of parents who abuse infants and small children. In R. E. Helfer and C. H. Kempe (Eds.), *The battered child.* 2nd ed. Chicago, Ill.: Univ. of Chicago Press, 1974, pp. 89–133.

Stein, J. Learning about learning. In H. E. Fitzgerald and T. H. Carr (Eds.), *Human development 82/83.* Guilford, Conn.: Dushkin Pub., 1982, pp. 136–140.

Stendler, C. B. Possible causes of overdependency in young children. *Child Devel.,* 1954, 25, 125–146.

Stevens, M. Coincidence or what? Cartoon in *The New Yorker,* June 22, 1981, p. 28.

Strauss, A., and Lehtinen, L. *Psychopathology and education of the brain-injured child.* Vol. 1. New York: Grune and Stratton, 1947.

Stroh, G. On the diagnosis of childhood psychosis. *J. Child Psychol. Psychiat.,* 1960, 1, 238–243.

Strupp, H. H., and Hadley, S. W. Specific and nonspecific factors in psychotherapy. *Arch. Gen. Psychiat.,* 1979, 36, 1125–1136.

Stuart, R. B. Critical reappraisal and reformulation of selected "mental health" programs. In L. A. Hamerlynck, P. O. Davidson, and L. E. Acker, *Behav-*

ior modification and ideal mental health services. Calgary, Alberta: Univ. of Calgary, 1969, pp. 5–100.

Stuart, R. B. *Trick or treatment: How and when psychotherapy fails.* Champaign, Ill.: Research Press, 1970.

Stuart, R. B.; Tripodi, T.; Jayaratne, S.; and Camburn, D. An experiment in social engineering in serving the families of predelinquents. *J. Abn. Child Psych.,* 1976, 4, 243–261.

Stumphauzer, J. S. (Ed.). *Behavior therapy with delinquents.* Springfield, Ill.: Charles C Thomas, 1973.

Sulzbacher, S. I., and Houser, J. B. A tactic to eliminate disruptive behaviors in the classroom: Group contingent consequences. *Amer. J. Ment. Defic.,* 1968, 73, 88–90.

Suran, B. G., and Rizzo, J. V. *Special children: An integrative approach.* Glenview, Ill.: Scott, Foresman and Co., 1979.

Szurek, S. A. Psychotic episodes and psychotic maldevelopment. *Amer. J. Ortho.,* 1956, 26, 519–543.

Taft, L. T., and Goldfarb, W. Prenatal and perinatal factors in childhood schizophrenia. *Develop. Med. Child Neurol.,* 1964, 6, 32–43.

Tarboroff, L. H., and Brown, W. H. A study of the personality patterns of children and adolescents with the peptic ulcer syndrome. *Amer. J. Ortho.,* 1954, 24, 602-610.

Taylor, R. L. Use of the AAMD classification system: A review of recent research. *Amer. J. Ment. Defic.,* 1980, 85, 116–119.

Telford, C. W., and Sawrey, J. M. *The exceptional individual.* 3rd ed. Englewood Cliffs, N.J.: Prentice-Hall, 1977.

Thomas, A.; Chess, S.; Birch, H. G.; Hertzig, M. E.; and Korn, S. *Behavioral individuality in early childhood.* New York: University Press, 1963.

Thomas, R. M. *Comparing theories of child development.* Belmont, Calif.: Wadsworth Pub., 1979.

Tieramaa, E. Psychosocial and psychic factors and age at onset of asthma. *J. Psychosom. Res.,* 1979, 23, 27–37.

Tolstrup, K. The necessity for differentiating eating disorders—discussion of Hilde Bruch's paper on the family background. In E. J. Anthony and C. Koupernik (Eds.), *The child in his family.* Vol. 1. New York: Wiley-Interscience, 1970, pp. 311–317.

Torgeson, J., and Goldman, T. Verbal rehearsal and short-term memory in reading-disabled children. *Child Devel.,* 1977, 48, 56–60.

Treffert, D. A. Epidemiology of infantile autism. *Arch. Gen. Psychiat.,* 1970, 22, 431–438.

Tuddenham, R. D. Jean Piaget and the world of the child. *Amer. Psychol.,* 1966, 21, 207–217.

Tyler, V. O., and Brown, G. D. Token reinforcement of academic performance with institutionalized delinquent boys. *J. Educ. Psych.,* 1968, 59, 164–168.

Ullman, L. P., and Krasner, L. *A psychological approach to abnormal behavior.* Englewood Cliffs, N.J.: Prentice-Hall, 1969.

Ultee, C. A.; Griffioen, D.; and Schellekens, J. The reduction of anxiety in children: A comparison of the effects of "systematic desensitization *in vitro*" and "systematic desensitization *in vivo.*" *Behav. Res. Ther.*, 1982, 20, 61–67.

Ungerer, J. A., and Sigman, M. Symbolic play and language comprehension in autistic children. *J. Amer. Acad. Child Psychiat.*, 1981, 20, 318–337.

U.S. Office of Education. Estimated number of handicapped children in the U.S., 1974–1975. Washington, D.C.: Bureau for the Education of the Handicapped, 1975. Cited in D. P. Hallahan and J. M. Kauffman, *Exceptional children: Introduction to special education.* Englewood Cliffs, N.J.: Prentice-Hall, 1978.

Uzgiris, I. C. and Hunt, J. McV. *Assessment in infancy: Ordinal scales of psychological development.* Urbana: University of Illinois Press, 1975.

Van Antwerp, M. The route to primary prevention. *Community mental health,* 1971, 7, 183–188. Cited in D. M. Wonderly, J. H. Kupfersmid, R. J. Monkman, J. M. Deak, and S. L. Rosenberg, Primary prevention in school psychology: Past, present, and proposed future. *Child Study J.,* 1979, 9, 163–179.

Van Evra, J. An ecological model of delivery for practicing clinicians. In A. I. Rabin (Ed.), *Clinical psychology: Issues of the seventies.* East Lansing, Mich.: Michigan State Univ. Press, 1974.

Van Evra, J.; Louis, A.; and Kays, D. A program evaluation follow-up in an adolescent treatment center. Unpublished study. Waterloo, Ontario, 1979.

Van Evra, J. P., and Rosenberg, B. G. Ego strength and ego disjunction in primary and secondary psychopaths. *J. Clin. Psych.*, 1963, 19, 61–63.

Van Riper, C. *Speech correction. Principles and methods.* 6th ed. Englewood Cliffs, N.J.: Prentice-Hall, 1978.

Vander Zanden, J. W. *Educational psychology in theory and practice.* New York: Random House, 1980.

Varsamis, J., and MacDonald, S. M. Manic-depressive disease in childhood. *Can. Psychiat. Ass'n. J.*, 1972, 7, 279–281.

Vasta, R. *Studying children.* San Francisco: W. H. Freeman, 1979.

Wahl, C. W. Commonly neglected psychosomatic syndromes. In S. Arieti (Ed.), *American handbook of psychiatry.* New York: Basic Books, 1966, pp. 158–165.

Waldfogel, S.; Tessman, E.; and Hahn, P. A program for early intervention in school phobia. *Amer. J. Ortho.*, 1959, 29, 324–333.

Wallace, G., and McLoughlin, J. A. *Learning disabilities: Concepts and characteristics.* Columbus, Ohio: Charles E. Merrill, 1975.

Wallick, M. M. Desensitization therapy with a fearful two-year-old. *Amer. J. Psychiat.*, 1979, 136(10), 1325–1326.

Warme, G. Childhood developmental problems. In P. D. Steinhauer and Q. Rae-Grant (Eds.), *Psychological problems of the child and his family.* Toronto: Macmillan, 1977, pp. 100–125.

Watson, J. B. *Behaviorism.* Chicago: University of Chicago Press, 1925.

Watson, J. B. *The ways of behaviorism.* New York: Harper and Row, 1928a.

Watson, J. B. *Psychological care of the infant and child.* New York: W. W. Norton, 1928b.

Watson, J. B. *Behaviorism* (rev. ed.). Chicago: Univ. of Chicago Press, 1980.

Watson, J. B., and Rayner, R. Conditioned emotional reactions. *J. Exper. Psych.,* 1920, 3, 1–14.

Weathers, L. R., and Liberman, R. P. Modification of family behavior. In D. Marholin II (Ed.), *Child behavior therapy.* New York: Gardner Press, 1978, pp. 150–186.

Wechsler, D. *Manual for the Wechsler Intelligence Scale for Children.* New York: Psych. Corp., 1949.

Wechsler, D. *Manual for the Wechsler Adult Intelligence Scale.* New York: Psych. Corp., 1955.

Wechsler, D. *Manual for the Wechsler Preschool and Primary Scale of Intelligence.* New York: Psych. Corp., 1967.

Wechsler, D. *Manual for the Wechsler Intelligence Scale for Children—Reivsed.* New York: Psych. Corp., 1974.

Weeks, E., and Mack, J. E. The child. In A. M. Nicholi, Jr. (Ed.), *The Harvard guide to psychiatry.* Cambridge, Mass.: Belknap Press of Harvard Univ. Press, 1978, Ch. 23.

Weinberger, G. Brief therapy with children and their parents. In H. H. Barten (Ed.), *Brief therapies.* New York: Behavioral Pub., 1971, pp. 196–211.

Weiner, H.; Thaler, M.; Reiser, M. F.; and Mirsky, I. A. Etiology of duodenal ulcer. *Psychosom. Med.,* 1957, 19, 1–10.

Weir, M. Mental retardation. *Science,* 1967, 157, 576–577. Cited in E. Zigler, Developmental versus difference theories of mental retardation and the problem of motivation. *Amer. J. Ment. Defic.,* 1969, 73, 536–556.

Weisberg, P. Operant procedures with the retardate: An overview of laboratory research. In N. R. Ellis (Ed.), *International review of research in mental retardation.* Vol. 5. New York: Academic Press, 1971, pp. 113–145.

Wender, P. H., and Klein, D. F. The promise of biological psychiatry. *Psychology Today,* Feb. 1981, pp. 25–41.

Werner, H., and Strauss, A. A. Pathology of the figure-ground relation in the child. *J. Abn. Soc. Psych.,* 1941, 36, 236–248.

Werry, J. S. The conditioning treatment of enuresis. *Amer. J. Psychiat.,* 1966, 123, 226–229.

Werry, J. S. Psychosomatic disorders (with a note on anesthesia, surgery and hospitalization). In H. C. Quay and J. S. Werry (Eds.), *Psychopathological disorders of childhood.* New York: John Wiley and Sons, 1972.

Werry, J. The use of psychotropic drugs in children. *J. Amer. Acad. Child Psychiat.,* 1977, 16, 446–468.

Werry, J. S. The childhood psychoses. In H. C. Quay and J. S. Werry (Eds.),

References

Psychopathological disorders of childhood. New York: John Wiley and Sons, 1979a.

Werry, J. S. Family therapy: Behavioral approaches. *J. Amer. Acad. Child Psychiat.*, 1979b, 18, 91–102.

Werry, J. S.; Sprague, R. L.; and Cohen, M. N. Conners' Teacher Rating Scale for use in drug studies with children—An empirical study. *J. Abn. Child Psych.*, 1975, 3, 217–229.

Whitehill, M.; DeMyer-Gapin, S.; and Scott, T. J. Stimulation seeking in antisocial preadolescent children. *J. Abn. Psych.*, 1976, 85, 101–104.

Wiig, E. H., and Roach, M. A. Immediate recall of semantically varied "sentences" by learning-disabled adolescents. *Percep. Motor Skills*, 1975, 40, 119–125.

Williams, G. J. The psychologist as child advocate: Reflections of a devil's advocate. *The Clinical Psychologist*, 1970, Summer, 7–8.

Windheuser, H. J. Anxious mothers as models for coping with anxiety. In C. M. Franks and G. T. Wilson (Eds.), *Annual review of behavior therapy theory and practice: 1978.* New York: Brunner/Mazel, 1978.

Windle, W. F. Brain damage by asphyxia at birth. In *The nature and nurture of behavior: Developmental psychobiology.* Readings from *Scientific American.* San Francisco: W. H. Freeman, 1973.

Wing, L. *Autistic children.* New York: Brunner/Mazel, 1972.

Wittkower, E. D., and Warnes, R. *Psychosomatic medicine: Its clinical applications.* New York: Harper and Row, 1977.

Wolberg, L. R. *Short-term psychotherapy.* New York: Grune and Stratton, 1965.

Wolff, H. G. Life stress and bodily disease—A formulation. *Proc. Ass. Res. Nerv. Ment. Dis.*, 1950, 24, 1059–1094. Cited in E. L. Lipton, A. Steinschneider, and J. B. Richmond, Psychophysiologic disorders in children. In L, W. Hoffman and M. L. Hoffman (Eds.), *Review of child development research.* Vol. 2. New York: Russell Sage, 1966, pp. 169–220.

Wolman, B. B. *Children without childhood.* New York: Grune and Stratton, 1970.

Wolpe, J. *Psychotherapy by reciprocal inhibition.* Stanford: Stanford Univ. Press, 1958.

Wolpe J. *The practice of behavior therapy.* New York: Pergamon Press, 1969.

Wolpe, J., and Lang, P. J. A fear survey schedule for use in behavior therapy. *Behav. Res. Ther.*, 1964, 2, 27–30.

Wolpe, J., and Lazarus, A. A. *Behavior therapy techniques: A guide to the treatment of neurosis.* New York: Pergamon Press, 1966.

Wonderly, D. M.; Kupfersmid, J. H.; Monkman, R. J.; Deak, J. M.; and Rosenberg, S. L. Primary prevention in school psychology: Past, present, and proposed future. *Child Study J.*, 1979, 9, 163–179.

Wong, B. Y. L. Strategic behaviors in selecting retrieval cues in gifted, normal achieving and learning-disabled children. *J. Lear. Dis.*, 1982, 15(1), 33–37.

Wright, L. Health care psychology: Prospects for the well-being of children. *Amer. Psychol.*, 1979, 34, 1001–1006.

Wulbert, M., and Dries, R. The relative efficacy of methylphenidate (ritalin) and behavior modification techniques in the treatment of a hyperactive child. In B. B. Lahey, *Behavior therapy with hyperactive and learning disabled children.* New York: Oxford Univ. Press, 1979, pp. 237–246.

Yates, A. J. *Behavior therapy.* New York: John Wiley and Sons, 1970a.

Yates, A. J. Tics. In C. G. Costello (Ed.), *Symptoms of psychopathology: A handbook.* New York: John Wiley and Sons, 1970b, pp. 320–335.

Yorkston, N. J. Behavior therapy in the treatment of bronchial asthma. In T. Thompson and W. S. Dockens, III (Eds.), *Applications of behavior modification.* New York: Academic Press, 1975.

Young, G. C., and Morgan, R. T. T. Rapidity of response to the treatment of enuresis. *Devel. Med. Child Neurol.,* 1968, 10, 465–470.

Zaslow, R. W., and Breger, L. A theory and treatment of autism. In L. Breger (Ed.), *Clinical-cognitive psychology.* Englewood Cliffs, N.J.: Prentice-Hall, 1969.

Zax, M., and Cowen, E. L. Early identification and prevention of emotional disturbance in a public school. In E. L. Cowen, E. A. Gardner, and M. Zax, *Emergent approaches to mental health.* New York: Appleton-Century-Crofts, 1967, pp. 331–351.

Zigler, E. Developmental versus difference theories of mental retardation and the problem of motivation. *Amer. J. Ment. Defic.,* 1969, 73, 536–556.

Zigler, E. The retarded child as a whole person. In H. E. Adams and W. K. Boardman (Eds.), *Advances in experimental clinical psychology.* New York: Pergamon Press, 1971, pp. 47–121.

Zimmerman, E. H.; Zimmerman, J.; and Russell, C. D. Differential effects of token reinforcement on instruction-following behavior in retarded students instructed as a group. *J. Applied Behav. Anal.,* 1969, 2, 101–112.

Glossary

affective: having to do with the expression of feelings and emotions.

anaclitic depression: the depressive behavior and attitude which Spitz described in institutionalized infants, including lethargy, poor appetite, and sadness.

anorexia nervosa: a severe disorder most frequently seen in adolescent girls and characterized by self-starvation to the point of life-threatening malnutrition.

anxiety attack: the experience of extremely intense and diffuse anxiety and panic, often with physiological concomitants.

attentional deficit: an inability to sustain directed attention and hence to stay with any one thought or task for a prolonged length of time.

attention-placebo: attention given a group that is being compared with other groups that receive treatment or that receive nothing in order to try to determine whether a specific treatment or nonspecific attention was responsible for any changes seen.

auditory blending: the ability to blend single sounds into more complex sounds, an important skill in learning to read.

auditory discrimination: the ability to distinguish one sound from another, particularly among those which are similar.

autonomic nervous system: the system responsible for such involuntary physiological events as salivation, breathing, and other automatic processes.

baseline data: the data collected at the beginning of the period of treatment or intervention for use as a reference against which to compare future levels of a given behavior.

behaviorism: the school of thought that developed out of learning theory and that stresses the study of observable behavior, experimental methodology, and the importance of reinforcement contingencies for the persistence of any behavior.

bell and pad: a device developed by Mowrer to treat enuresis through a classical conditioning process.

biofeedback: heightened awareness of bodily processes such as heart rate and gastric secretions, leading to greater control of them.

bonding: the development of an early, strong relationship or attachment between mother and infant.

charting: the careful monitoring and recording of behaviors that are being studied and that one is trying to change.

child advocacy: efforts made on behalf of children which are intended to ensure that basic needs are met and that basic rights are not violated.

classical (respondent) conditioning: the change of involuntary behavior through a process of conditioning which pairs previously neutral stimuli with a positive or negative present stimulus.

cognitive behavioral modification: an intervention approach which seeks to alter cognitive processes in order to effect behavior change.

compulsions: irrational, ritualistic, and repetitive actions which an individual feels compelled to engage in and is unable to stop or refrain from without experiencing considerable anxiety.

computer-assisted instruction (CAI): the use of computers to present programmed material to students who then proceed at their own rate and receive immediate feedback from the computer as to their success or failure.

control group: a group of subjects, matched with an experimental group on relevant variables, which does not receive the treatment that the experimental group receives.

conversion hysteria: the symbolic expression of unconscious conflict through bodily dysfunction, such as in the case of hysterical blindness.

correlational method: the comparison of two groups on specific variables or characteristics that are not manipulated experimentally, and from which causation cannot be inferred.

Cretinism (hypothyroidism): a disorder caused by thyroid gland dysfunction and usually associated with severe mental retardation.

critical period: a period of development during which certain events or agents have a maximum effect.

cross-modal perception: the process by which sensory information from one modality is converted into information in another, as when individuals visualize what they have been told.

cross-sectional studies: studies of certain behaviors or characteristics done simultaneously on several different age groups.

cultural-familial retardation: a form of mental retardation that is not a result of clear organic or physiological dysfunction. It accounts for three-quarters of those classified as retarded.

cumulative deficit: problems that become more complex and more extensive as the children grow because inadequate learning of concepts or skills that are basic to the mastery of other, higher-level ones causes them to get further and further behind.

cyclothymic personality: a personality type characterized by mood swings, or vacillations between strong feelings of well-being and depressive feelings.

decoding: the process of breaking down written or spoken communications in order to understand the meaning intended by the writer or speaker.

defectors: children or adolescents who are accepted for treatment and placed on a waiting list but who do not actually receive the treatment.

defense mechanisms: the psychological means by which individuals handle conflicts and anxiety.

deficit hypothesis: the hypothesis that retarded functioning reflects behavioral and cognitive functioning which is the same as that of normal children but is occurring at a slower developmental rate.

denial: a primitive defense mechanism by which an individual simply denies unpleasant or threatening aspects of reality.

dependent variable: the variable that is being studied for possible changes occurring as a function of the manipulation of experimental or independent variables.

developmental disturbance: disordered behavior that arises out of a child's difficulty with the mastery of normal developmental tasks.

Diagnostic and Statistical Manual of Mental Disorders, 3rd Ed. (DSM-III): the American Psychiatric Association's manual that defines and classifies psychological and organic mental disorders.

difference hypothesis: the hypothesis that retarded functioning reflects not only a slower rate but actual qualitative differences between the child's cognitive and behavioral functioning and that of normal children.

displacement: a defense mechanism by which anxiety or hostility is displaced from its original target onto a less threatening one, as in the case of a man who is angry with his boss but acts out his hostility at home with his wife or children.

distractibility: the inability to refrain from responding to many stimuli extraneous to the task at hand.

Down's syndrome (mongolism): a genetic disorder involving chromosomal abnormalities and associated with severe mental retardation.

DSM-III: see *Diagnostic and Statistical Manual of Mental Disorders, 3rd. Ed.*

dyslexia: a severe reading disorder, characterized by an inability to process auditory or visual information in the usual way.

early infantile autism: a severe disorder of infancy and early childhood which is characterized by stereotyped behavior, little if any use of language, inability to relate to other people, and severely withdrawn behavior, often accompanied by odd motor activity and mannerisms.

echolalia: a language or communication disorder in which an individual echos the words of others in a parroting, meaningless way.

eclectic: an approach to psychological disorders that draws on various theories and incorporates elements of several different approaches.

educable retarded: see *mildly retarded.*

elective mutism: an almost total absence of the use of any verbal language without any organic pathology to account for such nonuse.

electroencephalogram (EEG): a tracing of the electrical activity of the brain as recorded by an electroencephalograph, used to detect and assess possible brain damage or neurological dysfunction.

encoding: The process by which an individual puts thoughts into a communicable form such as written or spoken language to communicate ideas or meaningful information.

encopresis: continuing failure to achieve or exercise adequate sphincter control past the age when such control has ordinarily been mastered, resulting in uncontrolled bowel movements and soiling.

enuresis: persistent bedwetting either past the age when bladder control has ordinarily been mastered or after a period of continence.

etiology: the origins and causes of a disorder.

experimental method: a research method in which there is rigorous control of relevant variables and experimental manipulation of a behavior or characteristic *(independent variable)* to see what effects such manipulation has on another behavior or characteristic *(dependent variable).*

externalization: the acting out of symptoms, neurotic problems, anxiety, or hostility, often in an antisocial or aggressive way.

extinction: the decrease in, and eventual disappearance of, a response as a result of lack of reinforcement of that response.

factorial design: an experimental design that allows one to investigate the effects of and interactions among several variables simultaneously.

failure-to-thrive: a condition in which a delay in a child's development is associated with poor parenting, such as might occur in institutional settings or in homes where children are neglected.

false positive: the identification of someone as having a specific problem or disorder when in fact the person does not have it.

fetal alcohol syndrome: the appearance in a newborn infant of various symptoms, including retarded functioning, because of heavy alcohol intake of the mother.

field independence: the ability of individuals to use relevant cues in problem-solving while ignoring irrelevant ones.

flooding: see *implosive therapy.*

free association: a method used by psychoanalysts to investigate the unconscious of individuals by noting the content and sequencing of their uncensored thoughts and verbalizations.

functional analysis: an analysis of how variables interact and interrelate or covary.

genetic predisposition: a person's tendency, because of genetic inheritance, to be more likely than other individuals to develop certain diseases.

Gilles de la Tourette's disease: a specific tic disorder which is usually progressive and affects especially the coordination of the face and upper body.

group therapy: the inclusion of several people simultaneously in a therapeutic situation.

habit disorders: disorders that arise as a result of children's problems with behaviors which most children learn without undue difficulty, such as in the areas of eating, sleeping, and bowel training.

heterogeneous: mixed, or made up of different kinds of persons or problems.

homogeneous: made up of persons or problems that are very similar.

humanism: a school of thought among those dissatisfied with behaviorism and psychoanalysis. It arose as a "third force" that places great emphasis on growth, self-fulfillment, and the capacity to change and to solve one's own problems.

hydrocephaly: a condition that involves excess fluid accumulation in and enlargement of the head, usually associated with severe retardation.

hyperactivity: a common disorder of childhood marked by impulsive, poorly timed, often incessant verbal and motor behavior and associated with problems such as distractibility and a short attention span.

implosive therapy: a therapeutic technique in which an individual is exposed to high levels of feared stimuli on the assumption that the absence of aversive consequences will lead to extinction of anxiety response and avoidant behavior.

impulsivity: the tendency to act without thinking or reflecting on one's action.

incidence: the rate of occurrence of a problem or disorder.

independent variable: the variable that is manipulated in an experiment to see what measurable effect it has on other *(dependent)* variables.

individuation: the psychological and physical separation of an infant from the mother which is necessary for the development of an individual personality.

infant stimulation programs: programs designed to increase the early stimulation received by infants who are at risk, in order to prevent or lessen retarded functioning and enhance their overall development.

insight therapy: psychodynamically oriented psychotherapy intended to bring about insight in clients concerning the nature and meaning of their conflicts and behavior.

instrumental conditioning: see *operant conditioning.*

intellectualization: a defense mechanism by which individuals deal with anxiety and conflict by converting all of their concerns into intellectual terms and avoiding emotional, affective expression or involvement.

internalization: the expression of conflicts and anxiety through internal symptoms such as fears, phobias, depression, and somatic symptoms.

intrapsychic: having to do with psychological events or conflicts within the individual.

invulnerable children: children who have been able to resist disorders and who thrive and even excel despite a very disturbed and disorganized background; sometimes known as "stress-resistant" children.

kinesthetic cues: cues that give individuals feedback on their movements and allow them to develop judgments about balance, coordination, and other fluid movements.

least restrictive environment: an environment in which children receive help but which is as much like a normal environment as possible.

longitudinal studies: studies that follow the same individuals over a long period of time.

mainstreaming: the integration and education of children with special needs within a regular classroom.

malingering: conscious faking of illness or disability, usually to avoid some unpleasant task or responsibility.

manic-depressive psychosis: a severe disorder involving extreme mood swings, vacillating between euphoria and severe depression; rarely seen in children.

maturational lag: a delay in development in a specific area such as language or social development, which may interfere with a child's learning, peer relationships, or other development.

medical model: the view of behavior disorders as symptoms of underlying problems which need to be understood before the problem behaviors can be effectively changed or treated.

mental age: the intellectual age at which a child is actually functioning, which may or may not differ from the chronological age of that child.

mental retardation: intellectual functioning that is significantly below average and is associated with serious impairment of adaptive capacity as well.

microcephaly: a condition in which the head and the brain are abnormally small.

mildly retarded children: children so classified have test IQ's between 50 and 70 and, although somewhat impaired, have sufficient adaptive skills to attain functional literacy and to be somewhat self-supporting.

milieu therapy: therapy conducted in an environment in which all aspects of the setting are arranged or selected for their therapeutic impact.

minimal brain dysfunction: a term used to denote brain dysfunction inferred from such behavioral signs as poor coordination, reversal of letters, and other "soft signs" but not substantiated by such "hard" neurological equipment as EEGs.

modality: a channel for receiving sensory information, such as the auditory modality or visual modality; or, more broadly, any channel of communication, such as verbal modality.

modeling: the imitation and incorporation of behaviors exhibited by others in one's environment.

moderately retarded children: children so classified have test IQs between 35 and 49 and have poor social and adaptive skills, although they can communicate and can care for themselves with supervision.

motor theorists: a group of theorists who emphasize the role of good motor and perceptual-motor learning as fundamental and basic to higher learning and who attribute learning or academic problems to poor underlying motor skills or ability.

multiple baseline design: an experimental design which involves obtaining baseline data on a specific behavior as it occurs in a number of settings and then comparing that behavior as it changes in the various settings as a function of the introduction of specific techniques.

multisensory approach: an approach to remediation that may involve the use of visual, auditory, kinesthetic, and/or tactile stimuli simultaneously (for example, VAKT approach).

neurological impress method: a remedial method in which a teacher reads loudly and often directly into a child's ear at the same time that the child reads aloud and points to what is being read.

neurotic delinquent: a child who engages in antisocial or deviant behavior because of such problems as low self-esteem, overinhibited personality, guilt, or underlying conflicts.

nondirective therapy: a form of psychotherapy in which the therapist focuses on establishing an accepting atmosphere and lets the child lead the therapy.

objective tests: tests that provide objective data, which require minimum interpretation and about which there is fairly unanimous agreement; or sometimes tests that are objectively scored.

obsessions: irrational, ritualistic, and repetitive thoughts which intrude on an individual's consciousness and which the individual is unable to terminate without experiencing considerable anxiety.

operant (instrumental) conditioning: conditioning that is based on changing the reinforcement value of specific behaviors to encourage an individual to engage in new behaviors.

overinhibited delinquent: see *neurotic delinquent.*

partial reinforcement: the reinforcement of behaviors only part of the time according to either a fixed or a variable schedule.

pathogenic: contributing to the development of a disorder.

perceptual-motor age: the age level at which a child is functioning in the perceptual-motor sphere, which may or may not be the same as the chronological age of the child.

perceptual-motor integration: the ability to integrate information from various sensory modalities and to use that information efficiently in motor behavior, as in eye-hand coordination.

perseveration: the repetition of a behavior over a considerable period of time and a seeming inability to shift to other activities.

phobia: an extreme and irrational fear of something, the presence of which may lead an individual to extreme anxiety and panic.

pica: a disorder seen in young children, usually of deprived backgrounds with poor parenting, which is characterized by their ingestion of inedible objects or material such as lead and dirt.

placebo: a neutral substance that is administered as an alternative to a given treatment in experimental groups to unknowing subjects in order to test the actual effects of a drug as opposed to the expected effects; that is, to rule out possible effects due to expectation of effect.

premature termination: the cessation of therapy on the part of a patient before the whole course of therapy has been completed.

pretest-posttest format: a frequently used design for testing the effectiveness of a treatment in which individuals are tested before and after receiving treatment and any changes in the target behavior(s) are noted.

process training: a remedial approach that focuses on training underlying processes in which a child demonstrates a weakness, such as perception, rather than training in specific skills such as letter recognition.

profoundly retarded children: children with a severe level of retardation, characterized by extreme intellectual and social deficits and the need for constant supervision and care.

prognosis: the likelihood of significant improvement or recovery.

programmed learning: a highly structured approach in which material to be learned is set out in an orderly sequence of units to be mastered according to a definite plan.

projection: a defense mechanism by which individuals deny a certain quality or characteristic in themselves and attribute it to others in the environment, such as the projection of hostility by paranoid individuals onto others in the environment, and the consequent perception of others as behaving toward them in a hostile way.

projective tests: tests used in clinical assessment which presume that individuals will project their underlying conflicts and feelings onto ambiguous or neutral stimuli. Such tests require a high degree of interpretation.

psychoanalysis: a theoretical school of thought, as well as a form of therapy, that places heavy emphasis on an understanding of the unconscious conflicts which exist in individuals and how such conflicts can affect and motivate behavior in irrational and symbolic ways.

psychodynamic: having to do with psychological forces and events within the personality.

psychogenic: having to do with the operation or influence of psychological forces in the etiology of a disorder, as in psychogenically caused as opposed to organically caused or genetically caused.

psychopathic delinquent: see *unsocialized delinquent.*

psychosomatic: applied to disorders that are characterized by a complex interaction of physical and psychological factors.

rapid eye movement (REM): a later stage of sleep often associated with dreaming.

rationalization: a commonly used defense mechanism which excuses or provides an alibi for behavior with which an individual is not pleased.

reaction formation: a defense mechansim in which behavior opposite to one's impulse is engaged in, as when a very hostile person becomes very solicitous or overly kind in interactions with the person who is the focus or target of the hostile feelings.

recidivism: the degree to which criminal behavior recurs, or the rate at which individuals are reinstitutionalized.

refrigerator parents: parents who are cold, aloof, often highly intellectual, and, implicitly, unresponsive to their children's needs.

regression: a defense mechansim by which an individual, in the face of stress or anxiety, regresses or goes back to a much less mature, earlier form of behavior.

reinforcement: a consequence of one's behavior which either increases the likelihood of its recurrence *(positive reinforcement)* or decreases the likelihood of its occurring again *(negative reinforcement).*

REM: see *rapid eye movement.*

repression: a defense mechanism that involves making threatening or conflictual information or experiences unconscious.

residential treatment: treatment away from home, within an institution. The size and nature of the institution may vary widely.

resource room: a special education classroom to which children can go for part of the day for specific remedial help.

respondent conditioning: see *classical conditioning.*

response hierarchy: a ranking of responses according to the likelihood of their occurring for a given individual in response to specific stimuli.

reversal experimental design: an experimental design in which the experimental procedure is introduced, then withdrawn, and then reintroduced in order to assess the effects that the presence or absence of the procedure has on a specific behavior.

risk/benefit ratio: the ratio between the risks and the potential benefits of a proposed treatment, which needs to be weighed when one is deciding on a course of treatment.

ritalin: a central nervous system stimulant frequently used with hyperactive children to help them to focus their attention and improve their concentration, thus increasing the effectiveness of their behavior.

rubella: German measles, a disease that can have very serious, negative effects on a fetus if it is contracted by a woman during the first trimester of pregnancy.

schizophrenia: a severe cognitive-affective disorder frequently characterized by bizarre behavior, unusual use of language, disturbed relationships with others, disordered thought processes, and withdrawal from reality, and sometimes involving hallucinations and delusions.

school phobia: a refusal to attend school because of an apparent exaggerated fear of school and, frequently, of associated places or experiences, but which often also seems to involve a fear of leaving home.

secondary prevention: efforts made to intervene early, after problems have appeared, in order to prevent those problems from becoming more serious or to prevent additional ones from developing.

self-esteem: one's feelings about oneself and one's worth.

self-fulfilling hypothesis: occurrence of an event or appearance of a characteristic as a result of someone's belief that it does exist or expectation that it will appear.

self-report inventory: see *subjective tests.*

separation anxiety: an individual's fear of leaving a parent or a home, either physically or psychologically.

severely retarded children: children so classified have test IQs between 20 and 34 and demonstrate marked deficits in motor, language, and adaptive skills.

sheltered workshop: a protected environment in which individuals can learn skills and can work but which protects them from the stresses and decisions of a normal work situation.

socialized delinquents (subcultural): children who engage in antisocial behavior because of strong ties to a delinquent peer group.

social skills training: training in specific skills needed for adaptive functioning in society, including training in such areas as language and social relationship skills.

soft neurological signs: behaviors or characteristics from which one infers some kind of neurological or nervous system dysfunction that does not show up on such tests as an EEG.

somnambulism: sleepwalking.

spatial relations: the ability to understand the relationships of objects to one another in space.

specific learning disability: an inability to learn through the usual classroom procedures despite average or above-average intelligence and the absence of sensory impairment or emotional problems as causal factors.

spontaneous remission: an individual's improvement in the absence of any planned treatment or intervention.

standard deviation units: statistically derived deviation units used to evaluate the extent of the difference between an individual's score and the mean of the group with which a comparison is being made.

standardized norms: standards that have been derived from administering a particular test to large numbers of children of similar age, sex, and other characteristics.

stereotypy: the occurrence of repetitive, usually meaningless behavior over a significant period of time.

stress-resistant children: see *invulnerable children.*

subcultural delinquents: see *socialized delinquents.*

subjective tests: tests or inventories on which individuals make statements or answer questions about themselves and which are, therefore, open to bias or faking.

superego: according to psychoanalysts, the part of one's personality that is responsible for feelings of guilt and conscience, as well as one's ideals.

symbiotic infantile psychosis: a severe disturbance of early childhood which is characterized by an inability to separate from one's mother and develop one's own individual and separate identity.

symptom substitution: the appearance of a new symptom to replace one that has been removed, which occurs as a result of having treated the symptom without having eradicated the cause.

systematic desensitization: the procedure by which a person is exposed to a hierarchy of events, from least anxiety-provoking to most anxiety-provoking, while at the same time engaging in incompatible responses such as relaxation.

tactile cues: information and feedback originating from one's sense of touch.

target behavior: the specific behavior that is the focus for one's remedial or intervention efforts.

tertiary prevention: the efforts that are expended to minimize discomfort and pain from a serious and usually chronic disorder or condition.

test age: the level of test performance of a child, which may or may not be the same as the child's chronological age.

third-force psychology: see *humanism.*

tics: involuntary and repetitive muscular movements.

token reinforcement: the use of concrete rewards as reinforcements, including chips, points, money, and privileges.

trainable retarded: see *moderately retarded.*

unsocialized delinquents: individuals who engage in antisocial behavior because of a failure to incorporate society's values and norms and who therefore experience little anxiety, guilt, or remorse in relation to their deviant behavior.

verbal deficit: a disorder in one's language development, either of receptive language (input) or of expressive language (output).

verbal rehearsal: a process by which an individual rehearses specific problem-solving strategies.

visual discrimination: the ability to distinguish one letter from another, particularly those which are rather similar.

Author Index

Subject Index

419